T0192229

Mind–Body Medicine in Clinical Practice

Consumer demand for integrative medicine has increased over recent decades, and cutting-edge research in neuroscience has identified opportunities for new treatment options. This text outlines the evidence behind mind–body medicine and provides rich case-based examples. It is written by a clinician, for clinicians, to help practitioners stay current in this emerging field.

Including foundational chapters on the relevance of mind–body medicine, the physiologic effects of stress, communication skills, and methods for incorporating mind–body medicine into consultation, this book then introduces various mind–body therapies and considers their use in selected clinical conditions. The therapies are grouped into chapters on breath work and relaxation; hypnosis and guided imagery; meditation, mindfulness, spirituality, and compassion-based therapies; creative arts therapies; and movement therapies. Each chapter includes case studies, background and history, best use, training requirements, risks and benefits. The part focusing on specific conditions updates research and provides pediatric and adult examples in the areas of: anxiety and depression; acute and chronic pain; gastrointestinal and urologic conditions; autoimmune, inflammatory; and surgery, oncology, and other conditions.

Providing resources and practical tools to help clinicians incorporate evidence-based mind–body medicine therapies into patient care, this book is an invaluable reference for medical and nursing students, as well as for residents, fellows, nurse practitioners, and physician assistants across a wide variety of specialties.

Hilary McClafferty is board certified in pediatrics, pediatric emergency medicine, and integrative medicine. She is a founding member of the American Board of Integrative Medicine and Immediate Past Chair of the American Academy of Pediatrics Section on Integrative Medicine.

Mind–Body Medicine in Clinical Practice

Hilary McClafferty

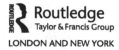

LONDON AND NEW YORK

First published 2018
by Routledge
2 Park Square, Milton Park, Abingdon, Oxon OX14 4RN

and by Routledge
52 Vanderbilt Avenue, New York, NY 10017

Routledge is an imprint of the Taylor & Francis Group, an informa business

© 2018 Taylor & Francis Group

British Library Cataloguing in Publication Data
A catalogue record for this book is available
from the British Library

Library of Congress Cataloging-in-Publication Data

Names: McClafferty, Hilary, author.
Title: Mind-body medicine in clinical practice / Hilary McClafferty.
Description: Abingdon, Oxon ; New York, NY : Routledge, 2018. | Includes bibliographical references and index.
Identifiers: LCCN 2018003033 | ISBN 9781498728317 (pbk.) | ISBN 9781315157238 (ebook)
Subjects: | MESH: Mind-Body Therapies | Mind-Body Relations, Metaphysical | Clinical Medicine
Classification: LCC RC489.M53 | NLM WB 880 | DDC 616.89/1--dc23
LC record available at https://lccn.loc.gov/2018003033

ISBN: 978-1-4987-2831-7 (pbk)

Typeset in Bembo
by Lumina Datamatics Limited

For Mary Greenan McClafferty and
James McClafferty, thank you, for everything

Contents

PART III
Clinical Application

Foreword

As I read Hilary McClafferty's *Mind–Body Medicine in Clinical Practice*, my overarching feeling, was "If only I had such a text when I was coming up through the ranks in my medical training!" Back then, in the 1970s, mind–body medicine was considered New Age woo-woo. If one practiced it, one certainly didn't tell one's colleagues about it. Indeed, as McClafferty points out, mind–body medicine is still considered fringe by many practitioners today, although the numbers of those naysayers are decreasing, largely due to the exponentially increasing wealth of scientific research providing evidence for how these practices work, that they work, and under what circumstances and for which conditions and diseases they work best. This book will go a long way toward dispelling any lingering doubts, both by providing the scientific evidence and clear practical step-by-step descriptions for practitioners of how and when to apply specific mind–body techniques. It is a handbook that every practitioner should carry.

McClafferty reviews all this and more in this clearly written and engaging guide to mind–body medicine. As the title of Part I indicates, she starts by providing an up-to-date systematic review of the foundations of mind–body medicine, including the science of stress, clinician self-care, and the language of the mind–body interview. While much has been written about stress, far less is available in textbooks on the latter two topics, both of which still bear some stigma. In the macho, 24-7 world of clinical medicine and medical training, some still consider the need for physician self-care an admission of weakness. However, as McClafferty points out, physician burnout is a very real and disturbing phenomenon, which leads to illness in the physician and could also potentially lead to medical errors. Thus, trainees and practicing physicians would do well to learn approaches to mitigate it, such as mind–body medicine. In a very real way, the book espouses the age old Biblical adage, "Physician heal thyself" (Luke 4:23). McClafferty addresses the issue of stigma for self-care head-on, with a real-world example of a medical resident experiencing derision and resistance from his superiors when he attempts to initiate a meeting for other residents interested in learning about mindfulness meditation. Through this example, McClafferty provides language and strategies for others to successfully overcome such barriers, just as her sample resident did.

McClafferty uses this approach throughout the book, in each chapter—starting with definitions of terms and a review of the science underlying the method or condition, then moving on to provide engaging examples from real life of patients or physicians applying the mind–body method to the situation or condition under discussion. These case studies make the book eminently readable and help the reader apply the method to their own experiences. But McClafferty goes beyond these case reports to provide clear, step-by-step descriptions for practicing each type of mind–body approach, both for adults and children.

One of the cleverest examples is her description of how to teach 4 year olds diaphragmatic breathing—by having them lie down, place a small stuffed beanbag animal on their bellies, and make the animal go up in the air and then down. One can easily visualize the children giggling and trying it over and over again until they master the technique! In addition to the descriptive case studies and bulleted step-by-step methods, she provides extensive practical lists at the end of chapters, including websites and references for more reading, for those who wish to take a deeper dive.

Chapter 4—"Language Use and the Mind–Body Interview"—is particularly compelling, providing precise wording for practitioners to use when approaching colleagues or patients who might be leery of trying out these techniques. Right up front, it addresses the conundrum of how to walk the fine line between truthfully delivering bad news to a patient without removing hope. During my training in the 1970s, the fashion was to be completely blunt in an effort to be truthful, unlike previous generations of physicians who might have colored the truth in order to maintain hope. But McClafferty provides a way forward—a way to be truthful while being mindful about one's language so that one doesn't *hex* the patient with a *nocebo* effect. Words do matter, and the application of the concept of mindfulness to also being mindful about one's words is a refreshing and important lesson. Again, in this chapter she illustrates the situation with a real-life description of an encounter by a resident who does *hex* the young patient and his family. She then provides alternate soothing wording, which could have been used to avoid this unfortunate effect. This is followed by a step-by-step guide to structuring the delivery of bad news, which every physician should carry with them until it becomes second nature. Finally, she provides specific interview questions—effectively several versions of a script, tailored to different situations— stress, school, work, family, and so on. Through these case descriptions, strategies, and scripts, the reader will be armed with specific approaches to presenting mind–body options and de-stigmatizing and de-mystifying mind–body approaches for their patients—even for those who might be anxious or skeptical about the benefits of mind–body therapies.

As the title indicates, Part II focuses on selected mind–body therapies, including breath work, biofeedback, hypnosis and guided imagery, mindfulness and compassion, and creative arts and movement therapies. McClafferty is careful to provide her reasons for selecting these and omitting others from this text. The therapies she reviews have been most rigorously studied and are best understood in terms of neuroscience and physiological mechanisms of action. They also have the largest body of evidence showing their effectiveness. McClafferty reviews this evidence in clear and accessible language. Again, as in the earlier chapters, she starts with a definition of the approach (e.g., "mindfulness" or "mindfulness-based stress reduction" developed and popularized by Jon Kabat-Zinn) and progresses to a review of the science underlying their effects, for example, increased neural connectivity related to mindfulness meditation. She then describes the applications of the technique to specific illnesses, in adults as well as children, and also to physician wellness.

The final section is an expanded review of the application of mind–body techniques to specific conditions or illnesses, with chapters addressing anxiety and depression, oncology and surgical conditions, gastroenterology, and pain—all of which have been shown to effectively respond to mind–body approaches.

This text is unique in that it addresses the use of mind–body medicine for the full spectrum of ages from young childhood through adolescence, to adults; in a range of applications from wellness to disease; and for a range of potential practitioners—patients and physicians. McClafferty is eminently qualified to advise on this spectrum, having trained and being board certified in pediatrics, pediatric emergency medicine, and integrative medicine and having led the University of Arizona's Center for Integrative Medicine's Integrative Medicine Fellowship as well as serving as founding director of the Pediatric Integrative Medicine in Residency program. Her years in clinical practice in pediatrics and certification in clinical hypnosis and acupuncture give her further hands-on experience and expertise in mind–body practices—experience that shines through in every word of her clear step-by-step practical descriptions. It is obvious that she is not only an academic, skilled at reviewing the literature—as important as that expertise is—but she also has extensive hands-on knowledge, which she imparts to readers on every page.

Esther M. Sternberg, MD
Director, University of Arizona Institute on Place and Wellbeing
Research Director, University of Arizona Center for Integrative Medicine
Professor, University of Arizona College of Medicine
University of Arizona, Tucson
Author of: *Healing Spaces: The Science of Place and Well-Being* and
The Balance Within: The Science Connecting Health and Emotions

Acknowledgments

I extend my sincere thanks to the many patients and families who initially led me to explore the mind–body therapies. Although my intention was to gain new skills to better serve their needs, in reality, I gained far more. In addition to expanding my scientific knowledge, my foray into this field of medicine has taught me to open my mind, look deeper, engage my humanity, and fully appreciate the individual's capacity to leverage their strengths in challenging circumstances.

It is my hope that this book will move my colleagues and students to extend their own exploration of this emerging field, learn to offer new treatment options, and share my sense of excitement and optimism at the rapidly unfolding research advances.

I would also like to thank Kathleen Kennedy for her expert assistance in preparing the manuscript and the many other women throughout my education, training, and professional life who have encouraged and supported my efforts and who have extended a hand back to pull me forward when I needed it the most.

Part I

Foundations

Part I provides an introduction to the field of mind–body medicine and a brief overview of its evolution, including a high-level review of early research advances foundational to the field. The physiology and impact of chronic stress is discussed with the intent of emphasizing the value of the mind–body therapies in buffering individuals from its heavy physiologic toll. An update on the placebo–nocebo response is provided to raise awareness about its role in mind-body medicine and the potential risks of precipitating unintended negative treatment responses Clinician self-care is deliberately included early in the book with the dual goals of piquing curiosity about the potential use of mind–body therapies in day-to-day practice, and of introducing mind–body tools that may help prevent burnout and promote preventive wellness. The importance of mindful language use in the medical encounter is discussed, with emphasis on its relevance in mind–body medicine. A recurring theme in the book, this is implemented using case-based examples to help the clinician expand skills in this important area.

1 Introduction

WHAT IS MIND–BODY MEDICINE?

Mind–body medicine describes a therapeutic approach used to harness the intricate connections between an individual's thoughts, emotions, and physiologic state. Many mind–body therapies have their origins in ancient cultures, and some, for example meditation, prayer, yoga, and imagery, are embedded in healing traditions around the world. Mind–body medicine has been accepted into modern medical practice gradually, with significant skepticism expressed by some clinicians practicing in the narrower biopsychosocial medical model, where the separation of mind and body is a central theme (Alonso 2004).

MIND–BODY THERAPIES IN MODERN MEDICINE

Seminal research by Walter B. Cannon, MD and colleagues in the early 1900s definitively established the existence of a powerful mind–body link. In 1926, Cannon coined the term *homeostasis* and demonstrated that challenges to the physiologic steady state resulted in activation of the sympathoadrenal axis (*fight or flight response*), leading to a surge in research around the stress response (Cannon 1929a, 1929b, 1939; Goldstein and Kopin 2007).

In the United States, Jon Kabat-Zinn, PhD, was the pioneer who introduced meditation into the medical mainstream through the program now known as Mindfulness-Based Stress Reduction, initially developed to help address the needs of chronic pain patients at the University of Massachusetts. Since its formation in the late 1970s, the program has evolved to include educational, training, and research initiatives housed in the Center for Mindfulness in Medicine, Health Care, and Society. Work at the Center has been instrumental in raising awareness about the field of mind–body medicine, catalyzing research, and opening doors for the introduction of other mind–body therapies into conventional practice models.

Early demonstration of the mind–body connection in children was published in *Pediatrics* by Olness et al. (1989) as a prospective randomized controlled study which demonstrated that salivary IgA concentrations could be acutely mediated in 57 children who received training in self-hypnosis with specific suggestions to increase salivary IgA concentrations versus a control group whose levels were unchanged ($p < 0.01$).

A groundbreaking study by Cohen et al. in the *New England Journal of Medicine* added further credibility to the field by demonstrating a correlation between a research subject's stress levels and immune function. In this innovative study, susceptibility to the common cold induced by nasal drops was measured in 394 healthy volunteers. Results showed a statistically significant dose–response relationship between stress and infection—independent of variables, including smoking, alcohol consumption, exercise, diet and sleep quality, baseline white blood cell counts, and total immunoglobulin levels (Cohen et al. 1991). These early studies, and others, were instrumental in turning the tide of skepticism, paving the way for new research initiatives that have led to the rich collection of studies supporting this rapidly evolving field.

MASTERY OF THE RELAXATION RESPONSE

One of the overarching goals of the mind–body therapies is activation of the relaxation response, roughly the physiologic opposite of *fight or flight*. Typically characterized by a decrease in heart rate, respiratory rate, blood pressure, and stress hormone secretion, it has been shown to buffer physiologic *wear and tear* on the body associated with both acute and chronic stress. Triggering of the relaxation response is central to the effective use of the mind–body therapies and can be achieved by children and adults from a spectrum of educational and developmental backgrounds, and in a surprising range of clinical settings. All the mind–body therapies discussed in Part II involve activation of the relaxation response, reinforcing the diversity of options available to interested patients. The selected mind–body therapies covered in Part II include: breath work, autogenics, progressive muscle relaxation, biofeedback, meditation, mindfulness, compassion-based cognitive therapy, yoga, tai chi, creative arts therapies, animal-assisted therapy, hypnosis, and guided imagery.

GOALS AND OBJECTIVES

The purpose of this work is to explore the wealth of research in the field and to highlight the potential of the mind–body therapies to promote health and healing in the clinical setting. These therapies describe a new approach to the patient and are foundational to the practice of integrative medicine, an emerging field that blends evidence-based complementary and conventional approaches (Maizes et al. 2015), that has been introduced into more than 70 highly respected academic medical institutions in the United States through the Academic Consortium for Integrative Medicine and Health, which promotes initiatives in education, research, and clinical work.

RELEVANCE OF MIND–BODY THERAPIES TO CLINICAL PRACTICE

The mind–body therapies are teachable skills and represent an important facet of *whole person care* that ideally emphasizes preventive health and healthy lifestyle practices in the form of stress management, quality nutrition, enjoyable regular physical activity, restorative sleep, awareness of environmental exposures, and cultivation of supportive relationships.

They also provide powerful, non-pharmacologic treatment options for a wide range of physical, mental, and behavioral conditions and can be used alone or in conjunction with conventional therapies to augment treatment or to reduce side effects. They may also help the physician leverage the placebo response—an area of active study discussed in Chapter 2.

Another important benefit is their flexibility, for example, they can be used in a range of clinical settings, from outpatient clinic to critical care unit, impacting an array of physical and mental measures. Their role in facilitating increased self-efficacy, self-regulation, and sense of agency in patients facing medical challenges is a further, and often underappreciated, strength.

A survey by the American Psychological Association reported that 44% of Americans reported an increase in their stress levels over the preceding 5 years, often a factor related to a chronic illness (American Psychological Association 2012). It has been estimated that a majority of adult primary care visits have a stress-related driver (Nerurkar et al. 2013), yet few physicians receive training in addressing stress in the primary care setting (Avey et al. 2003). Children and adolescents similarly experience frequent stressors with long-lasting physical and mental sequelae as described throughout the book, highlighting the urgent need for increased awareness of the utility of the mind–body therapies in clinical practice. In some cases, the mind–body therapies may be patient-initiated, further reinforcing the importance of clinicians becoming familiar with the range and application of these therapies and the need for an open-minded approach to their patient's curiosity about the therapies.

DEEPENING THE CLINICAL CONNECTION

Clinicians familiar with mind–body therapies also have the potential to create deeper connections with patients by exploring their experiences and strengths and helping them tap into their inner resources, reduce fear, offer hope, and reinforce realistic optimism. Use of the mind–body therapies may even indirectly benefit clinicians by adding to their available treatment options, especially in situations where conventional medicine has reached its limit of benefit, safety, or effectiveness. Evolving research around their direct use in clinician self-care is discussed in Chapter 3.

COST–BENEFITS

The ability to lower cost of treatment is an important driver in health care. Any therapy that can potentially reduce prescription drug use, decrease the post-operative length of stay, minimize pain, reduce stress-related health effects, or facilitate a successful procedure gains relevance in the business of modern health care.

POTENTIAL DOWNSIDES OF MIND–BODY THERAPIES

Potential downsides of mind–body medicine exist and include triggering or worsening of post-traumatic stress in a patient with a history of trauma of any type: physical, emotional, or sexual. This can be especially challenging if the patient has not disclosed their history, is young, or is unable to articulate their story. In a patient of any age who has experienced a trauma of any kind, or who has a diagnosis of post-traumatic stress disorder, the use of mind–body therapies should be carefully evaluated to avoid unintentional triggering of symptoms or additional distress (Section on Integrative Medicine 2016).

Ideally, these patients will already be under the care of an experienced mental health professional. Unfortunately, too often this may not be the case, and the use of mind–body therapies might precipitate unexpected emotions. In these situations, timely referral to a professional with expertise in mental health is warranted.

Other potential downsides of mind–body therapies include research gaps in some conditions, uncertainty about the best choice of therapy, and a relative paucity of trained practitioners. Unknowns in clinical outcome measurement tools and techniques are also potential downsides, although improvements in techniques, for example, use of functional magnetic resonance imaging (fMRI) has allowed significant advances in our understanding of the mechanism of action of certain therapies.

Additional potential pitfalls include unexpected worsening of a condition or symptom, inappropriate reliance on mind–body therapies as a primary treatment modality at the exclusion of proven conventional therapies in certain conditions, unrealistic expectations, resistance based on religious grounds, fear of trying something new, prohibitive cost, and lack of accessibility to therapies.

Gaps in national insurance coverage and reimbursement are further challenges, with wide variation seen in state-to-state and carrier-to-carrier coverage and a growing number of uninsured patients.

WHAT WILL NOT BE COVERED HERE

The rich philosophical debate related to the existence and nature of consciousness will not be covered here, although the topic is the focus of intense research interest. These questions are explored in a number of excellent works and lie beyond the intended scope of this book.

Some of the mind–body therapies not covered here fall into other fields, for example massage within the practice of manual medicine. Others lie outside the book's intended focus, and although popular, lack robust supporting evidence in the clinical setting.

References

Alonso, Y. 2004. The biopsychosocial model in medical research: The evolution of the health concept over the last two decades. *Patient Educ Couns* 53 (2): 239–244. doi:10.1016/S0738-3991(03)00146-0.

American Psychological Association. 2012. *Stress in America: Our Health at Risk.* Washington, DC: American Psychological Association.

Avey, H., K. B. Matheny, A. Robbins, and T. A. Jacobson. 2003. Health care providers' training, perceptions, and practices regarding stress and health outcomes. *J Natl Med Assoc* 95 (9): 833, 836–845.

Cannon, W. B. 1929a. *Bodily Changes in Pain, Hunger, Fear and Rage.* New York: D. Appleton & Company.

Cannon, W. B. 1929b. Organization for physiological homeostasis. *Am Physiol Soc* 9 (3): 399–431.

Cannon, W. B. 1939. *The Wisdom of the Body.* New York: W.W. Norton & Company.

Cohen, S., D. A. Tyrrell, and A. P. Smith. 1991. Psychological stress and susceptibility to the common cold. *N Engl J Med* 325 (9): 606–612. doi:10.1056/NEJM199108293250903.

Goldstein, D. S., and I. J. Kopin. 2007. Evolution of concepts of stress. *Stress* 10 (2): 109–120. doi:10.1080/10253890701288935.

Maizes, V., R. Horwitz, P. Lebensohn, H. McClafferty, J. Dalen, and A. Weil. 2015. The evolution of integrative medical education: The influence of the University of Arizona Center for Integrative Medicine. *J Integr Med* 13 (6): 356–362. doi:10.1016/S2095-4964(15)60209-6.

Nerurkar, A., A. Bitton, R. B. Davis, R. S. Phillips, and G. Yeh. 2013. When physicians counsel about stress: Results of a national study. *JAMA Intern Med* 173 (1): 76–77. doi:10.1001/2013.jamainternmed.480.

Olness, K., T. Culbert, and D. Uden. 1989. Self-regulation of salivary immunoglobulin A by children. *Pediatrics* 83 (1): 66–71.

Section on Integrative Medicine. 2016. Mind–body therapies in children and youth. *Pediatrics* 138 (3): e5, e7. doi:10.1542/peds.2016-1896.

UMass Medical School Center for Mindfulness. Retrieved from https://www.umassmed.edu/cfm/.

2 The science of stress

Why it matters in health care

WHAT IS STRESS AND WHY IS IT RELEVANT TO CLINICAL PRACTICE?

Stress in humans is generated when expectations of any kind, physiologic, emotional, situational, educational, and so on, do not match the individual's perceptions or anticipations, triggering compensatory responses that are often maladaptive (Goldstein and McEwen 2002).

As mentioned briefly in Chapter 1, it has been estimated that as many as 60%–80% of primary care visits have a stress-related component (Nerurkar et al. 2013), yet counseling about stress was rare in a survey study of 33,045 office visits with primary care physicians (3%) as compared to nutrition counseling (16.8%), physical activity counseling (12.3%), weight loss (6.3%), and tobacco cessation (3.7%).

Addressing stress effectively in the medical setting matters because, in excess, stress has been associated with significant mental and physical consequences in both children and adults. An overview by Chrousos (2009) provides insight into the origin and early work in the field of stress physiology and notes that the word stress stems from the Latin *strictus* drawn tight and the Greek *strangalizein* to strangle. The term is thought to have been introduced into medical research from the field of physics, where it describes the force applied to an object—for example, the force used to bend or shape metal.

In physiology, stress is defined as a state where homeostasis is challenged by mental or physical factors, requiring an adaptive response by the organism to reestablish equilibrium or steady state, a concept described by physiologist Walter Cannon in the early 1930s (Cannon 1963).

Failure to regain homeostasis through either excessive or insufficient correction has been associated with increased risks of morbidity or mortality (Chrousos 2009).

Work in the field was furthered by Hans Selye, MD, and others, who built on these findings and shaped the theory of allostasis (the process by which a state of internal, physiological equilibrium is maintained by an organism in response to actual or perceived environmental and physiological stressors) (Chrousos 2009).

Bruce S. McEwen, PhD, another pioneer in the field of stress research, has described allostasis as *maintaining stability through change* in which the body responds to stressors with the goal of reestablishing homeostasis. One of the underlying principles of allostasis is that the adaptive process is ongoing, based on information from a variety of inputs from the sympathetic and parasympathetic nervous systems and the hypothalamic–pituitary–adrenal (HPA) axis (Goldstein and McEwen 2002).

IS ALL STRESS BAD?

The concept of allostasis reminds us that, physiologically, not all stress is bad. In proper proportion, it can actually strengthen adaptive reserve. For example, stress to the immune system in the form of influenza infection causes upregulation of the proinflammatory cytokines necessary to fight the virus. Cytokines attack the invading organism and, in turn, activate the hypothalamic–pituitary–adrenal (HPA) axis readying the body systems for action in the form of fever, elevated cortisol release, increased blood flow, increased respiratory rate and so on, as seen in a typical reaction to infection with influenza. In a generally healthy host, once the virus has been subdued, cortisol forms a negative feedback loop, reining in the HPA-axis-driven inflammatory response and returning the system to equilibrium (Webster et al. 2002).

The adaptive reserve is increased in this scenario through the production of B lymphocyte memory cells which stand ready to deploy with a faster, more efficient response with the next exposure to a similar agent. Other examples of stressors increasing adaptive reserve include the building of muscle mass through repeated proportionate strength training and increasing cardiovascular endurance through incremental increase in speed and duration of training runs.

HOW DOES STRESS CAUSE ILLNESS?

The connection between stress and illness occurs because mediators of the stress response include a wide range of neuroendocrine hormones, neurotransmitters, cytokines, glucocorticoids, immune cells, and receptors involving peripheral and central nervous systems which influence essentially every part of the body, highlighting the real consequences of imbalance. Examples include neurologic, reproductive, endocrine, cardiac, pulmonary, gastrointestinal, urogenital, metabolic, circadian, and immune systems.

Work in stress physiology has also correlated release of proinflammatory cytokines with the sickness syndrome, which includes fatigue, social withdrawal, depressed mood, irritability, and poor cognition, seen in both adult and pediatric individuals suffering chronic stress (Elenkov and Chrousos 1999; Chrousos 2000).

It is widely recognized that stress can take a steep physiologic toll through upregulation of the inflammatory response, linked to an extensive list of conditions, including (Chrousos 2009):

- Asthma
- Allergies
- Migraine and other pain disorders
- Gastrointestinal conditions such as pain, diarrhea, constipation, reflux
- Cardiovascular abnormalities such as hypertension, angina, atherosclerotic disease
- Mental-emotional states such as depression, anxiety, panic attacks, psychotic breaks
- Insomnia and other sleep disorders

Chronic stress also drives metabolic disorders such as obesity, non-alcoholic fatty liver disease (NALFD), polycystic ovarian syndrome, and related conditions where upregulation of inflammatory pathways interfere with insulin receptors, glucose transport, and cholesterol and triglyceride metabolism (Hotamisligil 2006; Danese and McEwen 2012; Levine et al. 2014; Farr et al. 2015).

A comprehensive review by Hackett and Steptoe outlines the emerging literature linking stress and type 2 diabetes, and reviews the physiologic pathways involved, including dysregulation of the HPA axis and cardiovascular system, changes in cortisol secretion and effect, and upregulation of inflammation associated with increase in visceral adipose tissue, a well-established source of highly proinflammatory adipokines such as interleukin-6, tumor necrosis factor, and C-reactive protein, which are widely distributed via the circulatory system. Sympathetic nervous system induced increases in blood pressure, heart rate, and cardiac output have all been correlated with increased prevalence of type 2 diabetes, as has blunting of insulin sensitivity and flattening of diurnal cortisol concentrations after waking (Hackett and Steptoe 2017).

STRESS MODIFIERS

Variation in genetic, epigenetic, and individual susceptibility to stressors; the presence of compounding or buffering factors; and importantly *magnitude* and *duration* of the stressors play significant roles in the development of pathology. This is conveyed by the term *allostatic load*, which refers to the accumulated physiologic consequence of repeated stress to the system (Seeman et al. 1997; Goldstein and McEwen 2002).

STRESS AND THE LIFECYCLE, THE IMPACT OF ADVERSE CHILDHOOD EXPERIENCES

An important example of the cost of stress throughout the lifecycle can be found in research correlating adverse childhood experiences (ACEs) and adult health, which demonstrates the damage unmitigated stress, especially initiated early in life, can have on long-term health outcomes (Felitti et al. 1998).

Also known as *toxic stress*, it is associated with HPA axis dysregulation when the developing system is pressed into overdrive—compounded by blunting of the cortisol response, which allows the stress response to go unmitigated (Webster et al. 2002; Johnson et al. 2013).

Because the majority of immune system development occurs before birth and is refined and calibrated in the first year of life, it has been proposed that the maturational processes occurring in this time frame amplify the impact of early stress-related disruptions, "Like changing the course of a rocket at the moment of take-off" (Coe and Lubach 2003).

Children with these exposures are left in a state of *fight-fright-or-freeze*, with shunting of cognitive resources away from those involved in learning and memory. They exist in a state of perceiving constant danger, unable to focus on learning, failing to develop healthy relationships with peers, and unable to develop trust with adults and is correlated with a high prevalence of learning and/or behavioral problems in children who have experienced four or more adverse events (Johnson et al. 2013).

An understanding of the cascade of physiologic responses triggered by chronic stress in children, adolescents, and adults can help clarify the relevance of the mind–body therapies in clinical practice (Bethell et al. 2016; Liu 2017).

THE KAISER STUDY

Work in the field of adverse childhood events was initially documented by Dr. Vincent Felitti, chief of Kaiser Permanente's Department of Preventive Medicine, San Diego, CA, in the early 1980s, with colleagues David Williamson, PhD and Dr. Robert Anda, medical epidemiologist. They studied the association of childhood abuse and household dysfunction to leading causes of death in adults in 17,241 members of Kaiser Permanente (Felitti et al. 1998).

Results of this study showed that two-thirds of participants had at least one ACE, and 87% of those had more than one ACE. One-fourth had at least two categories of childhood ACE exposure, and a graded relationship was seen between the number of childhood exposures and each of the adult health risk behaviors and disease studies ($p < 0.001$). With an ACE score of 4 or more, the likelihood of disease increased exponentially:

- Chronic pulmonary lung disease increases by 390%
- Hepatitis by 240%
- Depression by 460%
- Suicide by 1,220%

Those with six or more ACEs died nearly 20 years earlier on average compared to those with no ACEs.

Seminal work by Shonkoff and colleagues has furthered our understanding of how HPA axis dysregulation occurs when the developing nervous system is pressed into overdrive. It demonstrated how chronic upregulation of interleukin-6, interleukin-1-beta, and tumor necrosis factor-alpha have been shown to have important roles in synaptic plasticity, neurogenesis, and neuromodulation—which affect learning, memory, and cognition (Shonkoff et al. 2009; Johnson et al. 2013; Shonkoff 2016).

OTHER PHYSIOLOGIC CONSEQUENCES OF CHRONIC STRESS

Telomere shortening

Pioneering work by Elizabeth Blackburn and Elissa Epel led to the discovery of the enzyme telomerase, associated with telomeres, which are short DNA sequences that cap the end of each chromosome. Telomere length has subsequently been established as a key biomarker of longevity and remains the subject of intense research activity (Blackburn and Epel 2012).

Reduction in telomere length has been associated with recent stressful life events in a 2015 study by Verhoeven involving 2,936 adults (Verhoeven et al. 2015), and a 2017 meta-analysis by Hanssen involving 16,238 participants found a significant correlation between higher levels of childhood stressors and shortened telomere length (Hanssen et al. 2017).

Cardiovascular complications

Large population studies in adults have demonstrated that cardiovascular complications, including the heightened risk of coronary artery disease and stroke, are significantly associated with long work hours described as more than 55 hours per week. A study in 603,838 adults showed an increase of incident stroke $p = 0.002$ (relative risk 1.33, 95% confidence interval 1.11–1.61) and of incident coronary artery disease $p = 0.02$, (relative risk 1.13, 95% confidence interval 1.02–1.26) (Kivimaki et al. 2015).

An earlier study in 197,473 adults found an association between job strain (psychological stress) and heart disease 1.23 (95% confidence interval 1.10–1.37) after controlling for sex, age groups, socioeconomic level, geographic region, lifestyle, and conventional risk factors (Kivimaki et al. 2012).

A subsequent study by Kang demonstrated a crossover effect correlating increased estimated 10-year risk of cardiovascular disease in individuals whose spouses worked above 30 hours per week. In this cohort of 16,917 adults, relative risk increased 2.52 for husbands of working women and 2.43 for wives of working husbands (Kang and Hong 2017).

Stress has also been shown to take a physiologic toll on the cardiovascular systems in younger generations. For example, low stress resilience, as determined by trained psychological evaluation, in young military conscripts in Sweden ($n = 1,547,182$) (Lilieblad and Stahlberg 1977; Falkstedt et al. 2013; Bergh et al. 2015) was found to be correlated with risk of adult hypertension when adjusted for body-mass index (BMI), family history, and socioeconomic factors, $p < 0.001$ (lowest vs. highest quintile: HR 1.43; 95% CI 1.40–1.46; $p < 0.001$; incidence rates, 278.7 vs. 180.0 per 100,000 person-years). In this large cohort, the men who had both low stress resilience and a high BMI also had a more than three times the risk of hypertension than those with normal BMI (Crump et al. 2016a).

Further analysis of the Swedish cohort ($n = 1,534,425$) found a statistically significant correlation between low stress resilience, as described in the aforementioned study, and risk of developing type 2 diabetes ($p < 0.0001$) adjusted for BMI, family history of diabetes, and a range of individual and socioeconomic factors. (HR for lowest vs. highest quintile: 1.51; 95% CI 1.46, 1.57) (Crump et al. 2016b).

BREAKING THE CYCLE OF TOXIC STRESS

Work by Shonkff and colleagues has distilled four themes for incorporation in policy and practice to educate and help to break the toxic stress cycle and emphasize how compounding factors such as socioeconomic status and cultural norms can contribute to the prevalence of chronic disease (Shonkoff 2016):

1 Early experiences affect lifelong health, not just learning.
2 Healthy brain development requires buffering from toxic stress, not simply enrichment.
3 Changing outcomes for at-risk children requires supporting their adult caretakers in their own life transformations.
4 The prenatal period through 3 years after birth is a time when more effective interventions are needed for the most disadvantaged.

MIND–BODY MEDICINE AND STRESS EFFECTS: ONLY FOR THE AFFLUENT?

Over time, encouraging research in the use of mind–body medicine is beginning to accumulate in underprivileged populations, for example, in a study by Gallegos et al. in 50 women with a history of trauma, family violence, childhood physical or sexual abuse, or family death who undertook an 8-week mindfulness-based stress reduction (MBSR) course consisting of weekly 120-minute sessions and one 4-hour retreat. Women received weekly phone reminders and evaluations were done at entry and 4, 8, and 12 weeks. Fifty-seven percent completed 50% or more of the classes, 43% completed 75% or more, and 21% completed all classes. Statistically significant improvements ($p < 0.001$) were seen in the following measures: perception of stress, depression, trait anxiety and state anxiety, emotional dysregulation, and post-traumatic stress. Participants had increased mindfulness, and session attendance was significantly associated with decreased interleukin-6 ($p = 0.03$) (Gallegos et al. 2015).

Another study in 27 female survivors of childhood sexual abuse who completed an 8-week MBSR course that included sitting meditation, body scan, walking meditation, gentle yoga, and informal day-to-day mindfulness showed a statistically significant decrease in all measured scales, including depression, anxiety, PTSD, avoidance, re-experiencing, and hyperarousal, and an improvement in mindfulness, all at $p <$ at least 0.0001, with 19 of the 27 women maintaining improvements in depression, anxiety, PTSD, and mindfulness at 2.5-year follow-up (Kimbrough et al. 2010).

Mindfulness interventions remain an area of active research for a range of groups including traumatized adults, adolescents, and children and adults and children living with chronic illness, including cancer (Ortiz and Sibinga 2017).

Studies such as these reinforce the utility of mind–body skills in the clinical setting and highlight the importance of gaining familiarity these non-pharmacologic tools for all clinicians, not simply those who work with the affluent or well educated (Liu 2017).

CHANGING THE APPROACH TO STRESS IN THE CLINICAL VISIT

Acknowledgment of the impact of stress on health in the clinical encounter destigmatizes the topic and sends an important message to the patient that the experience of stress is common and does not imply weakness, regardless of gender, culture, or socioeconomic status. The clinician who feels confident enough to initiate this discussion may also present an opening for patient's disclosure of adverse childhood experiences, creating an opportunity for education about how emerging research has linked these to adult health.

For example:

> "Research has determined that day-to-day stress impacts our long-term health. I'd like to talk with you about your stressors and how you're handling them—if you are open to discussion."

> "We are learning about new approaches to health that involve the mind–body connection especially with regard to stress. Would you like to know more?"

> "We now know that in some people, difficult experiences in childhood can impact adult health. Is this something you might like to talk more about?"

A familiar concern is that addressing complex topics such as stress in the clinic visit adds time pressure to an already burdened system. New approaches are being initiated nationally to address this in the form of a team-based approach that may include health coaches, group visits, and new methods of contact such as email, online educational material, text reminders, and phone calls (Bodenheimer et al. 2002).

CLOSING THE INFORMATION GAP

An informed approach to the impact of stress on health provides clinicians a way to help patients raise awareness of the presence and effect of stress in their day-to-day lives and how it impacts long-term health. With the clinician's guidance, patients can begin to recognize the gaps between their anticipated experience and actual experiences (perceptions), which can be the root cause of significant stress. By introducing new skills to help recognize and mitigate stressors, clinicians can open a new frontier to health for their patients and become valuable partners in supporting a patient's healthy lifestyle changes.

CASE-BASED LEARNING: PATIENT STORIES

Case examples of real-life patients (names changed for privacy) introducing mind–body therapies into clinical encounters are woven throughout the book with an emphasis in Part III "Clinical Application." In addition to learning from the successes and challenges these patients experienced, the intent is to encourage readers to become aware of potential opportunities for the use of mind–body therapies in their own lives, hopefully encouraging new pathways for experiential learning.

References

Bergh, C., R. Udumyan, K. Fall, H. Almroth, and S. Montgomery. 2015. Stress resilience and physical fitness in adolescence and risk of coronary heart disease in middle age. *Heart* 101 (8): 623–629. doi:10.1136/heartjnl-2014-306703.

Bethell, C., N. Gombojav, M. Solloway, and L. Wissow. 2016. Adverse childhood experiences, resilience and mindfulness-based approaches: Common denominator issues for children with emotional, mental, or behavioral problems. *Child Adolesc Psychiatr Clin N Am* 25 (2): 139–156. doi:10.1016/j.chc.2015.12.001.

Blackburn, E. H., and E. S. Epel. 2012. Telomeres and adversity: Too toxic to ignore. *Nature* 490 (7419): 169–171. doi:10.1038/490169a.

Bodenheimer, T., E. H. Wagner, and K. Grumbach. 2002. Improving primary care for patients with chronic illness. *JAMA* 288 (14): 1775–1779.

Cannon, W. B. 1963. *The Wisdom of the Body*, 2nd ed. Rev. and Enl. Ed edition (April 17, 1963). New York: W. W. Norton & Company.

Chrousos, G. P. 2000. The stress response and immune function: Clinical implications: The 1999 Novera H. Spector Lecture. *Ann N Y Acad Sci* 917: 38–67.

Chrousos, G. P. 2009. Stress and disorders of the stress system. *Nat Rev Endocrinol* 5 (7): 374–381. doi:10.1038/nrendo.2009.106.

Coe, C. L., and G. R. Lubach. 2003. Critical periods of special health relevance for psychoneuroimmunology. *Brain Behav Immun* 17 (1): 3–12.

Crump, C., J. Sundquist, M. A. Winkleby, and K. Sundquist. 2016a. Low stress resilience in late adolescence and risk of hypertension in adulthood. *Heart* 102 (7): 541–547. doi:10.1136/heartjnl-2015-308597.

Crump, C., J. Sundquist, M. A. Winkleby, and K. Sundquist. 2016b. Stress resilience and subsequent risk of type 2 diabetes in 1.5 million young men. *Diabetologia* 59 (4): 728–733. doi:10.1007/s00125-015-3846-7.

Danese, A., and B. S. McEwen. 2012. Adverse childhood experiences, allostasis, allostatic load, and age-related disease. *Physiol Behav* 106 (1): 29–39. doi:10.1016/j.physbeh.2011.08.019.

Elenkov, I. J., and G. P. Chrousos. 1999. Stress hormones, Th1/Th2 patterns, pro/anti-inflammatory cytokines and susceptibility to disease. *Trends Endocrinol Metab* 10 (9): 359–368.

Falkstedt, D., K. Sorjonen, T. Hemmingsson, I. J. Deary, and B. Melin. 2013. Psychosocial functioning and intelligence both partly explain socioeconomic inequalities in premature death: A population-based male cohort study. *PLoS One* 8 (12): e82031. doi:10.1371/journal.pone.0082031.

Farr, O. M., B. J. Ko, K. E. Joung, L. Zaichenko, N. Usher, M. Tsoukas, B. Thakkar, C. R. Davis, J. A. Crowell, and C. S. Mantzoros. 2015. Posttraumatic stress disorder, alone or additively with early life adversity, is associated with obesity and cardiometabolic risk. *Nutr Metab Cardiovasc Dis* 25 (5): 479–488. doi:10.1016/j.numecd.2015.01.007.

Felitti, V. J., R. F. Anda, D. Nordenberg, D. F. Williamson, A. M. Spitz, V. Edwards, M. P. Koss, and J. S. Marks. 1998. Relationship of childhood abuse and household dysfunction to many of the leading causes of death in adults: The adverse childhood experiences (ACE) study. *Am J Prev Med* 14 (4): 245–258.

Gallegos, A. M., M. C. Lytle, J. A. Moynihan, and N. L. Talbot. 2015. Mindfulness-based stress reduction to enhance psychological functioning and improve inflammatory biomarkers in trauma-exposed women: A pilot study. *Psychol Trauma* 7 (6): 525–532. doi:10.1037/tra0000053.

Goldstein, D. S., and B. McEwen. 2002. Allostasis, homeostats, and the nature of stress. *Stress* 5 (1): 55–58. doi:10.1080/102538902900012345.

Hackett, R. A., and A. Steptoe. 2017. Type 2 diabetes mellitus and psychological stress: A modifiable risk factor. *Nat Rev Endocrinol* 13 (9): 547–560. doi:10.1038/nrendo.2017.64.

Hanssen, L. M., N. S. Schutte, J. M. Malouff, and E. S. Epel. 2017. The relationship between childhood psychosocial stressor level and telomere length: A meta-analysis. *Health Psychol Res* 5 (1): 6378. doi:10.4081/hpr.2017.6378.

Hotamisligil, G. S. 2006. Inflammation and metabolic disorders. *Nature* 444 (7121): 860–867. doi:10.1038/nature05485.

Johnson, S. B., A. W. Riley, D. A. Granger, and J. Riis. 2013. The science of early life toxic stress for pediatric practice and advocacy. *Pediatrics* 131 (2): 319–327. doi:10.1542/peds.2012-0469.

Kang, M. Y., and Y. C. Hong. 2017. Crossover effect of spouse weekly working hours on estimated 10-years risk of cardiovascular disease. *PLoS One* 12 (8): e0182010. doi:10.1371/journal.pone.0182010.

Kimbrough, E., T. Magyari, P. Langenberg, M. Chesney, and B. Berman. 2010. Mindfulness intervention for child abuse survivors. *J Clin Psychol* 66 (1): 17–33. doi:10.1002/jclp.20624.

Kivimaki, M., M. Jokela, S. T. Nyberg, A. Singh-Manoux, E. I. Fransson, L. Alfredsson, J. B. Bjorner et al. 2015. Long working hours and risk of coronary heart disease and stroke: A systematic review and meta-analysis of published and unpublished data for 603,838 individuals. *Lancet* 386 (10005): 1739–1746. doi:10.1016/S0140-6736(15)60295-1.

Kivimaki, M., S. T. Nyberg, G. D. Batty, E. I. Fransson, K. Heikkila, L. Alfredsson, J. B. Bjorner et al. 2012. Job strain as a risk factor for coronary heart disease: A collaborative meta-analysis of individual participant data. *Lancet* 380 (9852): 1491–1497. doi:10.1016/S0140-6736(12)60994-5.

Levine, A. B., L. M. Levine, and T. B. Levine. 2014. Posttraumatic stress disorder and cardiometabolic disease. *Cardiology* 127 (1): 1–19. doi:10.1159/000354910.

Lilieblad, B., and Stahlberg, B. 1977. *Reliability of the Psychological Assessments at Conscription.* Stockholm, Sweden: Armed Forces Research Department.

Liu, R. T. 2017. Childhood adversities and depression in adulthood: Current findings and future directions. *Clin Psychol (New York)* 24 (2): 140–153. doi:10.1111/cpsp.12190.

Nerurkar, A., A. Bitton, R. B. Davis, R. S. Phillips, and G. Yeh. 2013. When physicians counsel about stress: Results of a national study. *JAMA Intern Med* 173 (1): 76–77. doi:10.1001/2013.jamainternmed.480.

Ortiz, R., and E. M. Sibinga. 2017. The role of mindfulness in reducing the adverse effects of childhood stress and trauma. *Children (Basel)* 4 (3): 16. doi:10.3390/children4030016.

Seeman, T. E., B. H. Singer, J. W. Rowe, R. I. Horwitz, and B. S. McEwen. 1997. Price of adaptation: Allostatic load and its health consequences—MacArthur studies of successful aging. *Arch Intern Med* 157 (19): 2259–2268.

Shonkoff, J. P. 2016. Capitalizing on advances in science to reduce the health consequences of early childhood adversity. *JAMA Pediatr* 170 (10): 1003–1007. doi:10.1001/jamapediatrics.2016.1559.

Shonkoff, J. P., W. T. Boyce, and B. S. McEwen. 2009. Neuroscience, molecular biology, and the childhood roots of health disparities: Building a new framework for health promotion and disease prevention. *JAMA* 301 (21): 2252–2259. doi:10.1001/jama.2009.754.

Verhoeven, J. E., P. van Oppen, E. Puterman, B. Elzinga, and B. W. Penninx. 2015. The association of early and recent psychosocial life stress with leukocyte telomere length. *Psychosom Med* 77 (8): 882–891. doi:10.1097/PSY.0000000000000226.

Webster, J. I., L. Tonelli, and E. M. Sternberg. 2002. Neuroendocrine regulation of immunity. *Annu Rev Immunol* 20: 125–163. doi:10.1146/annurev.immunol.20.082401.104914.

3   Clinician self-care

INTRODUCTION

The high prevalence of clinician burnout and its associated serious mental and physical comorbidities, including suicide, have been widely reported. At least 50% of physicians in the United States experience burnout. Between 2011 and 2014, burnout increased in all specialties in U.S. physicians, reinforcing the urgent need for change in the health care system (Dyrbye et al. 2017b).

Sustained initiatives at the personal, institutional, and cultural levels are needed to address ingrained behaviors, outdated beliefs, and to dissipate the *hidden curriculum* of medicine. Inaction is simply too costly (Dyrbye et al. 2015; Kulaylat et al. 2017; Shanafelt and Noseworthy 2017).

National initiatives are now shifting to prevention and to the identification of multisystem solutions needed to facilitate meaningful progress (Shanafelt et al. 2017).

This chapter will provide a brief background on burnout and resilience and narrow the focus to personal-individual approaches to burnout prevention and mitigation, with particular emphasis on the use of mindfulness and self-regulation in medicine.

UNDERSTANDING BURNOUT

Most commonly measured by the Maslach Burnout Inventory, burnout is assessed by measurement of emotional exhaustion, depersonalization, and sense of personal accomplishment (Maslach et al. 1996). Symptoms of burnout can be seen at every stage of medical training, peaking during training and in mid-career (Dyrbye et al. 2013).

CONTRIBUTING FACTORS

Many factors contribute to burnout, some of the most common include:

- *Individual stressors* such as fatigue, excessive work hours, difficult patients, patient death or poor outcomes, moral distress, malpractice suit threat, workplace bullying, financial duress, isolation, lack of coping skills, and competing family demands.
- *Personality traits*, paradoxically perceived positive traits, such as altruism, compassion, perfectionism, competitiveness, resiliency, and strong work ethic, valued in the quest for entry into medical school can predispose to burnout if pushed to extremes.

For example, manifesting as martyrdom, compassion fatigue, imposter syndrome, isolation, a sense of invincibility, workaholic behavior, and, ultimately, burnout.

- *Hospital- or practice-based stressors* such as competition, job insecurity, management conflicts, loss of personal control, time pressures, electronic medical records, productivity and performance demands, and unsupportive or hostile work environments. Organizational leadership has been shown to have a significant impact on physician burnout, especially the elements of good communication, efficiency of the organization, level of flexibility and autonomy, and workload expectations (Shanafelt et al. 2015).

- *Stressors embedded in the "culture of medicine"* such as expectation of unrealistic endurance, code of silence, vicarious traumatization (second victim phenomenon), academic pressures to publish or to obtain grant funding, fear of perceived vulnerability, and, paradoxically, increase in faculty stress and burnout due to reduction of resident duty hours (Blum et al. 2011; Wong and Imrie 2013).

MITIGATING FACTORS

Identifying effective approaches to burnout prevention and mitigation and promotion of well-being in health care professionals are areas of intense study. Factors associated with lower burnout have been identified and include (Maslach and Leiter 2008; Hinami et al. 2012):

- Greater sense of control
- Absence of role conflict
- A sense of fair treatment
- Positive social support
- Appropriate rewards (financial, institutional, and social)
- Alignment of values between individual and workplace
- Positive leadership

Emerging research from the field of positive psychology on the application of signature character strengths (ASCS) as related to well-being and burnout (especially emotional exhaustion) in medical training introduces new ideas about how medical trainees might leverage existing character strengths and cultivate their less-robust traits to help buffer the stressors of medical training and practice (Hausler et al. 2017).

WHOLE CLINICIAN WELLNESS

Accruing research on the serious physical, mental, and social effects of long-term stress, shift work, and sleep disruption reinforce the importance of a shift toward preventive clinician health that emphasizes *whole person health* (Dyrbye et al. 2017a; Hausler et al. 2017). Although no single approach has been identified as universally effective to combat burnout (West et al. 2016), some compelling research involves the mind–body therapies, particularly mindfulness and compassion training, discussed in more detail in the following and in Chapter 8, "Mindfulness."

Importantly, studies have shown that wellness behaviors in physicians are additive (Shanafelt et al. 2012), associated with increased telomere length (Sun et al. 2012) and can even impact patient outcome and the quality of patient counseling (Howe et al. 2010).

Given the rigors of medical training and practice, mastery of coping skills to reduce the detrimental mental and physical effects of chronic stress in health care workers and trainees should become a professional priority (Shonkoff 2012; Silverman and Sternberg 2012; Downs and Faulkner 2015).

BURNOUT PREVENTION

Maintaining a sense of self-efficacy and internal locus of control are critical to the development of professional values in medicine and are fundamentally important to cultivate early in training to anticipate the rigors that lie ahead and to build effective problem-solving skills in the professional setting (Warnock 2008). Cultural values and variations are also important to consider (Hamou-Jennings and Dong 2016).

A systematic review and meta-analysis of interventions to prevent physician burnout by West et al. found moderate positive effect in an array of individual measures taken by clinicians or trainees. These included: stress management training, facilitated small group meetings, and communication skills training. Organizational measures found to have benefit included duty-hour restrictions, changes to clinical work processes, and shorter length of inpatient attending rotation (West et al. 2016).

UNDERSTANDING RESILIENCE

The aforementioned factors tie into the growing literature on resilience in medicine, which is ideally characterized by a state of adaptive flexibility that builds on existing strengths (Howe et al. 2012).

Elements of resilience include: sense of self-efficacy, self-control, ability to ask for appropriate help and support, learning from challenging experiences, and persistence. Physical health and stamina are important parts of the equation, as are mastery of effective coping skills. It is important to qualify the goal here is *healthy resilience*, in the sense that even the hardiest individuals in medicine can be broken by a culture and practice that is consistently negative and unsupportive.

Much of the work in resilience research comes from the field of child psychology, through the study of children and their families who have faced extraordinary challenges. A summary of resilience characteristics by Martin and Marsh (2006) in students that linked academic performance with student self-perception, behaviors, and attitudes, categorized elements of individual resilience as *confidence, coordination (planning), control, composure,* and *commitment*. These traits exemplify the individual's internal sense of control and belief in their ability to shape and influence a situation despite setbacks.

Positive coping skills such as healthy social support, humor, managing negative emotions, learning from adversity, finding meaning in adverse circumstances, and finding motivation through one's moral beliefs have all been associated with resilience. Work in child psychology reinforces the message that resilience can be nurtured and learned, and a certain amount of challenge or adversity is needed for its development (Howe et al. 2012).

In the public health literature, community resilience has been seen to be cultivated by the development of social trust, reciprocity, neighborhood efficacy, and civic engagement (Zautra 2009; Reich et al. 2010).

These findings have immediate relevance to the medical community at large, as well as to faculty and trainees in a variety of clinical settings. Cultivating a sense of engagement, community, and common purpose can be highly protective, as can reframing a tough situation, cultivating coping skills, and focusing on problem solving rather than feeling victimized.

MORAL DISTRESS: A COMPOUNDING FACTOR

One issue complicating well-being in medicine is the high risk of *moral injury* or *moral distress*, documented in both military personnel and physicians. This can be caused by actions which run counter to individual values or to accepted societal behavior, such as frequent exposure to death and the need to deliberately cause pain to do good (bone setting, surgery, suturing, injections), which can take a heavy toll over time (Litz et al. 2009; Smajdor et al. 2011).

Other potential triggers of moral distress include (Fumis et al. 2017):

- Medical error
- Patient's suffering
- Prolongation of life
- Feeling of incompetence
- Conflict about treatment
- Poor team communication
- Perceived misalignment of values

In modern medical practice, these feelings may be compounded by the frustration of imposed organizational constraints such as electronic medical records, insufficient administrative support, or financial cutbacks.

BUILDING RESILIENCE IN MEDICAL TRAINEES

Shifts in medical education that align with resilience building in trainees include: a shift from didactic to case-based, self-directed learning, implementation of constructive feedback, and persistence in the setting and attaining of both short- and longer-term goals. Multiple tracks or increased flexibility in choosing rotations increases a sense of control, as do facilitated approaches to clinical learning that build resourcefulness and confidence in one's skills and abilities over time. Coaching and mentoring can be used to convey confidence in trainees and to reinforce the importance of persistence and commitment as core professional values that may help buffer the highly competitive culture fostered by some training programs (Dunn et al. 2008; Jensen et al. 2008; Smith et al. 2008; McAllister and McKinnon 2009; Epstein and Krasner 2013; Houpy et al. 2017).

A FOCUS ON MINDFULNESS

Mindfulness has drawn particular interest as a tool in clinician self-care as research continues to accrue delineating its benefits. Introduced into mainstream medicine in the late 1970s by Kabat-Zinn, Ph.D. (Kabat-Zinn 1982), research on mindfulness—often in the form of mindfulness-based stress reduction, or MBSR (discussed in detail in Chapter 8—"Mindfulness")—has revealed important benefits that can be applied to enhance clinician well-being. Some identified characteristics for clinicians include (West et al. 2014):

- Stress reduction
- Cognitive flexibility
- Emotional regulation
- Increased self-awareness
- Increased adaptive reserve
- Decrease in personal isolation
- More thoughtful decision making
- Improved attention and listening
- Effectiveness at addressing patient's concerns
- Improved patient outcomes

Mindfulness in the clinician may also help (Kabat-Zinn 2013):

- Cultivate a sense of calm
- Decrease rumination
- Maintain focus in the moment
- Invite curiosity and enhance resourcefulness
- Questions harsh self-judgment and negative internal dialogue
- Eliminate need for comparisons and pressure of need for *expert-mind*

Impact on brain structure, function, and inflammatory markers

The benefits of mindfulness include changes in both function and structure of the brain. It has been shown to enhance functional connectivity in brain areas associated with improvements in self-referential processing and positive effect as well as to decrease expression of some proinflammatory cytokines in small studies (Kilpatrick et al. 2011).

A systematic review of 30 studies on MBSR training found that mindfulness was associated with:

- Improved functional connectivity: prefrontal cortex, cingulate cortex, insula, hippocampus (associated with improved emotional regulation)
- Decreased functional activity in the amygdala (detection and response to perceived threats, fear) (Gotink et al. 2016)

And a randomized controlled study comparing an 8-week MBSR training versus relaxation training in ($n = 23$) elderly patients versus control relaxation-only group ($n = 22$) found that neural connectivity was more positive in the meditation group, and this enhanced connectivity correlated with increased self-awareness and regulation of negative affective processing (Shao et al. 2016).

The use of mindfulness and mindfulness-based stress reduction in addressing physician burnout has been shown to improve measures of empathy and sense of personal accomplishment, as well as reducing depersonalization and emotional exhaustion (Ludwig and Kabat-Zinn 2008; Fortney and Taylor 2010).

Studies investigating the use of abbreviated mindfulness interventions have shown benefit in reduction of burnout symptoms (Fortney et al. 2013), as have interventions designed using a hybrid in-person and group telephone approach (Bazarko et al. 2013). Other studies have used mindfulness or mindfulness-based stress reduction as part of a group-oriented intervention with encouraging success (West et al. 2014).

MINDFULNESS IN MEDICAL EDUCATION

Medical education in an area where acquisition of coping skills and mindfulness training are under active study. Research on the use of mindfulness in medical students reaching back to the late 1990s has shown consistent benefit in those who volunteered to be included in the training (Shapiro et al. 1998; Finkelstein et al. 2007; de Vibe et al. 2013; van Dijk et al. 2015; McConville et al. 2017), although results are not always positive. For example, in a more recent study of two cohorts of first-year medical students ($n = 54$) and ($n = 51$) enrolled in a required longitudinal stress management and resilience curriculum, results did not show overall benefit in those completing the surveys (44/54) and (22/51) in burnout measures, mental or physical quality of life, stress, resilience and happiness, or in empathy levels at the end of the first year of medical training. The intervention included: an introductory session; a curriculum on attention, gratitude, compassion, acceptance, meaning, forgiveness, relationships; and a conclusion with reflections (Dyrbye et al. 2017c).

CLINICAL APPLICATION: PHYSICIAN BURNOUT

Dr. Johnson is a 37-year-old internal medicine physician whose private practice was recently bought out by large health care organization. The new company has a proprietary EMR substantially different from the one the practice is currently using, implemented only a year ago. A new bonus-driven productivity system is also being rolled out. Salaries are under review, and staffing cutbacks are possible.

Dr. Johnson enjoys helping her patients and is dreading the upcoming corporate merger. She has two young children, substantial debt, and a husband who works full time. She has been fatigued since starting residency training. She is the primary caretaker of children and home due to her husband's long work hours. At a recent CME conference on burnout, she realized she met the criteria for several burnout measures. She has no desire to harm herself.

What approach is likely to be most helpful to this colleague?

Dr. Johnson is in a highly stressful situation, and her concerns need to be heard and validated. Reassurance and encouragement that she can be effective at changing her situation are also important.

With respect to the mind–body therapies, an initial approach would ideally include both acute and longer-term stress management skills, for example, learning a basic breath work exercise to immediately help reduce sympathetic overdrive (explored in detail in Chapter 5, "Breath Work, Autogenics, Progressive Muscle Relaxation"), followed by introduction of a skill such as mindfulness learned over several months. Taking time to fully assess her options and make conscious connection to her social and professional support networks to decrease sense of isolation would also be important. Taking stock of lifestyle habits (sleep, exercise, nutrition, physical health, relationships) will help identify strengths and weaknesses in these areas and encourages a *whole person* approach to her health.

Assessment of work flow issues, caliber of leadership, and support at work are also important and closely linked to burnout. Baseline screening for burnout with a validated scale (such as the Maslach Burnout Inventory) provides useful baseline measures and can be used to track progress. Any evidence of serious distress, such as suicidal ideation, should be promptly addressed.

Maslach's blueprint for positive progress in addressing burnout applies here and includes:

- Sense of personal control
- Absence of role conflict
- Feeling of being fairly treated
- Social support
- Appropriate reward (financial, institutional, social)
- An alignment of values between individual and workplace
- Good leadership

(Maslach and Leiter 2008)

Longer-term reduction of chronic stressors is also needed. She may benefit significantly from taking additional earned vacation time to rest, gain perspective, and decide if the job in its current form is meeting her needs. Professional coaching to hone skills in negotiation and communication as the merger moves forward may be both timely and helpful.

Physician coaching

Physician coaching is an emerging trend that can help physicians at all stages of training develop and implement a sustainable plan for long-term health (Schneider et al. 2014; Gazelle et al. 2015).

Some of the goals of a coaching relationship are to

- Grow beyond perceived limits.
- Expand your options.
- Provoke discussion and deeper understanding of career trajectory.
- Open to new approaches to health and healing.
- Increase adaptability.
- Tap into creativity and innovation.
- Create opportunities that enhance a sense of control and career gratification.

CLINICAL APPLICATION FOLLOW-UP

Based on information Dr. Johnson received at the conference on physician wellness and on results from her screening Maslach survey, she realized she would benefit from professional coaching. She spoke with her supervisor and arranged to take a 2-week vacation, the first she had taken since finishing residency training. Afterward, she identified an experienced physician coach and began bi weekly sessions to help her successfully navigate the upcoming practice merger. Through her work with the coach, Dr. Johnson tapped into latent leadership skills and was able to negotiate a more workable clinic schedule. A year later, Dr. Johnson was still employed with the company she had been on the verge of leaving, working 4 days per week, and had become the recognized physician well-being advocate in the organization.

SUMMARY

Clinician health and wellness are critical components of medical practice, ideally prioritized from the earliest stages of medical training. Every clinician, administrator, and member of the health care team can benefit from a conscious and organized approach to well-being with the goals of promoting individual's health and improving patient outcomes. Mind–body approaches that enhance self-regulation have significant potential to reduce burnout and to promote career satisfaction in conjunction with a well-rounded approach to healthy lifestyle measures.

RESOURCES

Stanford University

- Committee for Professional Satisfaction and Support (SCPSS)
- Well MD, Wellness Institute

National Academy of Medicine

- Action Collaborative on Clinician Well-Being and Resilience

Association of American Medical Colleges (AAMC)

- Well-Being in Academic Medicine

The Ohio State University, College of Medicine

- Mind–Body Stream (online mindfulness courses)

Schwartz Center for Compassionate Healthcare

- Schwartz Rounds

References

Bazarko, D., R. A. Cate, F. Azocar, and M. J. Kreitzer. 2013. The impact of an innovative mindfulness-based stress reduction program on the health and well-being of nurses employed in a corporate setting. *J Workplace Behav Health* 28 (2): 107–133. doi:10.1080/15555240.2013.779518.

Blum, A. B., S. Shea, C. A. Czeisler, C. P. Landrigan, and L. Leape. 2011. Implementing the 2009 Institute of Medicine recommendations on resident physician work hours, supervision, and safety. *Nat Sci Sleep* 3: 47–85. doi:10.2147/NSS.S19649.

de Vibe, M., I. Solhaug, R. Tyssen, O. Friborg, J. H. Rosenvinge, T. Sorlie, and A. Bjorndal. 2013. Mindfulness training for stress management: A randomised controlled study of medical and psychology students. *BMC Med Educ* 13: 107. doi:10.1186/1472-6920-13-107.

Downs, C. A., and M. S. Faulkner. 2015. Toxic stress, inflammation and symptomatology of chronic complications in diabetes. *World J Diabetes* 6 (4): 554–565. doi:10.4239/wjd.v6.i4.554.

Dunn, L. B., A. Iglewicz, and C. Moutier. 2008. A conceptual model of medical student well-being: Promoting resilience and preventing burnout. *Acad Psychiatry* 32 (1): 44–53. doi:10.1176/appi.ap.32.1.44.

Dyrbye, L. N., A. Eacker, S. J. Durning, C. Brazeau, C. Moutier, F. S. Massie, D. Satele, J. A. Sloan, and T. D. Shanafelt. 2015. The impact of stigma and personal experiences on the help-seeking behaviors of medical students with burnout. *Acad Med* 90 (7): 961–969. doi:10.1097/ACM.0000000000000655.

Dyrbye, L. N., D. Satele, and T. D. Shanafelt. 2017a. Healthy exercise habits are associated with lower risk of burnout and higher quality of life among U.S. medical students. *Acad Med* 92 (7): 1006–1011. doi:10.1097/ACM.0000000000001540.

Dyrbye, L. N., T. D. Shanafelt, C. A. Sinsky, P. F. Cipriano, J. Bhatt, A. Ommaya, C. P. West, and D. Meyers. 2017b. Burnout among health care professionals: A call to explore and address this underrecognized threat to safe, high-quality care. In National Academy of Medicine, Discussion Paper, Washington, DC.

Dyrbye, L. N., T. D. Shanafelt, L. Werner, A. Sood, D. Satele, and A. P. Wolanskyj. 2017c. The impact of a required longitudinal stress management and resilience training course for first-year medical students. *J Gen Intern Med* 32 (12): 1309–1314. doi:10.1007/s11606-017-4171-2.

Dyrbye, L. N., P. Varkey, S. L. Boone, D. V. Satele, J. A. Sloan, and T. D. Shanafelt. 2013. Physician satisfaction and burnout at different career stages. *Mayo Clin Proc* 88 (12): 1358–1367. doi: 10.1016/j.mayocp.2013.07.016.

Epstein, R. M., and M. S. Krasner. 2013. Physician resilience: What it means, why it matters, and how to promote it. *Acad Med* 88 (3): 301–303. doi:10.1097/ACM.0b013e318280cff0.

Finkelstein, C., A. Brownstein, C. Scott, and Y. L. Lan. 2007. Anxiety and stress reduction in medical education: An intervention. *Med Educ* 41 (3): 258–264. doi:10.1111/j.1365-2929.2007.02685.x.

Fortney, L., C. Luchterhand, L. Zakletskaia, A. Zgierska, and D. Rakel. 2013. Abbreviated mindfulness intervention for job satisfaction, quality of life, and compassion in primary care clinicians: A pilot study. *Ann Fam Med* 11 (5): 412–420. doi:10.1370/afm.1511.

Fortney, L., and M. Taylor. 2010. Meditation in medical practice: A review of the evidence and practice. *Prim Care* 37 (1): 81–90. doi:10.1016/j.pop.2009.09.004.

Fumis, R. R. L., G. A. Junqueira Amarante, A. de Fatima Nascimento, and J. M. Vieira Junior. 2017. Moral distress and its contribution to the development of burnout syndrome among critical care providers. *Ann Intensive Care* 7 (1): 71. doi:10.1186/s13613-017-0293-2.

Gazelle, G., J. M. Liebschutz, and H. Riess. 2015. Physician burnout: Coaching a way out. *J Gen Intern Med* 30 (4): 508–513. doi:10.1007/s11606-014-3144-y.

Gotink, R. A., R. Meijboom, M. W. Vernooij, M. Smits, and M. G. Hunink. 2016. 8-week mindfulness based stress reduction induces brain changes similar to traditional long-term meditation practice: A systematic review. *Brain Cogn* 108: 32–41. doi:10.1016/j.bandc.2016.07.001.

Hamou-Jennings, F. A., and C. Dong. 2016. Resilience training for healthcare providers: An Asian perspective. *Mhealth* 2: 25. doi:10.21037/mhealth.2016.06.01.

Hausler, M., C. Strecker, A. Huber, M. Brenner, T. Hoge, and S. Hofer. 2017. Associations between the application of signature character strengths, health and well-being of health professionals. *Front Psychol* 8: 1307. doi:10.3389/fpsyg.2017.01307.

Hinami, K., C. T. Whelan, R. J. Wolosin, J. A. Miller, and T. B. Wetterneck. 2012. Worklife and satisfaction of hospitalists: Toward flourishing careers. *J Gen Intern Med* 27 (1): 28–36. doi:10.1007/s11606-011-1780-z.

Houpy, J. C., W. W. Lee, J. N. Woodruff, and A. T. Pincavage. 2017. Medical student resilience and stressful clinical events during clinical training. *Med Educ Online* 22 (1): 1320187. doi:10.1080/10872981.2017.1320187.

Howe, M., A. Leidel, S. M. Krishnan, A. Weber, M. Rubenfire, and E. A. Jackson. 2010. "Patient-related diet and exercise counseling: dDo providers' own lifestyle habits matter?" *Prev Cardiol* 13 (4): 180–185. doi: 10.1111/j.1751-7141.2010.00079.x.

Howe, A., A. Smajdor, and A. Stockl. 2012. Towards an understanding of resilience and its relevance to medical training. *Med Educ* 46 (4): 349–356. doi:10.1111/j.1365-2923.2011.04188.x.

Jensen, P. M., K. Trollope-Kumar, H. Waters, and J. Everson. 2008. Building physician resilience. *Can Fam Physician* 54 (5): 722–729.

Kabat-Zinn, J. 1982. An outpatient program in behavioral medicine for chronic pain patients based on the practice of mindfulness meditation: Theoretical considerations and preliminary results. *Gen Hosp Psychiatry* 4 (1): 33–47.

Kabat-Zinn, J. 2013. *Full Catastrophe Living: Using the Wisdom of Your Body and Mind to Face Stress, Pain, and Illness*, Revised Edition. New York: Bantam Books.

Kilpatrick, L. A., B. Y. Suyenobu, S. R. Smith, J. A. Bueller, T. Goodman, J. D. Creswell, K. Tillisch, E. A. Mayer, and B. D. Naliboff. 2011. Impact of mindfulness-based stress reduction training on intrinsic brain connectivity. *Neuroimage* 56 (1): 290–298. doi:10.1016/j.neuroimage.2011.02.034.

Kulaylat, A. N., D. Qin, S. X. Sun, C. S. Hollenbeak, J. R. Schubart, A. J. Aboud, D. J. Flemming, P. W. Dillon, E. R. Bollard, and D. C. Han. 2017. Perceptions of mistreatment among trainees vary at different stages of clinical training. *BMC Med Educ* 17 (1): 14. doi:10.1186/s12909-016-0853-4.

Litz, B. T., N. Stein, E. Delaney, L. Lebowitz, W. P. Nash, C. Silva, and S. Maguen. 2009. Moral injury and moral repair in war veterans: A preliminary model and intervention strategy. *Clin Psychol Rev* 29 (8): 695–706. doi:10.1016/j.cpr.2009.07.003.

Ludwig, D. S., and J. Kabat-Zinn. 2008. Mindfulness in medicine. *JAMA* 300 (11): 1350–1352. doi:10.1001/jama.300.11.1350.

Martin, A. J., and H. W. Marsh. 2006. Academic resilience and its psychological and educational correlates: A construct validity approach. *Psychol Sch* (43): 267–281. doi:10.1002/pits.20149.

Maslach, C., S. E. Jackson, and M. P. Leiter. 1996. *Maslach Burnout Inventory Manual*, 3rd ed. Paloo Alton, CA: Consulting Psychologists Press.

Maslach, C., and M. P. Leiter. 2008. Early predictors of job burnout and engagement. *J Appl Psychol* 93 (3): 498–512. doi:10.1037/0021-9010.93.3.498.

McAllister, M., and J. McKinnon. 2009. The importance of teaching and learning resilience in the health disciplines: A critical review of the literature. *Nurse Educ Today* 29 (4): 371–379. doi:10.1016/j.nedt.2008.10.011.

McConville, J., R. McAleer, and A. Hahne. 2017. Mindfulness training for health profession students—the effect of mindfulness training on psychological well-being, learning and clinical performance of health professional students: A systematic review of randomized and non-randomized controlled trials. *Explore (NY)* 13 (1): 26–45. doi:10.1016/j.explore.2016.10.002.

Reich, J. W., A. Zautra, and J. S. Hall. 2010. *Handbook of Adult Resilience*. New York: Guilford Press.

Schneider, S., K. Kingsolver, and J. Rosdahl. 2014. Physician coaching to enhance well-being: A qualitative analysis of a pilot intervention. *Explore (NY)* 10 (6): 372–379. doi:10.1016/j.explore.2014.08.007.

Shanafelt, T. D., L. N. Dyrbye, and C. P. West. 2017. Addressing physician burnout: The way forward. *JAMA* 317 (9): 901–902. doi:10.1001/jama.2017.0076.

Shanafelt, T. D., G. Gorringe, R. Menaker, K. A. Storz, D. Reeves, S. J. Buskirk, J. A. Sloan, and S. J. Swensen. 2015. Impact of organizational leadership on physician burnout and satisfaction. *Mayo Clin Proc* 90 (4): 432–440. doi:10.1016/j.mayocp.2015.01.012.

Shanafelt, T. D., and J. H. Noseworthy. 2017. Executive leadership and physician well-being: Nine organizational strategies to promote engagement and reduce burnout. *Mayo Clin Proc* 92 (1): 129–146. doi:10.1016/j.mayocp.2016.10.004.

Shanafelt, T. D., M. R. Oreskovich, L. N. Dyrbye, D. V. Satele, J. B. Hanks, J. A. Sloan, and C. M. Balch. 2012. Avoiding burnout: The personal health habits and wellness practices of U.S. surgeons. *Ann Surg* 255 (4): 625–633. doi:10.1097/SLA.0b013e31824b2fa0.

Shao, R., K. Keuper, X. Geng, and T. M. Lee. 2016. Pons to posterior cingulate functional projections predict affective processing changes in the elderly following eight weeks of meditation training. *EBioMedicine* 10: 236–248. doi:10.1016/j.ebiom.2016.06.018.

Shapiro, S. L., G. E. Schwartz, and G. Bonner. 1998. Effects of mindfulness-based stress reduction on medical and premedical students. *J Behav Med* 21 (6): 581–599.

Shonkoff, J. P. 2012. Leveraging the biology of adversity to address the roots of disparities in health and development. *Proc Natl Acad Sci USA* 109 (Suppl 2): 17302–17307. doi:10.1073/pnas.1121259109.

Silverman, M. N., and E. M. Sternberg. 2012. Glucocorticoid regulation of inflammation and its functional correlates: From HPA axis to glucocorticoid receptor dysfunction. *Ann NY Acad Sci* 1261: 55–63. doi:10.1111/j.1749-6632.2012.06633.x.

Smajdor, A., A. Stockl, and C. Salter. 2011. The limits of empathy: Problems in medical education and practice. *J Med Ethics* 37 (6): 380–383. doi:10.1136/jme.2010.039628.

Smith, B. W., J. Dalen, K. Wiggins, E. Tooley, P. Christopher, and J. Bernard. 2008. The brief resilience scale: Assessing the ability to bounce back. *Int J Behav Med* 15 (3): 194–200. doi:10.1080/10705500802222972.

Sun, Q., L. Shi, J. Prescott, S. E. Chiuve, F. B. Hu, I. De Vivo, M. J. Stampfer, P. W. Franks, J. E. Manson, and K. M. Rexrode. 2012. Healthy lifestyle and leukocyte telomere length in U.S. women. *PLoS One* 7 (5): e38374. doi:10.1371/journal.pone.0038374.

van Dijk, I., P. L. Lucassen, and A. E. Speckens. 2015. Mindfulness training for medical students in their clinical clerkships: Two cross-sectional studies exploring interest and participation. *BMC Med Educ* 15: 24. doi:10.1186/s12909-015-0302-9.

Warnock, G. L. 2008. Reflecting on principles of professionalism. *Can J Surg* 51 (2): 84–87.

West, C. P., L. N. Dyrbye, P. J. Erwin, and T. D. Shanafelt. 2016. Interventions to prevent and reduce physician burnout: A systematic review and meta-analysis. *Lancet* 388 (10057): 2272–2281. doi:10.1016/S0140-6736(16)31279-X.

West, C. P., L. N. Dyrbye, J. T. Rabatin, T. G. Call, J. H. Davidson, A. Multari, S. A. Romanski, J. M. Hellyer, J. A. Sloan, and T. D. Shanafelt. 2014. Intervention to promote physician well-being, job satisfaction, and professionalism: A randomized clinical trial. *JAMA Intern Med* 174 (4): 527–533. doi:10.1001/jamainternmed.2013.14387.

Wong, B. M., and K. Imrie. 2013. Why resident duty hours regulations must address attending physicians' workload. *Acad Med* 88 (9): 1209–1211. doi:10.1097/ACM.0b013e31829e5727.

Zautra, A., J. Hall, and K. Murray. 2009. Community development an integrative approach. *Commun Dev* 39 (3): 130–147.

4   Language use and the mind–body interview

INTRODUCTION: MINDFUL LANGUAGE

A clinician's word choice matters. They are in an ongoing flow of communication with patients and families, have to think on their feet, perform painful or frightening procedures, and often need to deliver difficult news. Ideally, in each interaction, they would convey a sense of hope, encouragement, and conviction that the patient can successfully meet their challenges. (It is important to clarify that effective communication does not mean avoidance of truth but, rather, finding words that afford the patient realistic reassurance and support.) It is unrealistic to think that clinicians will always *get it right*, and despite best efforts even the most mindful may miss the mark. Few clinicians receive training in this area, yet word choice can be of significant benefit to those in our care and in delivery, and outcome may also have the potential to reduce a clinician's stress and burnout risk (Thirioux et al. 2016).

Similarly, use of skillful language in mind–body medicine can help patients leverage inner resources such as optimism, hope, determination, and courage. In addition to word choice, the tone and pace of the clinician's voice can be modulated to encourage calm confidence. People anticipate and perceive pain and stress in many different ways. Skillful word choice on the clinician's part can leave the door open for the patient to have a successful experience and prevent inadvertent medical hexing or the introduction of fear or doubt.

CLINICAL APPLICATION: INEXPERIENCE IN THE CLINIC

Consider this true story of a parent waiting for their child's test results in a busy clinic. The child is 6-years-old and has a chronic illness. He has been through years of complex treatments. Overall, he is doing well. The child has been through several hours of scheduled screening tests, and the family is anxiously awaiting the day's results.

Dr. Singh, the child's regular attending, has been called away to an emergency and an assigned first-year fellow steps in and relays the child's test results—all good news. On his way out of the exam room, the fellow pauses at the door, looks back, and says brightly, "Now we just have to wait for the cancer to develop," and leaves the room.

Fortunately, the child is too young to understand the comment, but the parent is shocked and leaves with a sense of anticipatory dread. This is a classic example of medical hexing.

The fellow was actually relaying the fact that routine screening would be needed going forward—which the family knew. However, his word choice foreshadowed a frightening complication that added significantly to the parents' stress after a very long day—despite the fact that the test results were good.

This true story is a powerful example of the importance of cultivating mindfulness and self-awareness in the clinical encounter. Consider the impact an alternative statement might have had.

> "I am glad to relay to you on behalf of your doctor, Dr. Singh, that the test results today look normal. He says to keep up the good work! He will call you later today to see if you have questions and apologizes for having to step away. Another child needed urgent attention. In the meantime, we will continue to monitor your child carefully and continue the periodic screening you have discussed with Dr. Singh. We will react to any changes as needed, and the team is standing by to help. Thank you, and let me know if you have any questions before you go."

Clinicians can learn to positively influence the medical encounter through thoughtful word choices and can make a significant difference in the perceived quality of care by using mindful and compassionate language, regardless of the medical setting.

MINDFUL LANGUAGE: EMPATHY AND COMPASSION

Empathy and empathic language are very important in the medical encounter and have been associated with increased patient satisfaction, improved diagnostic accuracy, treatment compliance, and even improved patient outcomes (Hojat et al. 2011).

Empathy stems from the Greek: em + pathos, *in, feeling*. The ability to relate to anther's pain vicariously, as if one has experienced the pain themselves. Literally *in feeling* with the other.

An appropriate measure of empathy may also serve as a buffer against clinician burnout (Thirioux et al. 2016), although an excess of empathy can actually predispose one to burnout.

Functional MRI (fMRI) studies have been done in humans measuring empathic brain responses for a variety of emotions, including pain, fear, anxiety, anger, sadness, and social exclusion, among others. Best studied in pain, an empathic response recruits brain areas in the observer that mirror neural activity in the subject who is experiencing the pain (Bernhardt and Singer 2012).

The benefit of empathy is that it can help one predict and understand the social and affective behavior of others (Hojat et al. 2017), but at an extreme, the *cost of caring* can exceed a clinician's ability to respond appropriately in stressful situations, which can lead to emotional depletion and burnout.

EMPATHY VERSUS COMPASSION

The distinction between empathy and compassion is nuanced and important to understand in this context. Compassion stems from the Latin: com +pati, to bear, suffer. It can be defined as a sympathetic consciousness of other's distress, together with a desire to alleviate it. In the clinical setting, this might involve seeking full understanding of the patient's situation, framing the conversation mindfully, generating the internal desire to ease the other's suffering, and taking the initiative to offer help.

Compassion has been shown to promote prosocial behavior. Even relatively brief compassion training delivered in a day has been shown to enhance prosocial helping behavior and activate brain areas associated with positive affect and reward (Bernhardt and Singer 2012). This is relevant in medical practice because it may buffer the development of burnout and increase resiliency related to aversive events by upregulating neural networks in the clinician associated with positive affect, reward, and attachment.

Cognitively based compassion training (CBCT) is now being offered to clinicians in academic centers such as Emory University through the Emory-Tibet Partnership, Emory Tibet Science Initiative, and through Stanford University's Center for Compassion and Altruism Research and Education, Stanford *CCare*.

This training helps the clinician focus on thoughtful word choices and emphasizes the skills of attentive and receptive listening so critical to the patient interaction. Ideally, this approach also encourages the patient to consider their answers more thoughtfully and hopefully gain a deeper understanding of their health-related fears, challenges, and motivations.

THE USE OF MINDFUL LANGUAGE IN DELIVERING DIFFICULT NEWS

Delivering bad news is a stressful and expected part of every clinician's work, yet few receive training in this skill, which can predispose to a variety of unwanted outcomes such as low patient satisfaction, poor patient compliance, and an increase in medical malpractice suits (Leone et al. 2017).

Training in the delivery of difficult news to patients and their families can help clinicians master effective word choices. An example that originated in oncology is the six-step (SPIKES) Buckman Protocol, which involves the following (Baile et al. 2000; Leone et al. 2017):

1 *Setting up*: Being prepared for bad news conversations, finding a private space, sitting down, and introducing oneself.
2 *Patient perception*: What does the patient already know, what they want to know, correct information, and assess understanding or denial.
3 *Invitation*: How much information is wanted, be available later if information is not wanted at present, determine the bare minimum needed to be shared, and start there.
4 *Knowledge*: Prior to relaying the bad news, signal that bad news is about to be conveyed. Avoid medical jargon, avoid being overly blunt, provide information in small packets, check for understanding, repeat key points frequently as needed.
5 *Emotions*: Respond to the patient's emotional responses, allow feelings to be expressed, name the patient's feelings, and provide an empathic response by acknowledging one's own emotions.
6 *Strategy and summary*: Summarize main points, if time is right to discuss available treatment options or follow-up. Frame information and future hope in terms of what is most meaningful to the patient and still able to be accomplished.

One can see where the use of mindful language and compassion throughout each of these steps could make an important difference to patient, family, and clinician in how difficult news is delivered, received, and perceived.

THE PLACEBO RESPONSE: RELEVANCY
TO MIND–BODY MEDICINE

Placebo comes from the Latin "I shall please" and refers to a positive change in clinical symptoms when an inert substance, typically a pill, liquid, or injectable, is used for treatment.

The most familiar use of placebo is probably its use in a control arm of a clinical trial where it is delivered in identical form as the agent under study. It has been established that the placebo response is associated with the release of endorphins and dopamine and that brain circuitry involved in placebo-related analgesic effects are involved in modulation of cognitive and emotional factors such as the stress response, mood, reward motivation, and neuroendocrine and autonomic regulation. The term *placebo response* may be used at times when unexpected treatment responses occur that are not explainable through the known action of the treatment (Amanzio and Benedetti 1999; Dodd et al. 2017).

The term *nocebo response* is used when an inert substance causes perceived harm (Chavarria et al. 2017).

The placebo–nocebo response is relevant in mind–body medicine in that word choice, for example, in the form of suggestions, can act as placebo. A study by Zubieta and Stohler demonstrated that specific neural circuits and neurotransmitter systems produce measurable change with the expectation of benefit during the administration of a placebo.

Leading theories regarding the placebo–nocebo responses involve conditioning and expectancy—that is, a response driven by memory, learning, and expectation. While understanding of the complexities of the placebo response has become more sophisticated over time, many questions remain, including a clear understanding of the range of influencing factors and the specific physiologic mechanisms involved. Personality characteristics such as hope and optimism may influence placebo response, whereas anxiety or uncertainty about tolerability or efficacy of treatment can drive the nocebo response. Choice and sense of control have both been shown to be important influencers of placebo–nocebo effects (Jakovljevic 2014).

Research is active into which part of the brain is involved in placebo–nocebo responses using fMRI and positron emission tomography (PET) scanning, which have shown that placebo and nocebo expectant responses use different brain networks when processing a pain stimulus (Dodd et al. 2017).

Studies have also shown that baseline brain connectivity can predict placebo responders and the magnitude of placebo analgesia they experience. This means that specific brain biology seems predictive of the clinical placebo effect originating from the *top down*, shaped by expectations and experience (Buchel et al. 2014; Tetreault et al. 2016).

A review by Dodd et al. (2017) concludes that placebo–nocebo responses are driven by a complex set of biological and psychological factors, and a wide range of individual variability is seen in studies using the same stimuli. Intangible factors such as expectancy, hope, desire to please, the quality of connection with the clinician, and personal beliefs are all factors in this complex area where research is still at a preliminary stage. This is relevant especially to the use of positive and encouraging language in the clinical setting, which may act to augment a positive treatment response in receptive patients. One obvious example is the use of therapeutic suggestion in clinical hypnosis, discussed in Chapter 7, "Hypnosis and Guided Imagery" (Pendergrast 2017).

INTRODUCING MIND–BODY THERAPIES
INTO THE CLINICAL VISIT

A framework for introducing mind–body therapies can help determine the most appropriate mind–body therapy for the situation at hand. Some clinicians will feel comfortable venturing into this territory with patients, while others may be reluctant or feel ill prepared for what may arise. Familiarity with the various mind–body therapies makes introducing the topics easier over time, and ideally both clinician and patient will enjoy exploring new treatment options and cultivating new skills.

MIND–BODY THERAPIES AND SPIRITUALITY

One of the guiding tenets of the use mind–body therapies in clinical work is that they are intended to be largely secular. This should reassure those who are uncomfortable with the idea of religion or spirituality intruding into health care, although accruing studies show that prayer is one of the most used complementary practices in the United States and can have a significant impact on a patient's experience of chronic illness and influence success in lifestyle change (Janssen-Niemeijer et al. 2017).

A large systematic literature review ($n = 12{,}327$) (Best et al. 2015) showed that a majority of patients actually express interest in discussing religion and spirituality in the medical visit. Those that did not feel questions about spirituality were intrusive or might imply a more serious illness. If the patient is amenable, raising the question of spirituality can allow the clinician to delve deeper and see what elements of the patient's character and social connections rise to the surface in times of trouble. The challenge lies in identifying which patients are open to this discussion and which are not. Spirituality has obvious overlapping themes with the mind–body therapies, and it is possible for the clinician to find the line between them based on intention, word choice, and patient preferences. One exception might be in palliative care, where spirituality and mind–body therapies have a more intuitive potential overlap. A rich body of literature exists exploring the use of spirituality in medicine which can serve as a useful resource for those interested in learning more (Graves et al. 2002; Puchalski et al. 2014a,b; Vitillo and Puchalski 2014).

Even if not formally presented as a spiritual inquiry, it can be very helpful for both patients and clinicians to reflect on what brings the patient strength and sustains them throughout a challenging situation and to identify where they go and what they do when they do not have all the answers and how they respond to conflict and to uncertainty.

DEVELOPING MIND–BODY INTERVIEW QUESTIONS

Development of a mind–body interview template serves several purposes: It allows the clinician to prepare and anticipate patient questions; it conveys the expectation that the patient has untapped inner resources and strengths; it helps lift the taboo of discussion of the deeper emotional issues related to health; and it prepares the clinician to offer expanded treatment options if the patient is receptive. It can be challenging to determine which type of mind–body therapy might appeal to the patient or be best suited to their needs, and being ready with more than one option is helpful. Patient preferences, expectations, cultural background, education level, and potential access to mind–body therapies can have a significant impact on their successful implementation.

The mind–body interview can cover a range of topics, including personal, health, work, family, long-term goals, and so on. Especially important are the identification of stressors and coping strategies. Mind–body interview questions can help patients better define challenges, obstacles, triggering events, and limiting beliefs and clarify their value systems. These questions might help them process pivotal events and identify support networks, champions, mentors, and pivotal relationships and might provide an insight into how their approach to health is impacting others.

With expanded understanding of the patient's situation, a clinician may be better able to tailor treatment options to the patient's needs. Introducing mind–body interview questions may also catalyze new ways of thinking about health challenges and encourage fresh approaches to problem solving. Simply the experience of undergoing a mind–body interview may stimulate the patient's imagination and help them identify previously unrecognized paths forward.

FRAMING THE QUESTIONS

Two broad approaches to asking the deeper questions involved in the mind–body interview include:

- Open-ended questions which invite reflection and processing
- Category-specific questions more similar to those used in a typical history of present illness

Open-ended questions slow the pace of questioning, are prompted by genuine curiosity, and use strategic pauses to enhance reflective listening and build a sense of trust and interest. They can also be very helpful in assessing the patient's readiness to change. Challenges with this type of approach include the need for the clinician to maintain a sense of direction to keep the interview on track.

Examples of open-ended questions include:

- How do you define health?
- When was the last time you felt really well?
- In what ways has the condition impacted your life?
- What do you feel may have contributed to your health condition?
- Are there things happening in your life that may be impacting your health?
- From where do you draw your strength?
- How do you think your emotional health impacts your physical health?
- What do you fear most about your illness?
- How else do you hurt?
- What thoughts or fears do you have about the treatment options that have been discussed so far?
- What keeps you from giving up?

Category-specific questions use a more structured approach and are geared toward obtaining specific data, similar to obtaining a history and review of symptoms. For example:

Category: Family and relationships

- Are there family events that you feel have impacted your illness?
- Are there relationships that might be contributing to your symptoms?
- If you have a partner, do you consider them supportive?

Category: Work/school

- Are there events or factors in your work/school life that may be contributing to your symptoms?
- Do you feel valued by others in your work or school environment?
- What would your ideal work or school situation look like?

Category: Stress management

- What do you feel are your greatest life stressors at the moment?
- What are you currently doing to manage stress?
- Are there stress management strategies you have used in the past that have been successful?
- What are your biggest challenges in managing stress?

Category: Mental health

- Are you experiencing anxiety, depression, or strong anger? If so, how do you feel this has impacted your health?
- Are there pivotal life events that have impacted your emotional health?

Category: Spirituality, meaning, and purpose

- Do you have a sense of your life's purpose?
- Is your life aligned well with this vision?
- Where do you find strength in challenging times?
- Where do turn for answers when you are unsure of your next step?

CLINICAL APPLICATION: INITIATING THE MIND–BODY INTERVIEW

Ms. Liu is a patient undergoing chemotherapy for breast cancer. In the follow-up visit after her first course of treatment, the physician could proceed through a routine visit or could add depth to the interview by exploring new perspectives that can help Ms. Liu recognize and tap into inner resources such as perseverance, patience, strength, hope, and optimism.

Ms. Liu, I respect the approach and attitude you are bringing to your treatment. Where do you find your strength?

Ms. Liu we are moving into the second cycle of your chemotherapy. Can you identify some inner resources that have served you well in the past that you could bring to bear to help you navigate this section of your treatment?

Ms. Liu, you have shown real strength through the first cycle of chemotherapy. What will you use to stay strong through the second cycle?

Ms. Liu, we are learning about new approaches to health that involve the mind–body connection, would you like to know more?

INTRODUCING MIND–BODY THERAPIES IN THE CLINICAL SETTING

The next challenge occurs in finding the best mind–body therapy *fit* for the patient at that time.

This is introduced briefly here and will be revisited in Part III, "Clinical Application."

Overview of steps in introducing the mind–body therapies in the patient visit (McClafferty 2011)

*   Frame the patient's situation and explain why mind–body therapies would have potential.
*   Ask about any prior use of mind–body therapies, good or bad.
*   Explore resistance or hesitation.
*   Offer a range of mind–body therapy options relevant to the case.
*   Remain open to the patient's interests, and be aware of supporting literature to help narrow the choices.
*   Evaluate potential obstacles, cost, accessibility, and patient interest.
*   Choose one to two therapies to explore.
*   Encourage and reinforce success, re-evaluate if first options do not work well.

SUMMARY

Many factors impact patient outcome. The goal of this chapter is to raise awareness about the importance of language, word choice, and delivery in the clinical setting. Although few clinicians receive training in these areas, learning how to interact mindfully, thoughtfully deliver difficult news, and to potentially engage the placebo response in eliciting positive treatment responses are useful skills that may help patients and potentially ease the burden of burnout and compassion fatigue in clinicians over time.

References

Amanzio, M., and F. Benedetti. 1999. Neuropharmacological dissection of placebo analgesia: Expectation-activated opioid systems versus conditioning-activated specific subsystems. *J Neurosci* 19 (1): 484–494.

Baile, W. F., R. Buckman, R. Lenzi, G. Glober, E. A. Beale, and A. P. Kudelka. 2000. SPIKES—A six-step protocol for delivering bad news: Application to the patient with cancer. *Oncologist* 5 (4): 302–311.

Bernhardt, B. C., and T. Singer. 2012. The neural basis of empathy. *Annu Rev Neurosci* 35: 1–23. doi:10.1146/annurev-neuro-062111-150536.

Best, M., P. Butow, and I. Olver. 2015. Do patients want doctors to talk about spirituality? A systematic literature review. *Patient Educ Couns* 98 (11): 1320–1328. doi:10.1016/j.pec.2015.04.017.

Buchel, C., S. Geuter, C. Sprenger, and F. Eippert. 2014. Placebo analgesia: A predictive coding perspective. *Neuron* 81 (6): 1223–1239. doi:10.1016/j.neuron.2014.02.042.

The Center for Compassion and Altruism Research and Education. Accessed March 17, 2018. Retrieved from http://ccare.stanford.edu/.

Chavarria, V., J. Vian, C. Pereira, J. Data-Franco, B. S. Fernandes, M. Berk, and S. Dodd. 2017. The placebo and nocebo phenomena: Their clinical management and impact on treatment outcomes. *Clin Ther* 39 (3): 477–486. doi:10.1016/j.clinthera.2017.01.031.

Dodd, S., O. M. Dean, J. Vian, and M. Berk. 2017. A review of the theoretical and biological understanding of the nocebo and placebo phenomena. *Clin Ther* 39 (3): 469–476. doi:10.1016/j. clinthera.2017.01.010.

Emory University Emory Tibet Partnership. Accessed March 17, 2018.Retrieved from https://tibet. emory.edu/.

Graves, D. L., C. K. Shue, and L. Arnold. 2002. The role of spirituality in patient care: Incorporating spirituality training into medical school curriculum. *Acad Med* 77 (11): 1167.

Hojat, M., J. DeSantis, and J. S. Gonnella. 2017. Patient perceptions of clinician's empathy: Measurement and psychometrics. *J Patient Exp* 4 (2): 78–83. doi:10.1177/2374373517699273.

Hojat, M., D. Z. Louis, F. W. Markham, R. Wender, C. Rabinowitz, and J. S. Gonnella. 2011. Physicians' empathy and clinical outcomes for diabetic patients. *Acad Med* 86 (3): 359–364. doi:10.1097/ACM.0b013e3182086fe1.

Jakovljevic, M. 2014. The placebo–nocebo response: Controversies and challenges from clinical and research perspective. *Eur Neuropsychopharmacol* 24 (3): 333–341. doi:10.1016/j.euroneuro. 2013.11.014.

Janssen-Niemeijer, A. J., M. Visse, R. Van Leeuwen, C. Leget, and B. S. Cusveller. 2017. The role of spirituality in lifestyle changing among patients with chronic cardiovascular diseases: A literature review of qualitative studies. *J Relig Health* 56 (4): 1460–1477. doi:10.1007/s10943-017-0384-2.

Leone, D., J. Menichetti, L. Barusi, E. Chelo, M. Costa, L. De Lauretis, A. P. Ferraretti et al. 2017. Breaking bad news in assisted reproductive technology: A proposal for guidelines. *Reprod Health* 14 (1): 87. doi: 10.1186/s12978-017-0350-1.

McClafferty, H. 2011. Complementary, holistic, and integrative medicine: Mind–body medicine. *Pediatr Rev* 32 (5): 201–203. doi:10.1542/pir.32-5-201.

Pendergrast, R. A. 2017. Incorporating hypnosis into pediatric clinical encounters. *Children (Basel)* 4 (3). doi:10.3390/children4030018.

Puchalski, C. M., B. Blatt, M. Kogan, and A. Butler. 2014a. Spirituality and health: The development of a field. *Acad Med* 89 (1): 10–16. doi:10.1097/ACM.0000000000000083.

Puchalski, C. M., R. Vitillo, S. K. Hull, and N. Reller. 2014b. Improving the spiritual dimension of whole person care: Reaching national and international consensus. *J Palliat Med* 17 (6): 642–656. doi:10.1089/jpm.2014.9427.

Tetreault, P., A. Mansour, E. Vachon-Presseau, T. J. Schnitzer, A. V. Apkarian, and M. N. Baliki. 2016. Brain connectivity predicts placebo response across chronic pain clinical trials. *PLoS Biol* 14 (10): e1002570. doi:10.1371/journal.pbio.1002570.

Thirioux, B., F. Birault, and N. Jaafari. 2016. Empathy is a protective factor of burnout in physicians: New neuro-phenomenological hypotheses regarding empathy and sympathy in care relationship. *Front Psychol* 7: 763. doi:10.3389/fpsyg.2016.00763.

Vitillo, R., and C. Puchalski. 2014. World health organization authorities promote greater attention and action on palliative care. *J Palliat Med* 17 (9): 988–989. doi:10.1089/jpm.2014.9411.

Zubieta, J. K., and C. S. Stohler. 2009. Neurobiological mechanisms of placebo responses. *Ann N Y Acad Sci* 1156: 198–210. doi:10.1111/j.1749-6632.2009.04424.x.

Part II

Selected Mind–Body Therapies

Review and Research Update

This section will introduce selected mind–body therapies with strong supporting research. It is not intended to be an exhaustive list of mind–body therapies. Case examples of adult and pediatric patients are included throughout to demonstrate clinical application of the therapies. The overlap of mind–body modalities is fairly common, which can be a confounding factor in mind–body research, and may present challenges in evaluating therapies for safety and efficacy. One approach to counter this is to use a hierarchy of evidence, which means the greater the potential harm, the better the strength of evidence required before the endorsement of the therapy can be made. Cohen and Kemper have developed a useful model to assess efficacy and safety of individual treatment approaches which can be easily applied to the mind–body therapies (Kemper and Cohen).

2 × 2 Table Illustrating an Approach to CAM Therapies in Children Based on Efficacy and Safety

		Efficacy	
		Yes	*No*
Safety	Yes	Recommend	Tolerate
	No	Monitor closely or discourage	Discourage

Source: O'Connor, K.G. and Kemper, K.J., *Ambul Pediatr* 4, 482–487, 2004.

Essentially, if a therapy is both safe and efficacious, recommendation is easy. If a therapy is safe but efficacy is uncertain, it can be accepted or *tolerated* with appropriate monitoring. If a therapy is thought not to be safe, but may be efficacious, monitoring is necessary, and the clinician may discourage the patient from pursuit of the therapy based on individual circumstances. If the therapy is both unsafe and not efficacious, the patient is discouraged from its use at any time. Mind–body therapies discussed in Part II include:

* Breath work
* Autogenics
* Progressive muscle relaxation
* Biofeedback
* Clinical hypnosis

- Guided imagery
- Mindfulness
- Creative arts therapies
- Yoga and other movement therapies

Part III—"Clinical Application," will go into more detail about determining how to choose an appropriate mind–body therapy and explores a range of conditions in adults, adolescents, and children, including anxiety and depression, oncology and surgical problems, gastroenterology, and pain, with the inclusion of case studies to better illustrate their use.

References

Kemper, K. J., and M. Cohen. Ethics meet complementary and alternative medicine: New light on old principles. *Contemp Pediatr.* 21(3): 61.

O'Connor, K. G., and K. J. Kemper. 2004. Pediatrician's recommendations for complementary and alternative (CAM) therapies. *Ambul Pediatr* 4: 482–487. doi:10.1367/A04-050R.1.

5 Breath work, autogenics, progressive muscle relaxation

BREATH WORK

Breath work is a fundamental tool in the practice of mind–body therapies and, ideally, would be taught to every patient, caretaker, and practitioner. In fact, in many cultures, the word for breath and spirit are the same, for example, the Sanskrit prana and the Latin spiritus. Breath work has ties to ancient practices in yoga and in meditation and is often taught by experienced teachers in these traditions.

Considered in the use of modern mind–body medicine, breathing is unique in several respects: It is one of the two functions in the human body that can be performed consciously as well as unconsciously. Similar to the eye blink, breath can be a completely voluntary or a completely involuntary act. Both are controlled by dual aspects of the nervous system, the voluntary nervous system, and the involuntary or autonomic nervous system, comprised of the sympathetic and parasympathetic branches. Breath has been shown to be a powerful conduit between the two systems, and research has demonstrated a sophisticated connection in its efficacy in mind–body therapies (Feldman et al. 2013).

Breath work is also:

- Accessible
- Portable
- Affordable
- Adaptable

It can be challenging to study breath as an individual element in mind–body therapies because it is frequently combined with other practices, including yoga, meditation, clinical hypnosis, and other therapies.

INVOLUNTARY BREATH CONTROL

Involuntary control of the breath is centered in the upper and lower brainstem. In simplified terms, the pons, located in the upper brainstem, regulates respiratory rate via the pneumotaxic center. The medulla oblongata, in the lower brainstem, uses chemoreceptors to sense levels of carbon dioxide, oxygen, and pH in the blood and interacts with the heart, lungs, intercostal muscles, and diaphragm to maintain equilibrium. Chemoreceptors present in the arch of the aorta and throughout the vascular system create a rapid feedback loop (Molkov et al. 2014).

A typical example of breath used to reestablish physiologic equilibrium would be a runner exerting themselves whose respiratory depth and rate increase in response to increased oxygen requirement, buildup of carbon dioxide, and lowering of blood pH due to the accumulation of lactic acid. These physiologic changes are instantly sensed by the chemoreceptors, signaling the respiratory center to stimulate pace and depth of respirations to reestablish physiologic equilibrium (Molkov et al. 2014).

VOLUNTARY BREATH CONTROL

Voluntary control of breath is based in the cortex. Common examples of triggering voluntary breath include swimming, playing a wind instrument, singing, and, in the mind–body therapies, consciously using the pacing and depth of the breath to shift the autonomic system away from sympathetic activation and toward parasympathetic activation (Kox et al. 2014).

Voluntary control of breath is a central element of ancient meditation and yoga practices.

Known as pranayama breathing, it has been associated with a reduction in blood pressure, improved heart rate variability, more diaphragmatic breathing, and reduction in perceived stress, among other things (Jerath et al. 2006).

Prana translates to *life force* or *energy*, ayama is defined as *extension* or *expansion*, so together they mean extension or expansion of prana or life force. Pranayama breathing generally consists of four stages: inhalation, internal retention of breath, exhalation, and external breath retention. One mechanism, proposed by Jerath et al. (2006) is that slow deep conscious breaths functionally reset the autonomic nervous system through stretch-induced inhibitory signals and hyperpolarized currents that synchronize neural signals in the organs (heart, lung, limbic system, and cortex).

A 2016 review by Nivethitha et al. of some of the many types of pranayama breathing (right nostril, left nostril, alternating techniques, duration, and depth of respirations) highlighted research gaps in understanding of the specific mechanism of action and specific applications of different techniques but found consensus that the slow types of yogic breathing (as opposed to fast) studied to date have been associated with more positive effect on cardiovascular and autonomic factors (Nivethitha et al. 2016).

As an example, a randomized controlled trial of healthy adult volunteers ($n = 39$) showed statistically significant lowering of both systolic and diastolic blood pressure after 5 minutes of slow pace Bhastrika pranayama breathing, which consists of inhalation through both nostrils for about 4 seconds and exhalation over about 6 seconds for a respiratory rate of six breaths per minute. Breathing instructions included a suggestion to *imagine the open blue sky* rather than over-focus on the timing of breath cycles. Ten volunteers who ingested oral hyoscine-N-butyl bromide (parasympathetic blocker) then undertook the same breathing exercises showed no significant drop in systolic or diastolic blood pressure or in heart rate in this study (Pramanik et al. 2009).

A similar study in 60 healthy adolescents mean age 14 years ($n = 30$ treatment group) evaluating the effect of Bhramari (humming bee breath) pranayama on resting cardiovascular parameters found significant reductions in heart rate ($p = 0.001$) and in mean arterial pressure, pulse pressure, and blood pressure indices in the treatment group. Bhramari pranayama was practiced for 45 minutes, or five cycles, of inhalation through both nostrils for about 5 seconds with a slow exhalation of about 15 seconds during which they said a mantra *A U Mmm* with a humming sound that is generated in the inner airway which resembles the humming of a bee, hence the name of the exercise. Students completed a 1-minute cycle at a respiratory rate of

3–4 breaths per minute, followed by a 1-minute rest, breathing normally, for up to five cycles (45 minutes) (Kuppusamy et al. 2016).

A prospective randomized controlled trial of 82 healthy volunteers age 18–27 ($n = 41$ study group) measuring lung function (peak expiratory flow, forced expiratory flow, and maximal voluntary ventilation) practiced Bhramari pranayama for 5 minutes (inhalation through both nostrils, exhale while producing humming sound) followed by OM chanting for 5 minutes (inhale through both nostrils, exhale producing OM chant until further exhalation is not possible) under supervision every morning for 6 days per week for 2 weeks. Results showed significant increases in peak expiratory flow, forced expiratory flow, and maximal voluntary ventilation in the treatment group ($p < 0.05$) (Mooventhan and Khode 2014).

Research is also actively examining the effect of voluntary breathing on inflammatory cytokine secretion. For example, a small randomized, controlled study by Twal measured salivary cytokines in healthy volunteers (intervention group $n = 10$) who performed two different ancient and well-described yoga breathing practices for 10 minutes each for an aggregated 20-minute session led by a trained yoga instructor. Breathing exercises in this study included a 10-minute exercise of OM chanting (Pranava pranayama) followed by an exercise with three components, inhalation through one nostril for two counts, breath holding for eight counts, and exhalation for four counts, repeated for 10 minutes. Samples were collected immediately after the breathing training and at 5-minute intervals until 20 minutes out. Results showed statistically significant reduction in multiple inflammatory cytokines (IL-1 beta, IL-8, MCP-1) compared to control (Twal et al. 2016).

One parallel randomized controlled study of 22 healthy volunteers ($n = 12$ intervention group) showed that subjects randomized to an intervention that included 10 days of training in meditation, breathing techniques (described as cyclic hyperventilation followed by breath retention) and exposure to cold had significant induction of anti-inflammatory IL-10, increase of epinephrine release, attenuation of proinflammatory innate immune response and fewer clinical symptoms of flu-like illness after intravenous administration of *Escherichia coli* endotoxin when they used the learned techniques (Kox et al. 2014).

The increase in epinephrine levels in the experiment mirrored the short-term elevation in epinephrine that has been associated with limiting production of proinflammatory cytokines in *in vivo* experiments with intravenous infusion of endotoxins in human volunteers (van der Poll et al. 1996).

A small study ($n = 15$) by Nivethitha et al. evaluated the effect of two different pranayamas, Bhastrika (bellows breath) and Kumbhaka (breath retention) on cerebral hemodynamics in young adults using continuous transcranial Doppler monitoring. The pranayamas were performed in two different orders for 1 minute each and showed significant opposing results on cerebral hemodynamics. Bhastrika (bellows) was correlated with significant reductions in end-diastolic velocity and mean flow velocity while Kumbhaka (breath retention) was associated with significant increase in peak systolic velocity, end-diastolic volume, and mean flow velocity (all $p < 0.01$). Holding breath is considered a very important element of pranayama and causes elevation of blood carbon dioxide, resulting in vasodilation and increased cerebral blood flow.

Conversely, hyperventilation (bellows breath) results in vasoconstriction and reduction of cerebral blood flow. These emerging studies offer further insight into the complexities of yogic breathing, and the authors suggest the future possibility of designing pranayama techniques tailored to the individual patient's requirements (Nivethitha et al. 2017).

CLINICAL RELEVANCE

It is apparent from the variability of studies and relatively small sample sizes that more information is needed before making generalized recommendations about pranayama (yogic breathing, the ancient art of breath control), long sustained inhalation (Puraka), exhalation (Rechaka), and holding breath (Kumbhaka). However, there is a sufficient body of research to confirm the positive reproducible effect of slow yogic breathing patterns on cardiovascular hemodynamics and inflammatory markers that would suggest the potential for benefit in the introduction of simple breathing exercises based on ancient teachings into modern practice.

Despite a lack of specific recommendations, many breath work options are relatively simple exercises and easily taught, even to children. (This does not include advanced pranayama practices, which are frequently paired with asanas (postures) in the practice of yoga and are taught by skilled practitioners.)

The goal of breathing exercises is for the individual to familiarize themselves with the sensations of breathing, especially pace and depth, and to practice periods of slowing down and exercising voluntary control of the breath. Ideally, practicing breath work would facilitate triggering of the relaxation response discussed in detail in Chapter 2. In addition to its use in yoga, meditation, and mindfulness practices, many other mind–body therapies emphasize breath awareness or breath counting as a core component and centering practice.

CAUTIONS

Hyperventilation causes excess loss of carbon dioxide and may cause lightheadedness, dizziness, numbness and tingling of extremities, muscle spasms, and syncope at its extremes.

Intentional hyperventilation, used to decrease carbon dioxide levels and slow the urge to breathe can cause *blackout* due to significant drops in the partial pressure in arterial oxygen. Hyperventilation is especially dangerous if used during swimming or diving. Breath work exercises are considered most effective if practiced regularly.

CLINICAL APPLICATION: BREATH WORK

Joe is a 42-year-old software salesman with chronic job stress and a hectic travel schedule. His wife is a pharmacist, and they have two children. He accepted a promotion last year that significantly increased his monthly travel and is regretting his decision. He would like to become an independent consultant; however, he has been experiencing high anxiety, bordering on panic, when he thinks of the possibility of failure and potential loss of his family's health benefits. He is not interested in any pharmaceutical treatment options for his escalating feelings of anxiety and would like to know what other options are available.

As an introduction to non-pharmacologic stress management, his integrative clinician reviewed some basic breath exercises and apps of potential interest with him during the visit.

Breath work exercises

- Ten to one (slowly count breaths down from 10 to 1).
- Breath count 4 up, 4 down (slowly count breaths 1,2,3,4—4,3,2,1).
- Count in the gap (slow inhale, slow exhale, hold, and count 1,2,3 after each out breath before next inhalation).

- Square breath (inhale for count of 4, hold for 4, exhale for 4, pause for count of 4).
- 4-7-8 breath (in for a count of 4, hold for 7, exhale for 8) up to four repetitions.
- Belly breath or diaphragmatic breath (inhale while relaxing belly, allowing the abdomen to protrude while lungs fully inflate, exhale, and relax abdomen) repeat slowly for 1–2 minutes.

Simple mantras or word prompts can be added to individualize the exercise

- Breathe in "I am," breathe out "at peace."
- Breathe in "calm," breath out "worry" or "tension."
- A, B, C breath: Bringing yourself to the moment, think "awareness," take a "breath," repeat "center" or "calm" with the exhale, pause.

Apps of potential interest

- Breathe2Relax
- Breathe Deep—Personal Assistant for Breathing Meditation
- Relax and Rest Guided Meditations

Integrative medicine clinicians are often trained to introduce breath work to patients and may have a card or handout with exercises listed. It can be very powerful for the clinician to take a moment to demonstrate a breath exercise and to practice breathing with the patient using one of the simple exercises mentioned earlier.

CLINICAL APPLICATION FOLLOW-UP: BREATH WORK

Joe was skeptical when breathing was introduced as a treatment option but open to suggestion, especially given his desire to avoid pharmaceuticals. He was interested in understanding the physiology of breathing and the reasons it might help him rebalance his sympathetic and parasympathetic nervous system. He liked the fact that he could use a variety of breathing techniques depending on the situation and that it did not require any special equipment that might complicate travel on his frequent business trips. In the office, he was very surprised to find himself practicing a square breath exercise with his physician but appreciated the few extra minutes taken to teach him a new skill. He left with a card that outlined four exercises: the square breath, the 4-7-8 breath, the count in the gap, and the belly breath. On the back of the card was a selection of recommended breath work apps which he was curious to try. He began using the square breath every morning for about 2 minutes and repeated that each evening before going to sleep. In stressful situations, he started using the simple *inhale calm, exhale tension* breath and over time noticed the benefit. Sometimes he would just count his breaths up to 5 and back to 1 to center himself.

Joe began to make other changes to slow the pace of his life and allow himself time to plan. He and his wife decided to move forward with his career change plan to consultant over the upcoming 12 months rather than making an abrupt change, giving the family time to adjust. This stepwise approach reduced everyone's stress and the transition ultimately went smoothly.

Other conditions where breath work may have benefit include:

* Insomnia
* Anxiety (social, test related, procedural)
* Heart arrhythmias (non–life-threatening tachycardias)

CLINICAL APPLICATION: BREATH WORK IN PEDIATRICS

Sophie is a 14-year-old girl with generalized anxiety disorder. Her symptoms are triggered by school, especially at the beginning of the year and after vacations. She also has exacerbations on Sunday evenings when preparing for Monday classes. Her symptoms include feeling out of control, inability to focus, irritability, and catastrophic thinking. She has missed a significant number of school days, and her grades are slipping. Both she and her family would like to avoid prescription medications.

In addition to preventive lifestyle measures such as reduction in caffeine, introduction of daily enjoyable exercise, moderating screen time, and inclusion of time in nature, Sophie was introduced to the 4-7-8 breath as a way to rebalance her sympathetic and parasympathetic nervous system. She began to practice the breath cycle (inhale for a count of 4, hold for 7, exhale for 8) repeating it no more than four times consecutively, every morning and evening, and anytime she felt symptoms of anxiety rising. Initially, she had a feeling of lightheadedness with the fourth cycle which gradually resolved when she slowed the pace.

Over time, she incorporated the 4-7-8 breath into her daily routine and began to use it in acute situations at school when she began feeling out of control. By the second month of practice, she was beginning to notice an encouraging difference in her symptoms of anxiety. She was able to successfully return to classes after the winter break for the first time since elementary school and saw an overall improvement in academic performance as the semester progressed. She found it especially helpful in reducing test anxiety. She continued to use the breathing technique at bedtime to help her fall asleep and when she woke in the night.

AUTOGENICS: AUTOGENIC RELAXATION TRAINING

Background

Auto (self) genics (generated) relaxation is a technique considered a precursor to modern biofeedback and has roots in clinical hypnosis and self-hypnosis. The goal of autogenics is to increase self-awareness of one's physical state, focus concentration on self-initiated therapeutic suggestions to induce the relaxation response, achieve physiologic relaxation, decrease stress, and increase one's overall sense of self-control in the process. It is a method of stress management widely used in Europe, especially Germany where it originated (Goldbeck and Schmid 2003).

Dr. Johannnes Schultz is credited with developing autogenic training in the early 1990s. Schultz was a German psychiatrist and neurologist whose work built on the work of Oskar Vogt's research in sleep, hypnosis, and self-hypnosis. The researchers noted that patients could learn to generate a state of deep relaxation, heaviness in the limbs, and warmth in the extremities during self-hypnosis (auto-hypnotic) exercises. This was associated with a reduction in stress and an improved feeling of well-being in patients who practiced the exercises several times per day. Schultz's work focused on identifying an approach that would lessen the need or dependence on a therapist to guide the patient (Lauche et al. 2013).

It is reported that Schultz developed his therapeutic suggestions based on what physiologic changes patients were experiencing during hypnosis, for example, heaviness in the limbs, slowing of the heart rate, and cooling of the forehead. This work resulted in the six classic autogenic phrases listed in the following.

Autogenics in practice

Six classic phases were developed by Schultz, typically repeated three times each in sequence.

Begin with sitting or lying in a comfortable position, scan the body for tension. Phrases can be read by the clinician or repeated silently by the individual.

1   My arms are heavy (heaviness, muscular relaxation).
2   My arms are warm (warmth, vascular dilation).
3   My heartbeat is calm and strong (heart function regulation).
4   My breathing is calm and relaxed (regulation of breathing).
5   My abdomen radiates warmth (regulation of the visceral organs).
6   My forehead is pleasantly cool (regulation of brain activity).

Finish by repeating a preferred mantra such as "I am at peace," or "I am calm."

The exercises are typically practiced twice a day and reinforce the ability to reliably trigger the relaxation response (Blodt et al. 2014). Each suggestion is also modifiable depending on the individual's needs, for example, in children with insomnia one might substitute a positive phrase such as "I will sleep through the night" (Klott 2013b).

Strengths of autogenic training

Autogenic training promotes self-regulation skills, self-efficacy, independence, and shift of sense of agency back to the patient rather than the clinician.

Challenges of autogenic training

The challenges of autogenic training include the need for proper training and need for consistency to see maximum effects. The hypothetical risk exists for hypotension or bradycardia based on individual physiology and response to the autogenic suggestions.

CLINICAL APPLICATION: AUTOGENICS

Patrick is a graduate student with a thesis to due in 6 months. He has a history of migraine headaches as a child. Now he is getting headaches which have been diagnosed by health service as tension-type headaches. Occurring two to three times per week, the headaches are causing delays in his research, and he has missed several important meetings with his mentor. He prefers to avoid medication and acknowledges that he is under considerable stress. He has read about autogenics and wonders if it is a recognized treatment for tension headache.

Autogenic training has been shown to be of potential benefit in tension headaches, although reviews of efficacy to date are mixed. For example, in a systematic review of seven controlled trials by Kanji et al., reviewers found variable study quality and size. Overall, autogenic training was found to have similar effects as self-hypnosis in this review, and small, non-significant benefits were seen for wait-list controls in one study of 337 patients. Adverse effects were rarely reported and were considered minor (Kanji et al. 2006).

Another review of 11 studies looking at the use of relaxation training (autogenic training, with two studies including biofeedback) in children with tension headaches again included studies of mixed quality and study size. Again, adverse events were not reported, and some clinical improvements were seen (Verhagen et al. 2005).

Autogenics has also been associated with a reduction in saliva amylase, measured as a stress biomarker. In the study of 43 adults ($n = 20$ patients with functional somatic syndromes, 23 control), patients with functional somatic syndrome had higher baseline salivary amylase prior to autogenic relaxation session and reduced following autogenic training (Kiba et al. 2015).

CLINICAL APPLICATION FOLLOW-UP: AUTOGENICS

Patrick's continued curiosity about autogenics and the low risk of reported adverse effects led him to seek out introductory training with a local practitioner. He also investigated mobile apps he could download onto his smartphone and found several that looked promising. He began to practice using the six classic phrases twice daily and tracked his symptoms using a headache diary. Over the next 3 months, he gradually experienced fewer headaches, although he had a setback with a cluster of headaches around one important project deadline. He recommitted to the practice and added a third autogenic practice session at lunchtime. He continued tracking his symptoms, and by the fifth month, he noticed a significant reduction in headache frequency.

USE OF AUTOGENICS IN OTHER CONDITIONS

Sleep

Autogenics was found to be efficacious in one prospective pre- and post-treatment study in 153 adults with sleep-related problems associated with their chronic health problem.

Participants received a standard 8-week training course in autogenics and showed improvement in sleep latency ($p = 0.049$), waking more refreshed ($p < 0.001$), and overall improvements in well-being, anxiety, and depression ($p < 0.001$) (Bowden et al. 2012).

Irritable bowel syndrome

Autogenic relaxation was studied in a small group of 21 adults with IBS ($n = 11$ treatment group) and was shown to be improve social functioning and bodily pain as compared to control group ($p < 0.05$), and improvements in emotional and general sense of overall health approached statistical significance at ($p = 0.051$) and ($p = 0.068$), respectively (Shinozaki et al. 2010).

Fibromyalgia

Autogenics was also shown to be of some benefit in fibromyalgia. In a study of 408 patients ($n = 108$) treatment group, patients received nine 2-hour sessions (five education and four sessions of autogenic training). The treatment group showed improvement in general fatigue, morning stiffness, anxiety, and depression. Absolute risk reduction was 36. 1% (95% confidence interval: 23.3–48.8). In this study, participants with lower trait anxiety showed the most benefit (Luciano et al. 2011).

Autogenics and meditation

Autogenics used during meditation was shown in a small study by Kim et al. to significantly influence heart rate variability, leading to significantly increased coherence scores. Heart coherence and electroencephalography (EEG) readings were measured in 14 adult volunteers during autogenic meditation, and results showed a significant increase in heart coherence during meditation compared to baseline. Participants had completed 8 weeks of standard autogenic training and had been meditating daily for a minimum of 1 month. Recordings of EEG output and heart rate variability were measured using a photoplethysmographic (PPG) sensor on a finger and used to calculate heart coherence that correlated heart coherence and meditative state measured by EEG. Authors postulated the potential for heart coherence could be used as an easily measured element that may provide a window into the meditative state (Kim et al. 2014).

Autogenic relaxation is also being studied in comparison to mindfulness meditation and guided imagery, with a variety of apps in development (Blodt et al. 2014).

CLINICAL APPLICATION: AUTOGENICS IN PEDIATRICS

Sanja is a talented 12-year-old violinist with a history of progressively worsening performance anxiety. She is skilled enough to compete in national and international youth competitions and plans to audition for the Julliard School in the upcoming year. Both she and her parents are adamant that no medication can be used, and she has tried a variety of botanical teas, aromatherapy, and cognitive behavioral therapy with no benefit. One of the main problems, in addition to a feeling of anticipatory anxiety, is tenseness of her shoulder, arm, and hand muscles, which is inhibiting her technique. Sanja is highly motivated to try a new approach and is curious to learn more about the mind–body therapies. You review the various mind–body options with them, and they express interest in autogenics because of its association with muscle relaxation. They ask if autogenics can be taught to children.

Autogenics can be taught to children with the use of modified language, relatable examples, and imagery. For example, in a study by Goldbeck and Schmidt, 50 children ($n = 35$ treatment group) ages 6–15 years were assessed for stress levels, psychosomatic complaints, and behavior symptoms before and after autogenic training. Training was done in small group sessions of 9–12 children, who received 8 weekly sessions lasting 30 minutes in the outpatient setting. The actual training sessions were delivered in 10-minute blocks of time interspersed with play activities and group conversation. Children received the classic suggestions from the therapist throughout the session. Home practice was encouraged, and children received written text of the exercises for home practice. Results showed small but clinically relevant reduced stress and psychosomatic complaints in the treatment group, although wide distribution of presenting complaints was a confounder. Authors concluded that 56% of children in the treatment group met their goals of increased relaxation, improvement in stress, and improved behavioral and emotional symptoms. No adverse effects were seen, and only one child dropped out of the study over the 8 weeks (Goldbeck and Schmid 2003).

One of the most important approaches to use in children is age and developmental-stage-appropriate language to realistically accommodate attention span. In Sanja's case, her educational level and discipline allowed her to master the technique using the six classic phrases in a series of a few visits with a trained practitioner. She began to practice the phrases every morning, after school, and before every practice session—especially focusing on her upper body, arms, hands, and fingers. She associated the sessions with a deep state of relaxation and enjoyment and found they helped her recapture the joy she found in music and the feeling that the music was coming through her effortlessly. Over time, she felt an overall lowering of baseline stress and found performances more enjoyable.

The experience of learning a stress management technique that was fully in her control was a very important element of her treatment plan. Over the following year, Sanja was able to gain enough confidence to tell her parents that she preferred to play music for enjoyment and was not interested in pursuing admittance to Julliard due to the high-stress application process. She continued to perform locally and regionally and after high school received a full scholarship to Northwestern University Bienen School of Music near her home.

PROGRESSIVE MUSCLE RELAXATION

Progressive muscle relaxation (PMR) is a type of relaxation therapy that consists of systematically tensing and relaxing muscle groups. It can be used to help highlight discrepancy between the tense and relaxed state and may be especially helpful in people new to relaxation techniques because of its straightforward technique. Progressive muscle relaxation was developed by Edmund Jacobson as an extensive exercise involving 30 muscle groups and has been shortened over time by various practitioners and in different applications to meet patients' needs (Jacobson 1938).

PMR objective: Develop discrepancy between tense and relaxed state (Salcedo).

Summary of steps:

- Brief body scan noticing areas of tension or relaxation
- Systematic tensing and relaxing of muscle groups
- Repeat brief body scan, compare to original state

Progressive muscle relaxation is often combined with other mind–body modalities, especially breath work, imagery, and music. PMR has a robust body of supporting data in anxiety (Manzoni et al. 2008) and has been shown to reduce frequency and severity of migraine headache (Meyer et al. 2016) and to significantly reduce salivary cortisol secretion in a study in 101 first-year university students as they navigated the stress of starting university (Chellew et al. 2015).

It has also been shown to be effective for non-specific neck pain in adults (Lauche et al. 2013). In Germany, PMR is recommended in national guidelines for the treatment of low back pain (Blodt et al. 2014).

Pediatric studies of PMR suggest that it can be reliably adapted to a variety of ages and settings. For example, the efficacy of progressive muscle relaxation was compared in 6- and 12-session interventions to teach techniques to reduce emotional stress, improve short-term memory, and improve attention in a randomized study of ($n = 132$) elementary school students. The PMR intervention in this study was delivered in a 30-minute pre-recorded CD designed for children, and the treatment group received either 6 or 12 sessions during health education class. Only short-term memory in the 12-session group showed a significant improvement in this study, although it was established that progressive muscle relaxation could be successfully administered in a school group setting (Hashim and Zainol 2015). Progressive muscle relaxation has been shown to improve mood in pediatric oncology patients (Tsitsi et al. 2017), and to improve sleep quality in a randomized pilot study of 20 hospitalized children with acute lymphoblastic leukemia (Zupanec et al. 2017).

TRAINING

There is no specific certification for progressive muscle relaxation, although training programs, scripts, and several apps are available to guide patients in its use.

Sample exercise: Allow 15–20 minutes in a quiet, undisturbed space

1   Sit or lie down comfortably.
2   Inhale and release, close your eyes if you choose.
3   Take a moment to scan the body, noticing how it feels and any areas of tension or discomfort.
4   The exercise can progress from head to toe or vice versa.

- In this example, begin with the feet, tense all the muscles in the feet, toes, arch, and sole, and hold until you feel muscles tiring, almost to the point of discomfort. With an out-breath, release all tension and completely soften and relax the foot muscles, allowing tension to flow out the toes, and notice any sensations you may be experiencing.
- Move on to the lower leg, and tense all the muscles in the lower leg. Hold until you feel muscle fatigue. Repeat the release of tension with the out-breath, allowing all muscles to soften and tension to release. Notice any associated sensations. As you continue, become aware of the difference in sensations before and after release of the muscle tension.
- Continue tensing and relaxing muscle groups as you work your way up the body, including: upper leg muscles, hips and buttocks, abdomen and lower back, chest and upper back, hands, lower arms, upper arms, shoulders, neck, face including the muscles surrounding the eye and the mouth and jaw, and the crown of the head. Tense and release each group of muscles in turn. After reach release of tension in a muscle group, take a moment to inhale and exhale fully,

releasing any remaining tension in the muscles and softening and loosening all the surrounding muscles involved.

- After completion of the exercise, scan through the entire body again, noticing feelings and sensations. Breath in and out slowly, enjoying the sensation of relaxation. This is the relaxation response. Progressive muscle relaxation is a useful way to demonstrate and reinforce it to patients and clinicians alike.

Any progressive muscle relaxation exercise can be tailored to age, setting, and time frame. For example, a PMR exercise in preschoolers may take just a few minutes, involve blowing bubbles, or *belly* breathing, that is, diaphragmatic breathing. PMR may also involve music and imagery, especially in children as they may benefit from a variety of means to release tension, for example, letting the tension float away in a balloon, or as a bubble, or as a warm wave leaving the body through the fingers or toes. Conversely, a PMR session in adults can be extended to 30–45 minutes and may involve a comprehensive tensing and relaxing of nearly every muscle group. PMR can also be used in a more focused manner in ambulatory settings, for example, limiting the tension to just the hand. The act of tensing the muscles, holding, and then releasing tension with the out-breath can be used to trigger the relaxation response when practiced. This can be a useful tool for clinicians as they move through a busy day or into a stressful situation that requires them to be fully present and ready to react.

RESOURCES

Apps

- Autogenic Training and Progressive Muscle Relaxation—Guided Rest and Meditation Techniques
- Relaxation App—Guided Relaxation

Free downloads

- Student Wellness Center Dartmouth: http://www.dartmouth.edu/~healthed/relax/downloads.html

Other resources

- Audio CD Progressive Muscle Relaxation: 20 Minutes to Total Relaxation, B. Salcedo, MD

References

B. Salcedo, MD. Progressive Muscle Relaxation: 20 Minutes to Total Relaxation.

Blodt, S., D. Pach, S. Roll, and C. M. Witt. 2014. Effectiveness of app-based relaxation for patients with chronic low back pain (Relaxback) and chronic neck pain (Relaxneck): Study protocol for two randomized pragmatic trials. *Trials* 15: 490. doi:10.1186/1745-6215-15-490.

Bowden, A., A. Lorenc, and N. Robinson. 2012. Autogenic training as a behavioural approach to insomnia: A prospective cohort study. *Prim Health Care Res Dev* 13 (2): 175–185. doi:10.1017/S1463423611000181.

Chellew, K., P. Evans, J. Fornes-Vives, G. Perez, and G. Garcia-Banda. 2015. The effect of progressive muscle relaxation on daily cortisol secretion. *Stress* 18 (5): 538–544. doi:10.3109/10253890.2015.1053454.

Feldman, J. L., C. A. Del Negro, and P. A. Gray. 2013. Understanding the rhythm of breathing: So near, yet so far. *Annu Rev Physiol* 75: 423–452. doi:10.1146/annurev-physiol-040510-130049.

Goldbeck, L., and K. Schmid. 2003. Effectiveness of autogenic relaxation training on children and adolescents with behavioral and emotional problems. *J Am Acad Child Adolesc Psychiatry* 42 (9): 1046–1054. doi:10.1097/01.CHI.0000070244.24125.F.

Hashim, H. A., and N. A. Zainol. 2015. Changes in emotional distress, short term memory, and sustained attention following 6 and 12 sessions of progressive muscle relaxation training in 10–11 years old primary school children. *Psychol Health Med* 20 (5): 623–628. doi:10.1080/13548506.2014.1002851.

Jacobson, E. 1938. *Progressive Relaxation: A Physiological and Clinical Investigation of Muscular States and Their Significance in Psychology and Medical Practice*. Chicago, IL: University of Chicago Press.

Jerath, R., J. W. Edry, V. A. Barnes, and V. Jerath. 2006. Physiology of long pranayamic breathing: Neural respiratory elements may provide a mechanism that explains how slow deep breathing shifts the autonomic nervous system. *Med Hypotheses* 67 (3): 566–571. doi:10.1016/j.mehy.2006.02.042.

Kanji, N., A. R. White, and E. Ernst. 2006. Autogenic training for tension type headaches: A systematic review of controlled trials. *Complement Ther Med* 14 (2): 144–150. doi:10.1016/j.ctim.2006.03.001.

Kiba, T., K. Kanbara, I. Ban, F. Kato, S. Kawashima, Y. Saka, K. Yamamoto et al. 2015. Saliva amylase as a measure of sympathetic change elicited by autogenic training in patients with functional somatic syndromes. *Appl Psychophysiol Biofeedback* 40 (4): 339–347. doi:10.1007/s10484-015-9303-z.

Kim, D. K., J. H. Rhee, and S. W. Kang. 2014. Reorganization of the brain and heart rhythm during autogenic meditation. *Front Integr Neurosci* 7: 109. doi:10.3389/fnint.2013.00109.

Klott, O. 2013. Autogenic training: A self-help technique for children with emotional and behavioural problems. *IJTC* 34 (4): 152–158.

Kox, M., L. T. van Eijk, J. Zwaag, J. van den Wildenberg, F. C. Sweep, J. G. van der Hoeven, and P. Pickkers. 2014. Voluntary activation of the sympathetic nervous system and attenuation of the innate immune response in humans. *Proc Natl Acad Sci USA* 111 (20): 7379–7384. doi:10.1073/pnas.1322174111.

Kuppusamy, M., D. Kamaldeen, R. Pitani, and J. Amaldas. 2016. Immediate effects of Bhramari Pranayama on resting cardiovascular parameters in healthy adolescents. *J Clin Diagn Res* 10 (5): CC17–CC19. doi:10.7860/JCDR/2016/19202.7894.

Lauche, R., S. Materdey, H. Cramer, H. Haller, R. Stange, G. Dobos, and T. Rampp. 2013. Effectiveness of home-based cupping massage compared to progressive muscle relaxation in patients with chronic neck pain: A randomized controlled trial. *PLoS One* 8 (6): e65378. doi:10.1371/journal.pone.0065378.

Luciano, J. V., N. Martinez, M. T. Penarrubia-Maria, R. Fernandez-Vergel, J. Garcia-Campayo, C. Verduras, M. E. Blanco et al. 2011. Effectiveness of a psychoeducational treatment program implemented in general practice for fibromyalgia patients: A randomized controlled trial. *Clin J Pain* 27 (5): 383–391. doi:10.1097/AJP.0b013e31820b131c.

Manzoni, G. M., F. Pagnini, G. Castelnuovo, and E. Molinari. 2008. Relaxation training for anxiety: A ten-years systematic review with meta-analysis. *BMC Psychiatry* 8: 41. doi:10.1186/1471-244X-8-41.

Meyer, B., A. Keller, H. G. Wohlbier, C. H. Overath, B. Muller, and P. Kropp. 2016. Progressive muscle relaxation reduces migraine frequency and normalizes amplitudes of contingent negative variation (CNV). *J Headache Pain* 17: 37. doi:10.1186/s10194-016-0630-0.

Molkov, Y. I., N. A. Shevtsova, C. Park, A. Ben-Tal, J. C. Smith, J. E. Rubin, and I. A. Rybak. 2014. A closed-loop model of the respiratory system: Focus on hypercapnia and active expiration. *PLoS One* 9 (10): e109894. doi:10.1371/journal.pone.0109894.

Mooventhan, A., and V. Khode. 2014. Effect of Bhramari pranayama and OM chanting on pulmonary function in healthy individuals: A prospective randomized control trial. *Int J Yoga* 7 (2): 104–110. doi:10.4103/0973-6131.133875.

Nivethitha, L., A. Mooventhan, and N. K. Manjunath. 2016. Effects of various Pranayama on cardiovascular and autonomic variables. *Anc Sci Life* 36 (2): 72–77. doi:10.4103/asl.ASL_178_16.

Nivethitha, L., A. Mooventhan, N. K. Manjunath, L. Bathala, and V. K. Sharma. 2017. Cerebrovascular hemodynamics during pranayama techniques. *J Neurosci Rural Pract* 8 (1): 60–63. doi:10.4103/0976-3147.193532.

Pramanik, T., H. O. Sharma, S. Mishra, A. Mishra, R. Prajapati, and S. Singh. 2009. Immediate effect of slow pace bhastrika pranayama on blood pressure and heart rate. *J Altern Complement Med* 15 (3): 293–295. doi:10.1089/acm.2008.0440.

Shinozaki, M., M. Kanazawa, M. Kano, Y. Endo, N. Nakaya, M. Hongo, and S. Fukudo. 2010. Effect of autogenic training on general improvement in patients with irritable bowel syndrome: A randomized controlled trial. *Appl Psychophysiol Biofeedback* 35 (3): 189–198. doi:10.1007/s10484-009-9125-y.

Tsitsi, T., A. Charalambous, E. Papastavrou, and V. Raftopoulos. 2017. Effectiveness of a relaxation intervention (progressive muscle relaxation and guided imagery techniques) to reduce anxiety and improve mood of parents of hospitalized children with malignancies: A randomized controlled trial in Republic of Cyprus and Greece. *Eur J Oncol Nurs* 26: 9–18. doi:10.1016/j.ejon.2016.10.007.

Twal, W. O., A. E. Wahlquist, and S. Balasubramanian. 2016. Yogic breathing when compared to attention control reduces the levels of pro-inflammatory biomarkers in saliva: A pilot randomized controlled trial. *BMC Complement Altern Med* 16: 294. doi:10.1186/s12906-016-1286-7.

van der Poll, T., S. M. Coyle, K. Barbosa, C. C. Braxton, and S. F. Lowry. 1996. Epinephrine inhibits tumor necrosis factor-alpha and potentiates interleukin 10 production during human endotoxemia. *J Clin Invest* 97 (3): 713–719. doi:10.1172/JCI118469.

Verhagen, A. P., L. Damen, M. Y. Berger, J. Passchier, V. Merlijn, and B. W. Koes. 2005. Conservative treatments of children with episodic tension-type headache: A systematic review. *J Neurol* 252 (10): 1147–11454. doi:10.1007/s00415-005-0940-7.

Zupanec, S., H. Jones, L. McRae, E. Papaconstantinou, J. Weston, and R. Stremler. 2017. A sleep hygiene and relaxation intervention for children with acute lymphoblastic leukemia: A pilot randomized controlled trial. *Cancer Nurs* 40 (6): 488–496. doi:10.1097/NCC.0000000000000457.

6 Biofeedback

INTRODUCTION

Biofeedback describes technology-assisted approaches to mind–body medicine that provides real-time interactive electronic physiological monitoring. During a biofeedback session, the individual is connected to electrical sensors or other types of electromechanical devices that provide auditory, visual, kinesthetic, or multimedia information about their physiologic state. The idea is to train individuals to control normally involuntary functions, for example, blood pressure, heart rate, respiratory rate, and skin temperature. Biofeedback can be especially helpful in individuals who are not able to objectively assess their stress levels—or who have become accustomed to living in a state of sympathetic overdrive. In a sense, it builds on the concept of progressive muscle relaxation by measuring physiologic response and relaying the information back to the patient in real time.

BACKGROUND AND HISTORICAL PERSPECTIVE

Early studies in biofeedback were based on the work of Benson and colleagues, initially using animals who were shown to be able to modulate systolic blood pressure in response to environmental stimuli (Benson et al. 1969).

Subsequent pilot studies were done in humans with essential hypertension who were taught using a series of positive feedback signals to lower their blood pressure (Benson et al. 1971; Kristt and Engel 1975).

Over time, more structured relaxation techniques were associated with reduction in blood pressure in study subjects, and the field of behavioral modification with physiologic feedback, now known as biofeedback, gained momentum and structure (Glasgow et al. 1982).

Biofeedback has modernized to the point where training equipment is portable and relatively affordable. Home biofeedback programs are commercially available as hand-held devices, smartphone apps, and virtual reality biofeedback training programs—among others.

BIOFEEDBACK STRENGTHS

The strengths of biofeedback include the ability to demonstrate the mind–body connection in a concrete manner for those who may be skeptical and the near-immediate positive reinforcement the individual receives when reaching their physiologic goal. Autonomy while interacting with technology may be another appeal of biofeedback for generations who have grown up using smartphones and video games. Some insurance companies cover biofeedback services; the 2017 International Classification of Disease (ICD)-10-Clinical Modification (CM) Procedure Code for Biofeedback is GZC9ZZZ.

RISKS AND POTENTIAL CHALLENGES

There are no particular risks or contraindications with biofeedback, although provider training specifications are less structured than with other mind–body therapies. It is incumbent upon the patient to be sure the biofeedback practitioner is properly trained and able to refer appropriately if needed. Variable training standards and programs may indirectly impact patient progress. Individuals must learn correct use of the modality, and some may need regular practice to maintain the physiologic benefits. Overdependence on technology is a potential risk, although, ideally, the patient learns to trigger their relaxation response independently and over time is able to minimize reliance on technology. The cost of equipment and access to appropriate therapies are also considerations, as is the financial impact if insurance does not cover services.

BIOFEEDBACK OVERVIEW

Commonly used forms of biofeedback include:

- Heart rate variability (HRV), beat-to-beat variability
- Electromyography (EMG), measures muscle tension
- Thermal biofeedback, skin temperature vasodilation (measures temperature change in hands or fingers)
- Neurofeedback or electroencephalography (EEG) (measures brainwave activity)
- Electrodermal activity (measures sweat gland activity)
- Pneumography (measures movement of chest and stomach associated with breathing)

HEART RATE VARIABILITY

Heart rate variability (HRV) is defined as the physiological phenomenon of variation in the time interval between heartbeats, measured by variation in the beat-to-beat interval (1996). The relevance of heart rate variability was recognized in the mid-1960s with relation to fetal distress when Hon and Lee (1996) recognized that fetal distress was preceded by variations in interbeat intervals before change occurred in the fetal heart rate itself (Hon and Lee 1963). Heart rate variability came into sharper focus in the late 1980s when it was recognized as an independent predictor of mortality after acute myocardial infarction (1996).

Researchers showed that in the QRS complex on the normal electrocardiogram, the RR interval between beats is considered an accurate representation of beat-to-beat control. Vagal stimulation leads to inhibition of sympathetic activity, and conversely, sympathetic stimulation upregulates sympathetic afferent activity. Both vagal and sympathetic efferent signals directed to the sinus node are characterized by synchronous discharge with each cardiac cycle that can be modulated by central vasomotor and respiratory centers and by peripheral oscillators found in arterial pressure and respiratory movements. These oscillators generate rhythmic fluctuations in neural discharge that manifest as short and long term oscillation in the heart rhythm (1996).

Modern companies such as HeartMath LLC have developed monitors, educational products, and training courses to teach individuals how to increase heart rate variability, primarily by adjusting their respiratory rate to approximately six breaths per minute, at which heart rate variability is maximized through action of the sinus node. This promotes the development of a sine-wave-like pattern in the heart rate variability measurement oscillating at a frequency of 0.1 Hz which HeartMath identifies as *coherence*. Desktop and hand-held heart rate variability monitors are now widely available.

ELECTROMYOGRAPHY

Electromyography (EMG) refers to the recording of electrical activity in muscle. In EMG, either surface electrodes or intramuscular electrodes can be used. Electromyography turns these signals into measurable values that can be recorded and measured, often visually as well as with auditory feedback. Nerve conduction studies are a type of EMG used to evaluate the speed and strength of motor neuron signal conduction and are not generally included in therapeutic biofeedback.

The primary drawback of surface sensors to measure changes in muscle tone include the ability to access only superficial muscles. Intramuscular EMG uses very fine wires or needles inserted into muscle attached to a surface electrode and allows measurement on a deeper level which provides a more reliable measurement. Intramuscular EMG is more involved and may be more uncomfortable for the patient.

EMG biofeedback has been used in treating a variety of conditions, including the following.

Essential hypertension

Classic articles, such as the 1981 study by McGrady et al. on the use of an 8-week biofeedback course administered to 38 adults, showed a statistically significant decrease in mean blood pressure in the treatment group. Significant changes were also seen in muscle tension and urinary cortisol which was also recorded in the treatment group (McGrady et al. 1981).

Long-term follow-up of patients trained in this 8-week biofeedback course showed sustained results in blood pressure reduction in responders at one, two, and three years follow-up, at rates of 31%, 38%, and 27%, respectively (McGrady et al. 1991).

Clinical guidelines in the management of primary hypertension in adults by the 2011 UK National Institute for Health and Clinical Excellence reviewed biofeedback and other relaxation therapies under lifestyle interventions and included 23 randomized controlled trials involving 1,481 adult participants. Most biofeedback interventions involved a median duration of 8 weeks of training, each session lasting an average of 60 minutes, over a range of 4 weeks to 6 months. In this review, although study size and design were variable, most relaxation interventions, including those delivering biofeedback, were associated with statistically significant reductions in both systolic and diastolic blood pressure (2011).

Migraine, tension-type, and medication-overuse headache

Electromyography biofeedback has been shown to be effective in reducing pain caused by migraine and tension-type headache and has been found to be as effective as medication in some patients. Biofeedback combined with medication has also been found to be very effective in facilitating reduction of medication use over time in some patient populations (Andrasik 2010).

EMG biofeedback is being investigated as a tool in the prophylactic treatment of medication-overuse headaches. For example, in a randomized pilot study by Rausa et al., EMG was used to measure frontalis muscle tension in 27 adults placed into EMG biofeedback and prophylactic pharmaceutical therapy ($n = 15$ treatment) or pharmaceutical therapy alone. The treatment group received 9 weekly sessions of frontalis muscle EMG biofeedback focused on decreasing muscle tension. Over the nine sessions, support on the biofeedback was gradually reduced by alternating presence and absence of sensors. Adults in the treatment group experienced significantly lower headache frequency, lower drug intake, and improved pain coping behaviors with results sustained at 4-month follow-up (Rausa et al. 2016).

Low back pain

The 2017 Annals of Internal Medicine *Non-Invasive Treatments for Acute, Subacute, and Chronic Low Back Pain: A Clinical Practice Guideline from the American College of Physicians* mention the use of electromyography biofeedback in their recommendations for patients with chronic low back pain, along with exercise, multidisciplinary rehabilitation, acupuncture, mindfulness-based stress reduction, tai chi, yoga, progressive relaxation, cognitive behavioral therapy, or spinal manipulation, among others (Qaseem et al. 2017).

Anxiety

A small study by Gholami Tahsini et al. used a combination of progressive muscle relaxation assisted EMG biofeedback, respiratory biofeedback measuring respiratory rate, and autogenic training measured by thermal biofeedback in a randomized trial of 29 university students with anxiety and depression. Students in the treatment group received eight 90-minute training sessions over a 4-week period and were also encouraged to practice at home for 30 minutes per day. The treatment group showed a significant reduction in emotional symptoms of stress and depression compared to controls (Gholami Tahsini et al. 2017).

Stroke rehabilitation

Electromyography biofeedback has been used in stroke rehabilitation to address a variety of functional deficits involving upper and lower extremities. For example, EMG biofeedback was used to beneficial effect in patients with hemiplegia in a controlled study of 30 patients ($n = 15$ treatment group) to address upper extremity function after stroke ($p < 0.01$) (Kim 2017). Other studies on EMG in stroke patients have shown benefit in patients with deficits in hand function (Rayegani et al. 2014) and improvement of gait (Del Din et al. 2014).

Dysfunctional voiding and pelvic pain

Electromyography biofeedback is widely used in the treatment of dysfunctional voiding and pelvic pain in children and adults, including fecal incontinence (Pager et al. 2002; Bartlett et al. 2011; Vonthein et al. 2013), urinary incontinence (Berghmans et al. 2013; Dumoulin et al. 2014), and pelvic pain (Schmitt et al. 2017). EMG biofeedback has also been used successfully in erectile dysfunction (Dorey et al. 2004; Prota et al. 2012).

THERMAL BIOFEEDBACK

Thermal biofeedback primarily reflects changes in blood flow and typically uses a temperature-sensitive sensor that measures change in Celsius or Fahrenheit. Patients can learn to warm or cool extremities using either vasodilation or vasoconstriction, depending on the desired clinical effect. Thermal biofeedback has been used in the treatment of a variety of conditions, including:

- Pain (Myrvik et al. 2012; Keppler et al. 2016)
- Migraine headache (Scharff et al. 2002)
- Raynaud's disease (Karavidas et al. 2006)

CLINICAL APPLICATION: BIOFEEDBACK

Dr. Larson is a 52-year-old physics professor with a history of hypertension. She is on two antihypertensives and continues to have intermittent blood pressure spikes with stress, which have been closely correlated to her headaches. Symptoms have become more frequent over the past semester. Sharice has a strong family history of hypertension and stroke, especially in female relatives. One of her greatest fears is having a stroke at a young age as her mother did. She dislikes the medication side-effects and is interested in exploring her therapeutic options. She is highly motivated to make lifestyle changes, is deeply religious, and draws great strength and comfort from her faith. On review of the various mind–body therapy options, she expresses interest in learning more about biofeedback.

ADULT BIOFEEDBACK: RESEARCH OVERVIEW

Biofeedback has been shown to be effective in adult headache and is used in two main approaches: biofeedback-assisted relaxation and more specific approaches. In assisted relaxation, electromyography and thermal feedback are commonly used to modulate sympathetic nervous system arousal. Music, imagery, breath pacing, and other mind–body therapies can be combined to augment relaxation. More specific approaches to target the underlying cause of the headache often focus on migraine headaches. Relaxation training, thermal biofeedback combined with relaxation training, and electromyographic biofeedback have Grade A evidence from U.S. Headache Consortium evidence-based guidelines for migraine headache (Silberstein 2000).

A meta-analysis of the use of biofeedback in tension headache included 52 trials and 1,532 patients. Results showed medium to large improvement in headache pain intensity, frequency, and duration (Nestoriuc et al. 2008b).

A further systematic review of the use of biofeedback in headache included 94 studies and more than 3,500 patients. Results showed that peripheral skin temperature feedback, blood-volume-pulse feedback, and electromyography feedback showed a statistically significant medium-sized effect on headache intensity, frequency, and duration over control groups. In patients with tension headache, EMG feedback had a large average size effect as compared to controls, placebo, and relaxation controls. Benefits persisted for several years after active therapy in many people (Nestoriuc et al. 2008a). And a randomized controlled pilot study in 25 people with migraine, 22 wait-list controls, found that use of a hand-held biofeedback device reduced headache intensity compared to controls ($p < 0.02$) (Odawara et al. 2015).

ELECTRODERMOGRAPHY

This type of biofeedback measures electrical conductance of the skin and can reflect levels of stress and anxiety. For example, when a person is experiencing stress, sweat gland activity may increase, which increases electrical conductivity. This is also called galvanic skin response—the same type of biofeedback typically used in lie detectors (Strofer et al. 2015).

Electrodermal biofeedback is being investigated as an aid in managing stress in crisis managers, professionals who are engaged in high-level decision making and coordination of personnel and resources in times of natural disaster, terror attacks, industrial disasters, and other similar events. It has also been used as a stress management tool by professionals such as pilots and athletes to reduce autonomic arousal. In a randomized study of 36 crisis managers, the treatment group received nine 45-minute electrodermal biofeedback training sessions over a 6-week period. Results showed a significant decrease in stress levels in the training group which persisted at 2-month follow-up (Janka et al. 2017).

Electrodermal biofeedback is also being explored as a tool in the anticipation and treatment of grand mal seizures, although specific mechanisms are not fully understood (Kotwas et al. 2015; Scrimali et al. 2015).

CLINICAL APPLICATION FOLLOW-UP: BIOFEEDBACK

After review of the current biofeedback data with her physician, Dr. Larson elected to begin EMG biofeedback sessions to learn to control her headaches. She enjoyed the challenge of understanding the physiology and applied a variety of relaxation tools to help her achieve her goals. She found breath work paired with a short faith-based phrase to be very effective in helping her trigger her relaxation response. Over time, she was able to recognize tension in its earliest stages and became adept at using her relaxation strategies to prevent progression to headache. She graphed her headache frequency on an Excel spreadsheet and found a consistent decrease over time. This correlated with a gradual decrease in systolic blood pressure, which she monitored at home on a daily basis. At 6-month follow-up, her systolic blood pressure had decreased by 10%, and she was beginning to wean one blood pressure medication. She was able to decrease biofeedback visits to monthly maintenance, with the goal of eliminating the need for them entirely, and was eventually able to wean off both antihypertensives, to her great satisfaction.

NEUROFEEDBACK

A comprehensive review by Sitaram et al. describes neurofeedback as "a psychophysiological procedure in which online feedback of neural activation is provided to the participant for the purpose of self-regulation." The field began when it was discovered that people could control their electroencephalogram (EEG) readings in real time and has progressed rapidly, aided by increasingly sophisticated measurement tools such as functional magnetic resonance imaging (fMRI) that show recruitment of functional networks integral to behavior, while providing real-time self-administered therapy (Sitaram et al. 2017).

Some of the practical applications of neurofeedback include application in paralyzed patients to learn how to coordinate movements of a robotic arm (Collinger et al. 2013) or a computer cursor (Hochberg et al. 2006) or to stimulate muscle movement able to address activities of daily living (Bouton et al. 2016).

Neurofeedback has also been studied in stroke rehabilitation, both with voluntary movement and with robotic or exoskeletal training. Once again, study heterogeneity precludes specific recommendations, although several studies show promising outcomes (Buch et al. 2008).

Neurofeedback has been shown to increase neuronal synchronization and boost visual attention to an object and to reduce mind-wandering and to improve musical performance (Sitaram et al. 2017).

Recent research has allowed imaging with portable EEG monitors and combines electro-physiological brain signals with monitoring of changes in brain blood oxygenation, called blood-oxygen-level-dependent (BOLD) activation. In some studies, authors describe trained participants who were able to downregulate EEG correlates of amygdala BOLD signals with resulting improvement in control of negative emotions (Zotev et al. 2014; Keynan et al. 2016).

Evaluating the potential of modulating neural networks rather than individual brain areas is an area of intense research in structural brain damage, for example stroke, and in neuropsychiatric disorders such as schizophrenia. This area of research uses functional connectivity and coherence as measurable markers. Connectivity-based neurofeedback is also being studied in harnessing *top-down* connectivity from areas in the prefrontal cortex to the amygdala to regulate emotional processing (Koush et al. 2017).

Neurofeedback-induced neuroplasticity is another area of active study and has been correlated with increases in white and gray brain matter volume—which have in turn been associated with significant improvements in visual and auditory attention in experimental subjects (Chein and Schneider 2005; Scholz et al. 2009).

Many questions remain about how neurofeedback learning determines performance, optimal length and type of training, and duration of neuroplastic change. Person-to-person variability in outcomes and varying learning capacity are also variables under study. Investigation of strategies in some studies seems to favor more successful learning when participants are in a state of focused relaxation rather than a *forced mastery* mode of learning—associated with the concepts of locus of control and sense of agency (Witte et al. 2013).

Research on the use of neurofeedback in attention deficit hyperactivity disorder (ADHD) originated from studies showing that children with ADHD and some other learning disabilities had high amplitudes of certain low-frequency EEG patterns compared to non-affected children—which were modifiable with medications in some children. Early work in neurofeedback determined that neurofeedback could address these low-amplitude frequencies and result in improvement in ADHD-related symptoms (Lubar and Lubar 1984; Chabot et al. 2001).

To date, meta-analyses of pediatric ADHD neurofeedback studies have highlighted study heterogeneity and treatment protocols, and specific guidelines for therapy type or duration do not yet exist (Sitaram et al. 2017).

Of interest, portable individual neurofeedback devices such as Muse are now commercially available.

PEDIATRIC BIOFEEDBACK RESEARCH OVERVIEW

Biofeedback has been studied in children since the late 1970s and has strong supporting evidence and a reassuring safety profile for a range of conditions. It is a commonly used mind–body modality in U.S. pediatric anesthesia programs, where a 2005 survey showed that 38 of 43 (83%) of programs surveyed offered biofeedback in their pain programs (Lin et al. 2005).

An overview of biofeedback in children in the 2016 American Academy of Pediatrics Clinical Report, Mind–Body Therapies in Children and Youth, shows that many children and adolescents are receptive to the use of biofeedback, and it has been used successfully in a variety of conditions, including (Section on Integrative Medicine 2016):

- Headache
- Asthma
- Enuresis
- Rehab applications
- Neurofeedback for ADHD
- Insomnia
- Chronic pain
- Anxiety
- Dysfunctional voiding and elimination

Conditions with supporting evidence in these age groups are discussed in the following sections.

Headache

EMG and thermal biofeedback have been used to help children mitigate and prevent recurrent symptoms of both migraine and tension-type headache (Andrasik and Schwartz 2006; Nestoriuc et al. 2008a; Faedda et al. 2016).

A 2016 meta-analysis of five studies including 137 pediatric patients with migraine found that biofeedback reduced migraine frequency (mean difference, −1.97 [95% confidence interval (CI), −2.72 to −1.21]; $P < .00001$), attack duration (mean difference, −3.94 [95% CI, −5.57 to −2.31]; $P < .00001$), and headache intensity (mean difference, −1.77 [95% CI, −2.42 to −1.11]; $P < .00001$) compared with a waiting-list control—although study variables and heterogeneity precluded definitive recommendations. No adverse events were reported in this meta-analysis (Parisi et al. 2011; Termine et al. 2011; Stubberud et al. 2016).

Asthma

Biofeedback has been explored in asthma due to the multifactorial etiologies (genetic, environmental, inflammatory, infectious, exercise, psychological factors) and has been shown to have some effectiveness in children with asthma (Lehrer et al. 2002).

In an early study by Peper and Tibbets (1992), biofeedback to help children release tension in neck and thorax muscles combined with a relaxed abdominal breathing technique resulted in increased inhalation volumes, reduction in asthma symptoms, reduced emergency room visits, and lower medication use.

Dysfunctional voiding

Often caused by vesicourethral reflux and recurrent urinary tract infections in children (Santos et al. 2017), biofeedback can be used to address symptoms of frequency, urgency, enuresis, and daytime incontinence by allowing the child to gain control of the pelvic floor and urethral sphincter (Tugtepe et al. 2015).

The optimal number of sessions and duration of biofeedback treatment are not known—a study by Sener et al. (2015) evaluated the efficacy of four sessions ($n = 20$) versus 6–10 sessions ($n = 20$) in school-aged children. Results showed that the shorter course of bio-feedback sessions was as effective as the longer ($p = 0.553$) with no adverse effects reported.

In younger children, the use of animated biofeedback using computer-animated characters has been used successfully in conjunction with pelvic floor retraining and dietary modification to address dysfunctional voiding and dysfunctional elimination syndrome (Kajbafzadeh et al. 2011).

Attention deficit hyperactivity disorder

EEG neurofeedback has proven to be a promising intervention in children with ADHD, as noted earlier. Unanswered questions about optimal number and type of sessions remain (Sitaram et al. 2017).

Children who received neurofeedback training in an in-school program sustained faster and more substantial gains in attention and behavior over a control group who received cognitive behavioral therapy in at-school sessions. Findings in the neurofeedback group were sustained 6 months following the 40-session treatment course (Steiner et al. 2014).

EEG neurofeedback is under study for other conditions such as seizures, symptoms of traumatic brain injury, chronic pain, autistic behaviors, headache, depression, anxiety, addictions, and sleep problems, although research is in relatively early stages in many of these areas, especially in children (Fovet et al. 2015). Brain–computer interface game applications for combined neurofeedback and biofeedback treatment for children on the autism spectrum are in active development (Friedrich et al. 2015).

CLINICAL APPLICATION: NEUROFEEDBACK IN PEDIATRICS

Seven-year-old Drew has been on psychostimulant medications for 2 years for a diagnosis of ADHD. His parents are concerned about the medication's long-term effects and are interested in exploring other options. Drew's schoolwork has improved on the medication, but he is not sleeping well and has lost weight, although linear growth has been maintained.

A full integrative intake history revealed that his diet consists of high-sugar, highly processed foods, and he spends an average of 4 hours on-screen time daily after school. He rarely exercises other than a brief recess after school lunch and has had trouble making friends this year. He takes no vitamins or dietary supplements. His parents estimate he is getting 6–7 hours of sleep a night and often has trouble winding down at night. His parents both work full time. Drew has one older sibling who is healthy.

In addition to a step-wise approach to lifestyle modification, including adjusting nutrition quality and meal timing, prioritizing organic foods when possible, and eliminating hidden caffeine, it was suggested that screen time be decreased and that enjoyable physical activity be introduced into Drew's daily activities—preferably with some supervised outdoor time.

Drew was also introduced to some animated game-based neurofeedback at the University Hospital. In the first session, he was not quite sure what to do, but when the clinician taught him some simple breathing exercises and he saw how that changed the characters on the screen as he relaxed, he understood and became more comfortable with the game.

Over the course of the next 4 months, Drew underwent 16 sessions of neurofeedback, gradually building his skill and learning several relaxation therapies during the sessions.

He found that the more he *tried*, the worse he did at the game, but when he let himself relax and get into the game, he did really well and felt better.

Drew's parents discovered that if the clinician used the EEG Biofeedback (Neurofeedback) code 90901 that several sessions would be covered by insurance, and they could also apply part of their flexible health savings account.

Drew's first ADHD medication was weaned slowly while he continued to attend weekly neurofeedback sessions. Parents and teachers gradually began to notice positive behavioral changes. Drew seemed more comfortable, his appetite improved, and he was falling asleep more easily. Over the summer, the pediatrician decided to wean his second medication. The dose was decreased gradually, and continued behavioral improvement was seen. The family continued to focus on improvement of his overall nutrition quality and together remained physically active. Overall, Drew had a very enjoyable summer and was medication free on entry to school in the fall. Plans were put in place for quarterly reassessments and maintenance neurofeedback sessions as needed.

BIOFEEDBACK CERTIFICATION

Biofeedback practitioners are not required by law to be certified in biofeedback, and most states do not restrict who can perform biofeedback services. Many state licensing boards do include the practice of biofeedback within the scope of practice of psychologists, physical therapists, nurses, physicians, occupational therapists, social workers, and others. It is important to note that having a professional license does not mean that the individual has any training in biofeedback.

The Association for Applied Psychophysiology and Biofeedback (AAPB) (Section on Integrative Medicine 2016) was founded in 1969 as the Biofeedback Research Society. It is an open membership non-profit organization dedicated to advancing development, dissemination, and utilization of biofeedback to improve health.

Regular membership requires:

• Persons engaged in the scientific and professional advancement of applied psychophysiology and biofeedback or related fields. Full members are required to hold an advanced degree, or the equivalent entry level degree, from an accredited school for the specific discipline in which the individual practices, does research, or teaches.
• Is a good resource for finding qualified biofeedback practitioners who have obtained board certification in biofeedback from organizations such as the Biofeedback Certification International Alliance (Andrasik and Schwartz 2006).

A statement on the Association for Applied Psychophysiology and Biofeedback website notes that the AAPB feels very strongly that anyone providing biofeedback-based services should meet at least the minimum standards of knowledge, training, and experience required to be certified by the Biofeedback Certification International Alliance (BCIA) (Andrasik and Schwartz 2006). If a provider is not so certified, they recommend due caution.

The Biofeedback Certification International Alliance is the recognized certification body for the clinical practice of biofeedback by the Association for Applied Psychophysiology and Biofeedback (AAPB), the Biofeedback Federation of Europe (BFE), and the International Society for Neurofeedback and Research (ISNR). Typically, practitioners must have a background in physiology and or psychology, an understanding of the mind–body connection, and proficiency in the use of biofeedback devices and technology.

RESOURCES

*   Biofeedback Certification International Alliance (Termine et al. 2011)
*   HeartMath LLC (Nestoriuc et al. 2008a)
*   Association for Applied Psychophysiology and Biofeedback (AAPB)
*   Biofeedback Certification International Alliance (BCIA)
*   International Society for Neurofeedback and Research (ISNR)
*   Biofeedback Foundation of Europe

References

1996. Heart rate variability: Standards of measurement, physiological interpretation and clinical use. Task Force of the European Society of Cardiology and the North American Society of Pacing and Electrophysiology. *Circulation* 93 (5): 1043–1065.

2011. Hypertension: The clinical management of primary hypertension in adults: Update of clinical guidelines 18 and 34, edited by National Clinical Guideline Centre (UK). London.

Andrasik, F. 2010. Biofeedback in headache: An overview of approaches and evidence. *Cleve Clin J Med* 77 (Suppl 3): S72–S76. doi:10.3949/ccjm.77.s3.13.

Andrasik, F., and M. S. Schwartz. 2006. Behavioral assessment and treatment of pediatric headache. *Behav Modif* 30 (1): 93–113. doi:10.1177/0145445505282164.

Bartlett, L. M., K. Sloots, M. Nowak, and Y. H. Ho. 2011. Biofeedback therapy for faecal incontinence: A rural and regional perspective. *Rural Remote Health* 11 (2): 1630.

Benson, H., J. A. Herd, W. H. Morse, and R. T. Kelleher. 1969. Behavioral induction of arterial hypertension and its reversal. *Am J Physiol* 217 (1): 30–34.

Benson, H., D. Shapiro, B. Tursky, and G. E. Schwartz. 1971. Decreased systolic blood pressure through operant conditioning techniques in patients with essential hypertension. *Science* 173 (3998): 740–742.

Berghmans, B., E. Hendriks, A. Bernards, R. de Bie, and M. I. Omar. 2013. Electrical stimulation with non-implanted electrodes for urinary incontinence in men. *Cochrane Database Syst Rev* (6): CD001202. doi:10.1002/14651858.CD001202.pub5.

Bouton, C. E., A. Shaikhouni, N. V. Annetta, M. A. Bockbrader, D. A. Friedenberg, D. M. Nielson, G. Sharma et al. 2016. Restoring cortical control of functional movement in a human with quadriplegia. *Nature* 533 (7602): 247–250. doi:10.1038/nature17435.

Buch, E., C. Weber, L. G. Cohen, C. Braun, M. A. Dimyan, T. Ard, J. Mellinger et al. 2008. Think to move: A neuromagnetic brain–computer interface (BCI) system for chronic stroke. *Stroke* 39 (3): 910–917. doi:10.1161/STROKEAHA.107.505313.

Chabot, R. J., F. di Michele, L. Prichep, and E. R. John. 2001. The clinical role of computerized EEG in the evaluation and treatment of learning and attention disorders in children and adolescents. *J Neuropsychiatry Clin Neurosci* 13 (2): 171–186. doi:10.1176/jnp.13.2.171.

Chein, J. M., and W. Schneider. 2005. Neuroimaging studies of practice-related change: fMRI and meta-analytic evidence of a domain-general control network for learning. *Brain Res Cogn Brain Res* 25 (3): 607–623. doi:10.1016/j.cogbrainres.2005.08.013.

Collinger, J. L., B. Wodlinger, J. E. Downey, W. Wang, E. C. Tyler-Kabara, D. J. Weber, A. J. McMorland, M. Velliste, M. L. Boninger, and A. B. Schwartz. 2013. High-performance neuroprosthetic control by an individual with tetraplegia. *Lancet* 381 (9866): 557–564. doi:10.1016/S0140-6736(12)61816-9.

Del Din, S., A. Bertoldo, Z. Sawacha, J. Jonsdottir, M. Rabuffetti, C. Cobelli, and M. Ferrarin. 2014. Assessment of biofeedback rehabilitation in post-stroke patients combining fMRI and gait analysis: A case study. *J Neuroeng Rehabil* 11: 53. doi:10.1186/1743-0003-11-53.

Dorey, G., M. Speakman, R. Feneley, A. Swinkels, C. Dunn, and P. Ewings. 2004. Randomised controlled trial of pelvic floor muscle exercises and manometric biofeedback for erectile dysfunction. *Br J Gen Pract* 54 (508): 819–825.

Dumoulin, C., E. J. Hay-Smith, and G. Mac Habee-Seguin. 2014. Pelvic floor muscle training versus no treatment, or inactive control treatments, for urinary incontinence in women. *Cochrane Database Syst Rev* (5): CD005654. doi:10.1002/14651858.CD005654.pub3.

Faedda, N., R. Cerutti, P. Verdecchia, D. Migliorini, M. Arruda, and V. Guidetti. 2016. Behavioral management of headache in children and adolescents. *J Headache Pain* 17 (1): 80. doi:10.1186/s10194-016-0671-4.

Fovet, T., R. Jardri, and D. Linden. 2015. Current issues in the use of fMRI-based neurofeedback to relieve psychiatric symptoms. *Curr Pharm Des* 21 (23): 3384–3394.

Friedrich, E. V., A. Sivanathan, T. Lim, N. Suttie, S. Louchart, S. Pillen, and J. A. Pineda. 2015. An effective neurofeedback intervention to improve social interactions in children with autism spectrum disorder. *J Autism Dev Disord* 45 (12): 4084–4100. doi:10.1007/s10803-015-2523-5.

Gholami Tahsini, Z., S. Makvand Hosseini, F. Kianersi, S. Rashn, and E. Majdara. 2017. Biofeedback-aided relaxation training helps emotional disturbances in undergraduate students before examination. *Appl Psychophysiol Biofeedback* 42 (4): 299–307. doi:10.1007/s10484-017-9375-z.

Glasgow, M. S., K. R. Gaarder, and B. T. Engel. 1982. Behavioral treatment of high blood pressure II. Acute and sustained effects of relaxation and systolic blood pressure biofeedback. *Psychosom Med* 44 (2): 155–170.

Hochberg, L. R., M. D. Serruya, G. M. Friehs, J. A. Mukand, M. Saleh, A. H. Caplan, A. Branner, D. Chen, R. D. Penn, and J. P. Donoghue. 2006. Neuronal ensemble control of prosthetic devices by a human with tetraplegia. *Nature* 442 (7099): 164–171. doi:10.1038/nature04970.

Hon, E. H., and S. T. Lee. 1963. Electronic evaluation of the fetal heart rate. Viii. Patterns preceding fetal death, further observations. *Am J Obstet Gynecol* 87: 814–826.

Janka, A., C. Adler, B. Brunner, S. Oppenrieder, and S. Duschek. 2017. Biofeedback training in crisis managers: A randomized controlled trial. *Appl Psychophysiol Biofeedback* 42 (2): 117–125. doi:10.1007/s10484-017-9360-6.

Kajbafzadeh, A. M., L. Sharifi-Rad, S. M. Ghahestani, H. Ahmadi, M. Kajbafzadeh, and A. H. Mahboubi. 2011. Animated biofeedback: An ideal treatment for children with dysfunctional elimination syndrome. *J Urol* 186 (6): 2379–2384. doi:10.1016/j.juro.2011.07.118.

Karavidas, M. K., P. S. Tsai, C. Yucha, A. McGrady, and P. M. Lehrer. 2006. Thermal biofeedback for primary Raynaud's phenomenon: A review of the literature. *Appl Psychophysiol Biofeedback* 31 (3): 203–216. doi:10.1007/s10484-006-9018-2.

Keppler, C., T. Rosburg, P. Lemoine, M. Pfluger, N. Gyr, and R. Mager. 2016. Functional somatic syndromes: Skin temperatures and activity measurements under ambulatory conditions. *Appl Psychophysiol Biofeedback* 41 (4): 363–373. doi:10.1007/s10484-016-9337-x.

Keynan, J. N., Y. Meir-Hasson, G. Gilam, A. Cohen, G. Jackont, S. Kinreich, L. Ikar et al. 2016. Limbic activity modulation guided by functional magnetic resonance imaging-inspired electroencephalography improves implicit emotion regulation. *Biol Psychiatry* 80 (6): 490–496. doi:10.1016/j.biopsych.2015.12.024.

Kim, J. H. 2017. The effects of training using EMG biofeedback on stroke patients upper extremity functions. *J Phys Ther Sci* 29 (6): 1085–1088. doi:10.1589/jpts.29.1085.

Kotwas, I., J. A. Micoulaud-Franchi, F. Bartolomei, and Y. Nagai. 2015. Commentary: Integrating electrodermal biofeedback into pharmacologic treatment of grand mal seizures. *Front Hum Neurosci* 9: 666. doi:10.3389/fnhum.2015.00666.

Koush, Y., D. E. Meskaldji, S. Pichon, G. Rey, S. W. Rieger, D. E. Linden, D. Van De Ville, P. Vuilleumier, and F. Scharnowski. 2017. Learning control over emotion networks through connectivity-based neurofeedback. *Cereb Cortex* 27 (2): 1193–1202. doi:10.1093/cercor/bhv311.

Kristt, D. A., and B. T. Engel. 1975. Learned control of blood pressure in patients with high blood pressure. *Circulation* 51 (2): 370–378.

Lehrer, P., J. Feldman, N. Giardino, H. S. Song, and K. Schmaling. 2002. Psychological aspects of asthma. *J Consult Clin Psychol* 70 (3): 691–711.

Lin, Y. C., A. C. Lee, K. J. Kemper, and C. B. Berde. 2005. Use of complementary and alternative medicine in pediatric pain management service: A survey. *Pain Med* 6 (6): 452–458. doi:10.1111/j.1526-4637.2005.00071.x.

Lubar, J. O., and J. F. Lubar. 1984. Electroencephalographic biofeedback of SMR and beta for treatment of attention deficit disorders in a clinical setting. *Biofeedback Self Regul* 9 (1): 1–23.

McGrady, A., P. A. Nadsady, and C. Schumann-Brzezinski. 1991. Sustained effects of biofeedback-assisted relaxation therapy in essential hypertension. *Biofeedback Self Regul* 16 (4): 399–411.

McGrady, A. V., R. Yonker, S. Y. Tan, T. H. Fine, and M. Woerner. 1981. The effect of biofeedback-assisted relaxation training on blood pressure and selected biochemical parameters in patients with essential hypertension. *Biofeedback Self Regul* 6 (3): 343–353.

Myrvik, M. P., A. D. Campbell, and J. L. Butcher. 2012. Single-session biofeedback-assisted relaxation training in children with sickle cell disease. *J Pediatr Hematol Oncol* 34 (5): 340–343. doi:10.1097/MPH.0b013e318253f0ba.

Nestoriuc, Y., A. Martin, W. Rief, and F. Andrasik. 2008a. Biofeedback treatment for headache disorders: A comprehensive efficacy review. *Appl Psychophysiol Biofeedback* 33 (3): 125–140. doi:10.1007/s10484-008-9060-3.

Nestoriuc, Y., W. Rief, and A. Martin. 2008b. Meta-analysis of biofeedback for tension-type headache: Efficacy, specificity, and treatment moderators. *J Consult Clin Psychol* 76 (3): 379–396. doi:10.1037/0022-006X.76.3.379.

Odawara, M., M. Hashizume, K. Yoshiuchi, and K. Tsuboi. 2015. Real-time assessment of the effect of biofeedback therapy with migraine: A pilot study. *Int J Behav Med* 22 (6): 748–754. doi:10.1007/s12529-015-9469-z.

Pager, C. K., M. J. Solomon, J. Rex, and R. A. Roberts. 2002. Long-term outcomes of pelvic floor exercise and biofeedback treatment for patients with fecal incontinence. *Dis Colon Rectum* 45 (8): 997–1003.

Parisi, P., L. Papetti, A. Spalice, F. Nicita, F. Ursitti, and M. P. Villa. 2011. Tension-type headache in paediatric age. *Acta Paediatr* 100 (4): 491–495. doi:10.1111/j.1651-2227.2010.02115.x.

Peper, E., and V. Tibbetts. 1992. Fifteen-month follow-up with asthmatics utilizing EMG/incentive inspirometer feedback. *Biofeedback Self Regul* 17 (2): 143–151.

Prota, C., C. M. Gomes, L. H. Ribeiro, J. de Bessa, Jr., E. Nakano, M. Dall'Oglio, H. Bruschini, and M. Srougi. 2012. Early postoperative pelvic-floor biofeedback improves erectile function in men undergoing radical prostatectomy: A prospective, randomized, controlled trial. *Int J Impot Res* 24 (5): 174–178. doi:10.1038/ijir.2012.11.

Qaseem, A., T. J. Wilt, R. M. McLean, M. A. Forciea, and Physicians Clinical Guidelines Committee of the American College of. 2017. Noninvasive treatments for acute, subacute, and chronic low back pain: A clinical practice guideline from the American College of Physicians. *Ann Intern Med* 166 (7): 514–530. doi:10.7326/M16-2367.

Rausa, M., D. Palomba, S. Cevoli, L. Lazzerini, E. Sancisi, P. Cortelli, and G. Pierangeli. 2016. Biofeedback in the prophylactic treatment of medication overuse headache: A pilot randomized controlled trial. *J Headache Pain* 17 (1): 87. doi:10.1186/s10194-016-0679-9.

Rayegani, S. M., S. A. Raeissadat, L. Sedighipour, I. M. Rezazadeh, M. H. Bahrami, D. Eliaspour, and S. Khosrawi. 2014. Effect of neurofeedback and electromyographic-biofeedback therapy on improving hand function in stroke patients. *Top Stroke Rehabil* 21 (2):137–151. doi:10.1310/tsr2102-137.

Santos, J. D., R. I. Lopes, and M. A. Koyle. 2017. Bladder and bowel dysfunction in children: An update on the diagnosis and treatment of a common, but underdiagnosed pediatric problem. *Can Urol Assoc J* 11 (1–2Suppl1): S64–S72. doi:10.5489/cuaj.4411.

Scharff, L., D. A. Marcus, and B. J. Masek. 2002. A controlled study of minimal-contact thermal biofeedback treatment in children with migraine. *J Pediatr Psychol* 27 (2): 109–119.

Schmitt, J. J., R. Singh, A. L. Weaver, K. C. Mara, R. R. Harvey-Springer, F. R. Fick, and J. A. Occhino. 2017. Prospective outcomes of a pelvic floor rehabilitation program including vaginal electrogalvanic stimulation for urinary, defecatory, and pelvic pain symptoms. *Female Pelvic Med Reconstr Surg* 23 (2): 108–113. doi:10.1097/SPV.0000000000000371.

Scholz, J., M. C. Klein, T. E. Behrens, and H. Johansen-Berg. 2009. Training induces changes in white-matter architecture. *Nat Neurosci* 12 (11): 1370–1371. doi:10.1038/nn.2412.

Scrimali, T., D. Tomasello, and M. Sciuto. 2015. Integrating electrodermal biofeedback into pharmacologic treatment of grand mal seizures. *Front Hum Neurosci* 9: 252. doi:10.3389/fnhum.2015.00252.

Section on Integrative Medicine. 2016. Mind-body therapies in children and youth. *Pediatrics* 138 (3): e2–e5. doi:10.1542/peds.2016-1896.

Sener, N. C., A. Altunkol, U. Unal, H. Ercil, O. Bas, K. Gumus, H. Ciftci, and E. Yeni. 2015. Can a four-session biofeedback regimen be used effectively for treating children with dysfunctional voiding? *Int Urol Nephrol* 47 (1): 5–9. doi:10.1007/s11255-014-0837-4.

Silberstein, S. D. 2000. Practice parameter: Evidence-based guidelines for migraine headache (an evidence-based review): Report of the Quality Standards Subcommittee of the American Academy of Neurology. *Neurology* 55 (6): 754–762.

Sitaram, R., T. Ros, L. Stoeckel, S. Haller, F. Scharnowski, J. Lewis-Peacock, N. Weiskopf et al. 2017. Closed-loop brain training: The science of neurofeedback. *Nat Rev Neurosci* 18 (2): 86–100. doi:10.1038/nrn.2016.164.

Steiner, N. J., E. C. Frenette, K. M. Rene, R. T. Brennan, and E. C. Perrin. 2014. In-school neurofeedback training for ADHD: Sustained improvements from a randomized control trial. *Pediatrics* 133 (3): 483–492. doi:10.1542/peds.2013-2059.

Strofer, S., M. L. Noordzij, E. G. Ufkes, and E. Giebels. 2015. Deceptive intentions: Can cues to deception be measured before a lie is even stated? *PLoS One* 10 (5): e0125237. doi:10.1371/journal.pone.0125237.

Stubberud, A., E. Varkey, D. C. McCrory, S. A. Pedersen, and M. Linde. 2016. Biofeedback as prophylaxis for pediatric migraine: A meta-analysis. *Pediatrics* 138 (2): 1–13. doi:10.1542/peds.2016-0675.

Termine, C., A. Ozge, F. Antonaci, S. Natriashvili, V. Guidetti, and C. Wober-Bingol. 2011. Overview of diagnosis and management of paediatric headache. Part II: Therapeutic management. *J Headache Pain* 12 (1): 25–34. doi:10.1007/s10194-010-0256-6.

Tugtepe, H., D. T. Thomas, R. Ergun, T. Abdullayev, C. Kastarli, A. Kaynak, and T. E. Dagli. 2015. Comparison of biofeedback therapy in children with treatment-refractory dysfunctional voiding and overactive bladder. *Urology* 85 (4): 900–904. doi:10.1016/j.urology.2014.12.031.

Vonthein, R., T. Heimerl, T. Schwandner, and A. Ziegler. 2013. Electrical stimulation and biofeedback for the treatment of fecal incontinence: A systematic review. *Int J Colorectal Dis* 28 (11): 1567–1577. doi:10.1007/s00384-013-1739-0.

Witte, M., S. E. Kober, M. Ninaus, C. Neuper, and G. Wood. 2013. Control beliefs can predict the ability to up-regulate sensorimotor rhythm during neurofeedback training. *Front Hum Neurosci* 7: 478. doi:10.3389/fnhum.2013.00478.

Zotev, V., R. Phillips, H. Yuan, M. Misaki, and J. Bodurka. 2014. Self-regulation of human brain activity using simultaneous real-time fMRI and EEG neurofeedback. *Neuroimage* 85 (3): 985–995. doi:10.1016/j.neuroimage.2013.04.126.

7   Hypnosis and guided imagery

INTRODUCTION: WHAT IS CLINICAL HYPNOSIS?

As defined by the American Society of Clinical Hypnosis (ASCH), hypnosis is a state of inner absorption, concentration, and focused attention, often referred to as a trance state. ASCH further defines hypnotic trance as focused consciousness that enables mind and body to accept and share intentions, beliefs, and expectations as true by magnifying the power and capacity of one's belief to cause the subconscious mind to accept and act upon them. It has been described as having three specific aspects: focused attention, dissociation from the usual state of awareness, and heightened responsiveness to suggestions (McBride et al. 2014).

The majority of medical hypnosis encounters involve elements of guided relaxation, information exchange, counseling, psychotherapy, and tapping into the placebo effect. Hypnosis may be incorporated into cognitive behavioral therapy and has become the focus of active research in medicine (Entwistle 2017).

HYPNOSIS AND NEURAL NETWORKS: EMERGING THEORIES

One of the great controversies in hypnosis is whether it can be considered an altered state of consciousness. Some studies suggest that hypnosis is associated with decreased default mode network activity, with high hypnotizability correlating with increased functional connectivity between the executive control network and the salience network, regions of the brain that determine which stimuli are most relevant. A 2016 study by Jiang et al. used functional MRI (fMRI) imaging to examine brain activity and functional connectivity between brain regions in 57 individuals tested and grouped based on high versus low hypnotizability using the Harvard Group Scale for Hypnotic Susceptibility. Participants underwent scanning in four states: resting, memory retrieval, and two different hypnotic experiences (Jiang et al. 2016).

During hypnosis in those in the high hypnotizability group only, reduced activity was seen in the dorsal anterior cingulate cortex and posterior cingulate cortex. The dorsal anterior cingulate cortex is a central node in the salience network and has been correlated with attentional control—differentiating what should we pay attention to and what can be ignored. The decrease in dorsal anterior cingulate activity was linearly correlated with the individual's feeling hypnotized while in the scanner, which indicates a selective reduction in activity in this region during hypnosis. This is consistent with a state of suspension of critical judgment and the ability to immerse oneself into a task. This state has also been associated with a will to persevere through challenges (Parvizi et al. 2013).

Jiang's study also showed that those with high hypnotizability had increased connectivity between bilateral dorsolateral prefrontal cortex and the ipsilateral insula during hypnosis as compared to low hypnotizable controls. Subjects with the highest levels of hypnotic trance showed the highest connectivity. One point of interest here is that the insula is involved in processing of body control and experience, emotion, empathy, and time through a wide range of connections to both cortical and limbic structures. The insula is also involved in spatial and temporal elements of pain processing, and empathic perception of pain in others. Authors note that the insular cortex is also involved in self-reflection, self-monitoring, and self-regulation (Jiang et al. 2016).

A further finding in highly hypnotizable subjects in the study showed uncoupling of connectivity between the executive control network and the default mode network during hypnosis, with the subjects reporting highest intensity of hypnosis showing the least coupling. Authors surmised that dissociation between the executive control network and the default mode network indicates that hypnosis is a different state of consciousness, not consistent with a decreased level of arousal. In addition, while the executive control network and default mode network were less connected, increases in other brain areas related to task management and somatic surveillance were seen in highly hypnotizable subjects (Jiang et al. 2016). Research is very active in this area, and many questions remain. A 2017 systematic review of the neuroimaging literature on hypnosis by Landry et al. (2017) concludes that studies still show substantial inconsistency and consensus has not yet been reached on the exact neural mechanisms involved in hypnosis. The high variability in hypnotic induction and treatments and lack of standardized methodological approaches are associated with heterogeneity of study results to date.

BRIEF HISTORICAL BACKGROUND

Reviews by Entwistle and Kauders offer background into the origins of hypnosis, which can be traced back at least as far as the use of hypnotic suggestion in the Asklepian sleep healing temples in approximately 1300 B.C. In the 1800s Franz Mesmer, an Austrian physician, promoted the theory that magnetism existed around each person and that interacting with magnets could produce a healing response, a theory met with understandable skepticism in the medical field. In the 1840s, James Braid and James Esdaile, British surgeons, concluded that rather than exposure to the magnets, Mesmer's results were likely in response to the suggestions offered. The field was renamed hypnosis by Braid and became the focus of active study with a focus on attention and distraction of patients rather than *magnetism*. Eventually, it became more widely accepted that the trance state was in the patient's control, rather than something that was being done to them, and the field gradually gained wider acceptance (Entwistle 2017; Kauders 2017).

In 1949, the Society for Clinical and Experimental Hypnosis was founded and began publication of the *International Journal of Clinical and Experimental Hypnosis*. The ASCH was founded by psychiatrist Milton Erickson in 1957, with membership initially limited to physicians. It remains the only recognized professional accreditation that is based on successful completion of a very rigorous standard of training and testing.

WHAT STEPS ARE INVOLVED IN HYPNOSIS THERAPY?

There are six classic stages to a hypnosis session: introduction, induction, deepening, therapeutic suggestions, awakening, and debriefing, although each session is unique to the individual patient. While in the trance state of inner absorption, the individual is offered guided hypnotic suggestions via words, visualizations, and imagery. The goal is to have the individual's mind to accept and act on the idea as true and real. Self-hypnosis, where individuals learn to access the trance state independently using simple physical triggers such as a breath or a finger tap, has been shown to be very effective in adults and in children at even very young ages. Self-hypnosis is often taught to patients in the first session so they can begin to practice at home (Kohen et al. 1984).

INCORPORATING HYPNOSIS INTO CLINICAL PRACTICE

Introducing hypnosis into the clinical setting requires the basic elements of time, appropriately trained specialists, and (ideally) a quiet consult room, although with children, hypnosis has been administered in playrooms, emergency rooms, and radiology suites successfully (Pendergrast 2017). Hypnosis sessions in a clinic or office setting are often recorded by the clinician for future use by the patient (Entwistle 2017).

Traditionally, hypnosis has been used to address a wide variety of physical and mental conditions and symptoms such as pain or anxiety, but more recent perspectives from leaders in the field, Alter and Sugarman (2017), suggest that hypnosis has a unique and important place in modern health care based on the premise that one's health is ultimately based on the condition of constant adaptive self-regulating systems, and as such hypnosis can be very effective in helping individuals adapt to change and modify behavior to best serve their desired health outcomes. They propose that adaptation of hypnosis training to best serve this approach may be needed, with more focus on the individual and their ability to effect the changes they need and want and adoption of a less prescriptive approach than traditionally taught. The authors propose reorienting hypnosis training around six principles to better meet individuals' needs in modern health care:

- Rather than rely on formulaic approaches expecting *hypnotic phenomena* (for e.g., use of prescriptive inductions and therapeutic suggestions), the focus in beginner and intermediate training should be on adjustment and adaptation strategies that will help people be more effective when facing external and internal stressors.
- Exposure to novelty and uncertainty in life activates a trance-like state (*disorientation and reorientation*), and so it should be more widely recognized that trance, especially in the health care setting, always starts before the clinical encounter. An example is a conscious patient in the emergency room. These individuals are almost universally in a state of mental disorientation, sometimes recognized as *trauma trance*, on arrival and therefore in a potentially very receptive state to suggestions of calming, pain control, and stabilization of some physiologic functions, for example, respiratory rate.
- The individual's inner resources exist as potentials which can be effectively activated by the use of hypnosis in the clinical setting. The authors equate the human potential for change with neuroplasticity, now widely recognized as an inherent part of neurophysiology.
- To be most effective, the clinician should be highly tuned into the presenting behavioral cues demonstrated by the patient—which typically reflect their

approach to adaptive and effective solutions and can act as guide posts for the clinician who is paying close attention.

- This encourages curiosity on the part of the clinician, rather than a focus on diagnostic labels, and can give clues about approaches that may or may not have been effective for the patient to date.
- In effect, they advocate for a paradigm shift from a "what should be done" approach to a "what can emerge" approach that honors and encourages viewing the patient (individual) as a person with expansive capacity for self-reorganization and self-expression—and by corollary in the health care setting the ability to handle challenges and modify behaviors successfully to enhance health (Alter and Sugarman 2017).

CAUTIONS AND CAVEATS

Historically, hypnosis has been viewed with skepticism or portrayed as a way to manipulate vulnerable patients. This comes in part from a history of the use of hypnosis as a *stage show* and not from its use in the clinical setting. It is important to reinforce that the individual always remains in control and under their own control. The patient is the one *doing the hypnosis*. It is the work of the patient's unconscious mind that determines the content and direction of any given hypnosis session (Reid 2016).

Cautions include early referral to or consultation with a mental health specialist for any child or adult with a history of abuse or pre-existing mental illness or history of a conversion reaction to avoid unintended triggering of old symptoms or precipitation of new problems. Response to hypnosis can be variable and can be situational, practitioner related, or part of a person's genetic *wiring*. Assessments of hypnotizability remain a source of discussion and debate, which has contributed to variability in research results. One of the challenging elements of hypnosis is its lack of controllability in terms of the patient's inner experience. For example, some patients will move in and out of trance even during the length of one session regardless of whether specific scripts or planned approaches are used.

Informed consent is obtained prior to any hypnosis, similar to psychotherapy. Agreements are made that assure confidentiality except in cases of immediate harm to self or others or other high-level threat.

OVERVIEW OF ADULT HYPNOSIS RESEARCH

A 2017 review by Entwistle on the use of hypnosis in the clinical setting points to its successful use in several areas, including acute and chronic pain, asthma, insomnia, irritable bowel syndrome (IBS), and weight management. Additional studies support its use in the peri-operative setting and in the management of dental anxiety. In the mental health arena, studies have supported the use of hypnosis in depression, attention deficit disorder, anorexia, anxiety, and post-traumatic stress disorder (Entwistle 2017).

Pain

A review by Jensen exploring the use of hypnosis in chronic pain reinforces findings that pain is not centralized in the brain or nervous system, but fMRI and positron emission tomography (PET) scans show that pain is associated with activity in a range of areas, including the prefrontal cortex, thalamus, and anterior cingulate cortex and others. Hypnosis has also been associated with increased alpha brain activity in those experiencing relief of pain. Imaging studies on the impact of hypnosis for pain management have shown that various areas of the brain involved in pain processing respond to hypnosis. Pain intensity, quality, degree of unpleasantness, sense of comfort, and the ability to screen out unpleasant sensations and allow in comfortable sensations have each been shown to be modifiable with hypnosis. In addition to pain reduction, hypnosis was shown to be associated with improved sleep, greater overall well-being, and a greater sense of control in many patients (Jensen and Patterson 2014).

A review of the use of clinical hypnosis for reducing labor and delivery pain included 13 studies and 5,914 women found that the use of clinician or partner directed hypnosis or self-hypnosis was found to be consistently more effective than standard medical care, supportive counseling, and childbirth education classes in reducing pain. Infants in the maternal hypnosis groups also had improved Apgar scores and shorter Stage 1 labor. Authors conclude further randomized controlled trials and standardization of therapeutic approaches are needed (Landolt and Milling 2011).

A later randomized controlled trial examining the use of self-hypnosis for pain relief during labor and delivery included 343 women who received either two antenatal self-hypnosis training sessions or supportive CD for home use each day from 32-weeks gestation until delivery. Women in the self-hypnosis group who were interviewed found self-hypnosis to organize into several themes, including calmness, confidence, focused relaxation, and empowerment (Finlayson et al. 2015).

A 2016 Cochrane Database Systematic review including nine trials randomizing 2,954 women undergoing labor and childbirth found study variability too high to make definitive recommendations and reiterated the need for larger, controlled randomized trials (Madden et al. 2016).

A review by Potié et al. (2016) examining the benefit of hypnosis in patients undergoing breast cancer surgery showed a positive impact on distress and post-operative pain.

And a systematic review of randomized controlled trials in women undergoing breast cancer treatment and those in survivorship, (and three studies of women not in breast cancer treatment but experiencing hot flashes) showed benefit in a variety of symptoms, although study size and design variability impacted results. The review included 13 randomized controlled trials and 1,357 women. In women undergoing diagnostic breast biopsy, hypnosis had a positive effect on pain and distress. One trial on women undergoing surgery found benefits for hypnosis related to pain, distress, fatigue, and nausea. In women undergoing radiation therapy, hypnosis combined with cognitive behavioral therapy improved fatigue and distress. And three studies in women with metastatic breast cancer also showed benefit on pain and distress. Overall safety was excellent with no adverse events reported. Interventions varied across studies. Seven of the studies used only one hypnosis session; the studies on hot flashes used a once-weekly session lasting 50–60 minutes. Two studies in the metastatic cancer group combined hypnosis or self-hypnosis with support groups, and the third study in this group used self-hypnosis over a period of 4 weeks (Cramer et al. 2015).

Insomnia

Hypnosis has also been shown to be an effective tool in addressing insomnia, in part because preparing for sleep is enhanced by relaxation, increased suggestibility, and post-hypnotic suggestion (sleep deeper), and imagery rehearsal (allow yourself to let go and drift into welcome, restorative sleep), which has been correlated with increase in recorded slow-wave sleep in a study of 70 college-aged women where listening to an auditory text with hypnotic suggestions versus a control tape led to an 81% increase in slow-wave sleep in a midday nap in those rating high on the Harvard Group Scale of Hypnotic Suggestibility (Cordi et al. 2014).

Other components of hypnosis in sleep include access to preconscious cognitions and emotions that can be helpful in addressing somnambulism (sleepwalking) and pavor nocturnus (sleep terrors) in both adults and children (Becker 2015).

A study by Hurwitz et al. in 27 sleepwalking adult patients found that 74% experienced much or very much improvement after training in self-hypnosis which they practiced in the home setting. The range of clinic visits required was one to six, with a mean of only 1.6 visits to achieve symptom improvement or resolution (Hurwitz et al. 1991).

Hypnosis has also been used in the treatment of parasomnias, for example, a study of 36 patients, four children, mean age 32.7 years with parasomnias found that at 1-month follow-up 45.4% were symptom free or significantly improved after 1–2 hypnotherapy sessions with a trained practitioner. Nearly half (42.2%) had sustained improvement at 18-month follow-up, and 40.5% remained symptom free at 5-year follow-up (Hauri et al. 2007).

CLINICAL APPLICATION: ADULT HYPNOSIS

June is an 80 year old generally healthy and active retired school teacher scheduled for knee replacement surgery in 6 weeks. She is undergoing the surgery in order to maintain the ability to play golf, a significant social activity for her in her active retirement community. She has a history of a bad experience (extreme nausea, vomiting, frightening dream/nightmare) emerging from anesthesia during a Caesarean section when she had her last child years ago and is hoping to avoid a similar experience with this surgery. She is also experiencing pre-procedural anxiety which is building by the day. She is interested in exploring the use of clinical hypnosis and has received clearance from her surgical and anesthesia team to use a CD and earphones in pre-operative preparation, during surgery, and in the recovery room.

The initial approach is to review the basics of hypnosis and invite June to identify a mental image or scenario that signifies a safe and relaxing space to her. Using a simple technique involving use of a deep breath and systematic tensing and relaxing of her muscles starting at the feet, she is able to transition into a light trance state which can be identified by seeing her shoulder muscles relax, her breathing slow and deepen, and by smoothing of the lines on her forehead. June is then invited to bring to mind her safe and relaxing space and to add anything that would make it even more inviting and safe for her. She is in full control of what enters or leaves the space and takes some time to mentally enhance every aspect, for example, light, sound, sensations, temperature, people or animal companions, and so on until it is optimized.

The trance state is deepened by inviting her to sink deeper into relaxation with each outbreath, and she is then invited to visualize herself preparing in a very relaxed and focused manner for her surgery. She is invited to visualize herself in the pre-operative suite extending her sense of calm and centering to the entire medical team. She then visualizes herself during the actual surgery with vital signs strong and steady, allowing her body to experience the surgery with minimal discomfort and scant blood loss, facilitating the success of the surgery in partnership with her medical team. She visualizes the completion of the surgery and sees herself moving very comfortably into the post-operative recovery area, always surrounded by her expert team. She is invited to add feelings, sensations, and words that will cue her body to comfortably and effortlessly move into gradual awakening in the post-operative period with no excess pain or distress. She sees herself surrounded by support and uses the sensations and memory of her safe space to remain relaxed and confident as she moves into a fully awake state, surgery successfully completed. A recording is made of the session, which June listens to daily in the lead up to the procedure as she practices self-hypnosis. In a follow-up visit before surgery, June reports a growing sense of ease about the procedure and growing confidence in her ability to use self-hypnosis.

In fact, June's surgery went very well, and she was moved onto the surgical post-operative floor without incident where she required only minimal oral medication (acetaminophen) post-operatively. She was ambulatory by the same afternoon and became a minor sensation on the ward due to her rapid recovery.

HYPNOSIS IN PEDIATRICS

Clinical hypnosis has strong support for a variety of medical conditions in children. An excellent overview of the use of hypnosis in pediatrics can be found in a classic article by Karen Olness, MD, a widely recognized pioneer in the field (Olness and Gardner 1978).

Children as young as 2–3 years old have been taught hypnosis and self-hypnosis, which in children very commonly incorporates rich visual and sensory imagery and is facilitated by their ability to slip almost spontaneously into fantasy, make believe, and role playing—often while maintaining eyes open and remaining engaged in play activity while the session unfolds. Incorporating hypnosis into pediatric clinical encounters can be facilitated by being observant to the periods of natural trance, when a child might be more amenable to positive suggestions and can benefit from reinforcement and acknowledgment of their powerful inner resources.

Hypnosis has important utility in helping to address underlying psychological issues, such as school or home stressors, or prior events that may be driving current symptoms. Hypnosis has the ability to reinforce a child or adolescent's capacity for self-regulation and help them to learn to control attentional focus and responses related to their emotions, behaviors, and physiologic measures. These strengths are ideally fostered by parents or caretakers that support the child's developing independence and mastery of typical age-appropriate stressors, incrementally increasing their internal locus of control (Kaiser 2011).

A 2005 a survey of 43 pediatric anesthesia fellowship programs in the United States showed that 44% of the 38 responding programs offered hypnosis for treatment of pain (Lin et al. 2005).

Advances in pediatric training have continued through refinement of the curriculum delivered in the National Pediatric Hypnosis Training Institute curriculum which includes direct teaching by expert faculty, clinical training videos, individualized learning, and emphasis on personalized goal-oriented sessions with a focus on developmental and self-regulation strategies. Faculty development is an integral part of the training (Kohen et al. 2017).

CAVEATS AND CAUTIONS

As mentioned, one of the surprising things about hypnosis in children is that they may continue to play or engage in a creative activity such as drawing while undergoing hypnosis as opposed to adults who may appear extremely drowsy. In fact, children often demonstrate spontaneous trance during play or while reading—or while avoiding a difficult or painful situation.

Cautions regarding the use of hypnosis in children, as with other mind–body therapies—include referral or consultation with a mental health specialist for any child with a history of abuse or pre-existing mental illness and the use of only fully trained practitioners. Any hypnosis must be directed and delivered at the appropriate developmental level to meet the child's needs.

Hypnosis should not be offered as a substitute for a directly treatable illness, for example, an acute infection such as pneumonia or a serious toothache (Pendergrast 2017).

PEDIATRIC RESEARCH OVERVIEW

Kohen et al. (1984) reported on 505 hypnotic interventions in children as young as 3 years old with a variety of conditions, including: enuresis, pain, asthma, habit disorders such as cough or tic, encopresis, and anxiety. In this group of patients, a reported 51% had complete resolution of symptoms, typically after four or fewer visits.

A 2014 review by Kohen and Kaiser confirms research support for hypnosis in the pediatric population, especially in acute and chronic pain, physical and mental discomfort around cancer treatment, self-regulation skills in a variety of medical settings, and as an adjunct treatment in psychotherapy in pediatric obesity interventions (Kohen and Kaiser 2014).

For example, self-hypnosis was found to be highly effective in the treatment of insomnia based on chart review of 84 children (mean age 12 years range 7–17). The majority of children, 68%, required two or fewer sessions to reduce time of sleep onset. Of the 70 children reporting a sleep delay of more than 30 minutes, 90% of those reported reductions in sleep onset following hypnosis. A significant majority, 87% of children, reported improvement or resolution of somatic complaints, such as functional abdominal pain, headache, and habit cough, following hypnosis (Anbar and Slothower 2006).

Hypnosis has also been used successfully for enuresis (bedwetting). For example, in a controlled study of 50 children aged 5–16 years children were randomized to 3 months of imipramine ($n = 25$) or hypnosis ($n = 25$). Patients in the hypnosis group received training then were encouraged to use self-hypnosis in the home setting daily. Children in the imipramine group had 72% positive symptom resolution at 6-month follow-up as compared to 72% in the hypnosis group. In comparison at the 9-month follow-up, 24% in the imipramine group had full symptom resolution versus 68% of those treated with hypnosis (Banerjee et al. 1993).

A review by Brown showed a range of respiratory conditions, including asthma, as receptive to clinical hypnosis in both children and adults (Brown 2007).

Improvements were seen in symptom frequency and severity, improvement in forced expiratory volume, reduction in inflammatory markers, reduced medication use, and reduced fear and anxiety during acute attacks.

Hypnosis has been shown to help with other respiratory conditions such as cystic fibrosis, habit cough, and vocal cord dysfunction, via both physical and psychological approaches. One of the most important approaches in this patient population is a focus on relaxation through hypnosis, often with the addition of relaxing imagery (McBride et al. 2014).

In a study by Anbar and Hall (2004), 56 pediatric patients (mean age 10.7 years) treated with hypnosis for longstanding habit cough, it was shown that 78% had full resolution of cough during or immediately after their first hypnosis training session, and an additional 12% had resolution by one month after the first session of hypnosis therapy.

Hypnosis has been shown to be effective in both acute and chronic pediatric pain. A review of randomized controlled trials by Accardi showed that hypnosis was effective in reducing pain experienced by children undergoing painful invasive medical procedures such as bone marrow aspirations, lumbar punctures, voiding cystourethrograms, and post-surgical pain (Silove et al. 1997).

Pediatric procedural pain and anxiety

One hour of instruction in self-hypnosis was shown to be highly effective for procedural pain and stress in a randomized controlled trial of 44 children undergoing voiding cysto-urethrography (VCUG) for dysfunctional voiding. In the prospective randomized study, 44 children aged 4–15 years ($n = 21$ hypnosis group) were assigned to a 1-hour training session in self-hypnotic visual imagery by a trained therapist the day before the scheduled procedure. They were instructed to practice at home several times before the procedure. The therapist was present during the procedure to conduct similar exercises with the child. Results indicated significant benefits to the hypnosis group. Parents reported the procedure to be significantly less traumatic for their child as compared to prior VCUG, observational assessments by staff reported significantly less distress than controls, medical staff also reported significantly less difficulty in completing the procedure in the hypnosis group, and procedure time was shortened by 14 minutes for hypnosis versus control group (Butler et al. 2005).

The use of home-based hypnosis self-therapy in pediatric functional abdominal pain was shown to be effective compared to individually delivered hypnotherapy by a trained therapist in a randomized controlled trial of 260 children aged 8–18 years. Home CD self-hypnosis was used by 132 children 5 days per week or more for 3 months. Individualized therapy was done in six 50–60-minute sessions over 3 months. The CD used standardized scripts that were exactly the same as the exercises delivered in the individual sessions.

Directly after treatment, 36.8% of children in the CD group and 50.1% of children in the individualized therapy group were successfully treated. Results were maintained at 12-month follow-up for 62.1% in the CD group and 71% in the individualized group, (difference, −8.9%; 90% CI, −18.9% to 0.7%; $P = 0.002$). Authors concluded that use of clinical hypnosis in a self-directed home CD format provides a viable option for treatment of functional abdominal pain in children and adolescents (Rutten et al. 2017).

Clinical application: Pediatric hypnosis

Koa is an 8-year-old boy with a history of long-standing enuresis. He has never experienced more than 2–3 dry nights in a row. There is a family history of enuresis in the father into his early adolescence. Koa has had a full workup to rule out any contributing medical or psychologic condition related to enuresis. No abnormality was found. He has tried a fluid-sensing bed alarm and a brief trial of medication without success. He did not like the side effects of the medication. Koa wants to attend a summer camp with friends but is too embarrassed to go while he continues to require pull ups at night. They are interested in non-pharmacologic options, and Koa is highly motivated to succeed.

An initial discussion in a child with enuresis would typically include an age and developmentally appropriate discussion of the anatomy involved in urination with a brief description of the kidneys, ureters, uretovesical (ureter–bladder) junction, bladder, and urethral sphincter. This often involves a simple drawing to demonstrate how the kidneys drain urine into the holding container for the urine (bladder) and shows the control valve (urethral sphincter) that allows urine to drain out of the bladder. The clinician can then invite the child to imagine how they might arrange a signal from their bladder to wake them up at night if they need to urinate. The child will also typically develop ideas with the clinician about how to turn off the valve (urethral sphincter) at night so no fluid passes through until morning awakening.

Koa viewed a drawing and model of the kidneys and bladder and expressed understanding about how the system worked. He then agreed to learn about hypnosis and learn self-hypnosis. The session started with a brief relaxation exercise that included relaxing imagery and some simple progressive muscle relaxation. Koa was then invited to relax even more deeply and bring to mind an image of his own bladder and valve. During hypnosis, he developed the plan that if his bladder was so full it had to be emptied while he was asleep, it would send an instant message to his brain that would wake him up so he could go to the restroom. To help the urine stay safely in his bladder until he woke up, (or ideally hold until morning), he imagined himself using a tiny screwdriver to tighten the valve (urethral sphincter) so no fluid would leak out until he let it out.

While learning self-hypnosis, Koa practiced a simple physical trigger that would help him remember to go back into a deeply relaxed state whenever needed. He made a circle with his right thumb and first finger, pushing his fingers together, then on cue with the breath released the tension in his fingers, dropping easily into trance.

In this relaxed state, he could check on bladder and the valve to the outside (urethral sphincter). Koa practiced moving into and out of trance in the session and quickly mastered the technique of self-hypnosis. The clinician recorded the session for Koa's home use and encouraged him to practice every day before bed. Koa was given a simple diary and stickers to track dry nights, planting further expectations for success.

Koa practiced the self-hypnosis nightly and in a 4-week follow-up visit reported only five wet nights. Further discussion found that these nights were often associated with a later dinner and less careful attention to fluid intake in the evening. A brief reinforcing session for the self-hypnosis was done and a second diary with stickers given. At the next month follow-up, Koa reported no wet nights. He continued to practice self-hypnosis nightly and was able to attend summer camp 4 months later. Although he took pull ups with him to use if needed, he maintained success and had no further wet nights. This had a significant impact on his overall confidence and self-esteem, especially at school.

TRAINING AND CERTIFICATION

In the United States, ASCH currently offers a formal certification process for professionals in medicine, psychology, dentistry, social work, and nursing:

- American Society of Clinical Hypnosis: http://www.asch.net/
- The National Pediatric Hypnosis Training Institute offers ASCH certified pediatric specialization: http://www.nphti.org/

RESOURCES

- American Society of Clinical Hypnosis: http://www.asch.net/
- Society for Clinical and Experimental Hypnosis: http://www.sceh.us/
- American Journal of Clinical Hypnosis: http://www.asch.net/Public/American JournalofClinicalHypnosis.aspx
- International Journal of Clinical and Experimental Hypnosis: http://www.ijceh.com/

PEDIATRIC RESOURCES

- National Pediatric Hypnosis Training Institute: http://www.nphti.org/
- *Hypnosis and Hypnotherapy with Children* by Karen Olness and Daniel Kohen, 1996, Guilford Press, New York, NY
- *Harry the Hypnopotomous: Metaphorical Tales for the Treatment of Children* by Linda Thompson, 2005, Crown House Publishing, Wales, UK

GUIDED IMAGERY

The use of imagery can be found in healing as part of many cultures and religions across history. It has been described as a process of deliberately using the imagination to help the mind and body heal, stay well, or perform well. The use of imagery came into use in the medical arena in the United States in the 1970s, primarily in work with oncology and burn patients (Naparstek 1994).

An important point regarding the successful use of guided imagery is that the name can be quite misleading. In fact, effective imagery draws on all the senses, sight, sound, smell, taste, and touch. This is important, because a substantial portion of people are not primarily visual and need a multidimensional sensory approach to have a successful experience with guided imagery.

Guided imagery has been compared to a directed sort of daydream which taps into the power of imagination to promote healing. It is often paired with music to reinforce a multi-sensory experience. There is an obvious overlap of imagery and clinical hypnosis, especially in children where the use of imagery in hypnosis is prevalent. Overlap with other mind–body therapies such as progressive muscle relaxation and meditation or mindfulness is also common.

The idea in imagery is that, in the body, sensory images are experienced almost like actual events.

Combining this with deep relaxation and being in essentially a trance state (relaxed receptivity similar to the hypnotic trance) allows learning and change on a very deep level, and this combined with a strong sense of internal control provides individuals the needed components to make significant progress in a wide variety of areas, including physical and mental health.

STRENGTHS OF GUIDED IMAGERY

- Portable
- Flexible
- Affordable
- Effective when delivered by audio recording
- Immediately available whenever skills are called upon

GUIDELINES FOR SUCCESS USING GUIDED IMAGERY

Ideally listen to the same imagery daily for 2–3 weeks. Waking and just before sleep are times when people may be especially receptive. People can use hand positioning during the time listening to imagery to help the trigger the feelings and helpful sensations of guided imagery when they are not actually listening to it. Falling asleep during guided imagery does not detract from the benefit. In general, guided imagery has been shown to have a cumulative effect (Naparstek 1994).

CONTRAINDICATIONS

- Trauma survivors
- PTSD
- Abuse
- Serious mental health diagnosis

ADULT RESEARCH OVERVIEW

An early randomized study examining the use of guided imagery in 130 patients undergoing elective colorectal surgery showed that those in the treatment group ($n = 65$), who listened to guided imagery tapes for 3 days before surgery, during induction of anesthesia, intraoperatively, in recovery, and for 6 days after surgery experienced significantly less pre- and post-operative anxiety and pain, and required nearly 50% less narcotic medications post-operatively than controls. Additional findings in the study were an increase in sense of self-worth, comfort, solace, and hope—intangible factors that are critical to the healing process (Rutten et al. 2017).

Another early study on the use of guided imagery showed more rapid wound healing in 24 surgical patients undergoing cholecystectomy who were randomized to an audiotape, entitled "Relaxation with Guided Imagery," or a quiet period and underwent measurements of state anxiety, urinary cortisol levels, and wound inflammatory response. Results showed that the guided imagery group showed significantly less state anxiety and lower cortisol levels 1 day following surgery and less surgical wound erythema than the control group (Holden-Lund 1988).

A later study on the use of guided imagery in wound healing randomized 60 patients to receive either standard care or standard care with a 45-minute intervention that included relaxation and guided imagery directed at preparation for surgery with additional CDs for home use 3 days prior to surgery and 7 days after surgery focused on healing after surgery. Patients were evaluated for perceived stress and speed of wound healing. Patients in the intervention group had more significant progress in wound healing ($p = 0.03$) and reduced perceived stress ($p = 0.048$). Those in the intervention group who listened to the CD more frequently reported greater stress reduction ($p = 0.026$). In this study, reductions in perceived stress were not directly correlated to wound healing (Broadbent et al. 2012).

A blinded, randomized, placebo controlled pilot study on the use of guided imagery in 58 adults ($n = 29$ guided imagery group) undergoing total knee replacement showed that those in the imagery group had significantly improved gait velocity and lower pain scores at 3 weeks post-surgery compared to controls and significantly lowered hair cortisol concentration at 6 months post-surgery compared to control (Jacobson et al. 2016).

Guided imagery has been studied in adults with arthritis and other rheumatic diseases. A systematic review of randomized controlled trials included seven studies and 287 participants who completed the interventions. All of the interventions were recorded guided imagery scripts and were delivered in time frames ranging from a one-time exposure up to 16 weeks. Impact of imagery on pain, function, anxiety, depression, and quality of life were measured. All studies reported statistically significant improvements in the observed outcomes. Authors call for further well-designed, randomized controlled trials to inform definitive treatment guidelines (Giacobbi et al. 2015).

Guided imagery has also been used in the treatment of symptoms of IBS on the basis that visceral pain sensation experienced in IBS is heightened by emotional stress. In a study in 34 adults ($n = 15$ treatment group) received eight 3-hour, individualized sessions once weekly with a board-certified therapist experienced in gut-directed psychotherapy with *homework* between sessions. Patients in the treatment group experienced significant improvement in symptom severity as compare dot controls ($p = 0.04$) and significant improvement in IBS quality of life score ($p < 0.01$) compared to control group (Boltin et al. 2015).

PEDIATRIC RESEARCH OVERVIEW

Positive effects of guided imagery have been reported in a number of pediatric conditions, including a randomized lifestyle intervention pilot study designed to support weight loss in 35 overweight Latino adolescents. Use of the scripted Interactive Guided Imagery recordings over the course of the 12-week program in the treatment group was associated with reduction in sedentary behavior ($p < 0.05$), and increase in physical activity ($p < 0.05$). Significant reductions in salivary cortisol were recorded during the time span of the 45-minute recording ($p < 0.01$), which was independently associated with improved insulin sensitivity ($p = 0.03$) (Weigensberg et al. 2014).

Guided imagery was also shown to be effective in small studies in patients with sickle cell disease (Dobson and Byrne 2014), asthma (Section on Integrative Medicine 2016), and during venipuncture (Forsner et al. 2014).

Another successful use of guided imagery in children has been reported in patients with functional abdominal pain, which is estimated to effect up to 19% of children and is one of the most common types of chronic pain. The functional gut disorders lend themselves to mind–body therapies due to their multifactorial etiologies, including hypersensitivity of the intestines to pain stimuli, hyperactive gut wall smooth muscle, and dysfunctions in processing brain–gut communications, and susceptibility to amplification by stress and depression. A review by Palsson and van Tilburg (2015) highlights the efficacy of scripted protocols which have been developed at the University of North Carolina for both gut-directed hypnosis and for functional abdominal pain in children. Sessions are typically delivered in seven sessions approximately once every 2 weeks in 30–40-minute increments for the adult hypnosis group and repeated on audio tapes for home use at least five times per week. The scripts include language that encourages healthy and normal movement of the bowel and includes extended relaxation protocols, vivid imagery, and a focus away from bowel discomfort and toward a state of well-being and comfort.

Scripts for the functional abdominal pain in children were directed at those in the 6–12 age range and include more active imagery, simple instructions, and in three 20-minute audio sessions once every other week in a fixed sequence. In between these sessions, children are asked to use one of the audios daily. Imagery includes floating on a cloud, going down a slide, swinging on a swing, and flying a magic carpet, among others. Goals are to produce a general feeling of well-being, shift attention away from abdominal discomfort, protect the gut from unpleasant stimuli, and weaken the sensations of pain and discomfort over time. In the recordings, therapeutic suggestions are provided once full relaxation has occurred and include an image of a warm and healing light radiating from the child's hand which is used to soothe and heal abdominal pain and discomfort. Another image used in the North Carolina Protocol is for the child to imagine drinking a favorite beverage which is then visualized coating and protecting the stomach and intestines (belly) and the suggestion that each time the child drinks the beverage they will make the protective layer stronger (Palsson and van Tilburg 2015).

The pediatric scripts were tested in a clinical trial in 34 children aged 6–15 years. Children in the treatment group ($n = 19$) attended one training session then completed the protocol at home using recordings. The treatment group showed a higher response to treatment (goal 50% reduction in abdominal pain) 73.3% versus 26.7% in controls, with improvements maintained over a 6-month follow-up period in 62.3% in the treatment group. Compliance with home treatment in the study was high at 98.5% compliance overall (van Tilburg et al. 2009).

Imagery has also been used in the pediatric post-operative setting. A study by Huth et al. included 73 children aged 7–12 undergoing tonsillectomy and or adenoidectomy. The treatment group ($n = 36$) watched a professionally developed videotape on imagery and listened to a 30-minute audio tape of imagery 1 week prior to their surgery then audio tape only 1–4 hours after surgery and audio tape at 22–27 hours after discharge. Pain and anxiety were measured, and the amount of analgesics used at home was recorded. Significant reduction in pain and anxiety were recorded in the treatment group at 1–4 hours after surgery but not at the 22–27-hour time window. No difference in pain medication was seen in this study (Huth et al. 2004).

TRAINING

There is no licensed training in guided imagery at this time in the United States.

RESOURCES

Academy for Guided Imagery: 150-hour, mentored, long distance learning, certificate program for health professionals: http://www.academyforguidedimagery.com

- Health Journeys: http://www.healthjourneys.com
- Kaiser Guided Imagery Resources (free to all) in cooperation with Health Journeys Podcasts: https://healthy.kaiserpermanente.org

References

Academy for Guided Imagery. Accessed March 18, 2018. Retrieved from http://academyforguided-imagery.com/.

American Society of Clinical Hypnosis (ASCH). Accessed March 18, 2018. Retrieved from http://www.asch.net/.

Alter, D. S., and L. I. Sugarman. 2017. Reorienting hypnosis education. *Am J Clin Hypn* 59 (3): 235–259. doi:10.1080/00029157.2016.1231657.

Anbar, R. D., and H. R. Hall. 2004. Childhood habit cough treated with self-hypnosis. *J Pediatr* 144 (2): 213–217. doi:10.1016/j.jpeds.2003.10.041.

Anbar, R. D., and M. P. Slothower. 2006. Hypnosis for treatment of insomnia in school-age children: A retrospective chart review. *BMC Pediatr* 6: 23. doi:10.1186/1471-2431-6-23.

Banerjee, S., A. Srivastav, and B. M. Palan. 1993. Hypnosis and self-hypnosis in the management of nocturnal enuresis: A comparative study with imipramine therapy. *Am J Clin Hypn* 36 (2): 113–119. doi:10.1080/00029157.1993.10403053.

Becker, P. M. 2015. Hypnosis in the management of sleep disorders. *Sleep Med Clin* 10 (1): 85–92. doi:10.1016/j.jsmc.2014.11.003.

Boltin, D., N. Sahar, E. Gil, S. Aizic, K. Hod, R. Levi-Drummer, Y. Niv, and R. Dickman. 2015. Gut-directed guided affective imagery as an adjunct to dietary modification in irritable bowel syndrome. *J Health Psychol* 20 (6): 712–720. doi:10.1177/1359105315573450.

Broadbent, E., A. Kahokehr, R. J. Booth, J. Thomas, J. A. Windsor, C. M. Buchanan, B. R. Wheeler, T. Sammour, and A. G. Hill. 2012. A brief relaxation intervention reduces stress and improves surgical wound healing response: A randomised trial. *Brain Behav Immun* 26 (2): 212–217. doi:10.1016/j.bbi.2011.06.014.

Brown, D. 2007. Evidence-based hypnotherapy for asthma: A critical review. *Int J Clin Exp Hypn* 55 (2): 220–249. doi:10.1080/00207140601177947.

Butler, L. D., B. K. Symons, S. L. Henderson, L. D. Shortliffe, and D. Spiegel. 2005. Hypnosis reduces distress and duration of an invasive medical procedure for children. *Pediatrics* 115 (1): e77–e85. doi:10.1542/peds.2004-0818.

Cordi, M. J., A. A. Schlarb, and B. Rasch. 2014. Deepening sleep by hypnotic suggestion. *Sleep* 37 (6): 1143–1152, 1152A–1152F. doi:10.5665/sleep.3778.

Cramer, H., R. Lauche, A. Paul, J. Langhorst, S. Kummel, and G. J. Dobos. 2015. Hypnosis in breast cancer care: A systematic review of randomized controlled trials. *Integr Cancer Ther* 14 (1): 5–15. doi:10.1177/1534735414550035.

Dobson, C. E., and M. W. Byrne. 2014. Original research: Using guided imagery to manage pain in young children with sickle cell disease. *Am J Nurs* 114 (4): 26,36 doi:10.1097/01.NAJ.0000445680.06812.6a.

Entwistle, P. A. 2017. A pragmatic guide to the setting up of integrated hypnotherapy services in primary care and clinical settings. *Int J Clin Exp Hypn* 65 (3): 257–295. doi:10.1080/00207144. 2017.1314720.

Finlayson, K., S. Downe, S. Hinder, H. Carr, H. Spiby, and P. Whorwell. 2015. Unexpected consequences: Women's experiences of a self-hypnosis intervention to help with pain relief during labour. *BMC Pregnancy Childbirth* 15: 229. doi:10.1186/s12884-015-0659-0.

Forsner, M., F. Norstrom, K. Nordyke, A. Ivarsson, and V. Lindh. 2014. Relaxation and guided imagery used with 12-year-olds during venipuncture in a school-based screening study. *J Child Health Care* 18 (3): 241252. doi: 10.1177/1367493513486963.

Giacobbi, P. R., Jr., M. E. Stabler, J. Stewart, A. M. Jaeschke, J. L. Siebert, and G. A. Kelley. 2015. Guided imagery for arthritis and other rheumatic diseases: A systematic review of randomized controlled trials. *Pain Manag Nurs* 16 (5): 792–803. doi:10.1016/j.pmn.2015.01.003.

Hauri, P. J., M. H. Silber, and B. F. Boeve. 2007. The treatment of parasomnias with hypnosis: A 5-year follow-up study. *J Clin Sleep Med* 3 (4): 369–373.

Holden-Lund, C. 1988. Effects of relaxation with guided imagery on surgical stress and wound healing. *Res Nurs Health* 11 (4): 235–244.

Hurwitz, T. D., M. W. Mahowald, C. H. Schenck, J. L. Schluter, and S. R. Bundlie. 1991. A retrospective outcome study and review of hypnosis as treatment of adults with sleepwalking and sleep terror. *J Nerv Ment Dis* 179 (4): 228–233.

Huth, M. M., M. E. Broome, and M. Good. 2004. Imagery reduces children's post-operative pain. *Pain* 110 (1–2): 439–448. doi:10.1016/j.pain.2004.04.028.

Jacobson, A. F., W. A. Umberger, P. A. Palmieri, T. S. Alexander, R. P. Myerscough, C. B. Draucker, S. Steudte-Schmiedgen, and C. Kirschbaum. 2016. Guided imagery for total knee replacement: A randomized, placebo-controlled pilot study. *J Altern Complement Med* 22 (7): 563–575. doi:10.1089/acm.2016.0038.

Jensen, M. P., and D. R. Patterson. 2014. Hypnotic approaches for chronic pain management: Clinical implications of recent research findings. *Am Psychol* 69 (2): 167–177. doi:10.1037/a0035644.

Jiang, H., M. P. White, M. D. Greicius, L. C. Waelde, and D. Spiegel. 2016. Brain activity and functional connectivity associated with hypnosis. *Cereb Cortex* 27 (8): 4083–4093. doi:10.1093/cercor/bhw220.

Kaiser, P. 2011. Childhood anxiety, worry, and fear: Individualizing hypnosis goals and suggestions for self-regulation. *Am J Clin Hypn* 54 (1): 16–31. doi:10.1080/00029157.2011.575965.

Kaiser Guided Imagery Resources in cooperation with Health Journeys. Accessed March 18, 2018. Retrieved from https://healthy.kaiserpermanente.org

Kauders, A. D. 2017. The social before sociocognitive theory: Explaining hypnotic suggestion in German-speaking Europe, 1900–1960. *Am J Clin Hypn* 59 (4): 422–439. doi:10.1080/00029157. 2016.1239062.

Kohen, D. P., and P. Kaiser. 2014. Clinical hypnosis with children and adolescents: What? Why? How?—Origins, applications, and efficacy. *Children (Basel)* 1 (2): 74–98. doi:10.3390/children1020074.

Kohen, D. P., P. Kaiser, and K. Olness. 2017. State-of-the-art pediatric hypnosis training: Remodeling curriculum and refining faculty development. *Am J Clin Hypn* 59 (3): 292–310. doi:10.1080/0002 9157.2016.1233859.

Kohen, D. P., K. N. Olness, S. O. Colwell, and A. Heimel. 1984. The use of relaxation-mental imagery (self-hypnosis) in the management of 505 pediatric behavioral encounters. *J Dev Behav Pediatr* 5 (1): 21–25.

Landolt, A. S., and L. S. Milling. 2011. The efficacy of hypnosis as an intervention for labor and delivery pain: A comprehensive methodological review. *Clin Psychol Rev* 31 (6): 1022–1031. doi:10.1016/j.cpr.2011.06.002.

Landry, M., M. Lifshitz, and A. Raz. 2017. Brain correlates of hypnosis: A systematic review and meta-analytic exploration. *Neurosci Biobehav Rev* 81: 75–98. doi:10.1016/j.neubiorev.2017.02.020.

Lin, Y. C., A. C. Lee, K. J. Kemper, and C. B. Berde. 2005. Use of complementary and alternative medicine in pediatric pain management service: A survey. *Pain Med* 6 (6): 452–458. doi:10.1111/j.1526-4637.2005.00071.x.

Madden, K., P. Middleton, A. M. Cyna, M. Matthewson, and L. Jones. 2016. Hypnosis for pain management during labour and childbirth. *Cochrane Database Syst Rev* (5): CD009356. doi:10.1002/14651858.CD009356.pub3.

McBride, J. J., A. M. Vlieger, and R. D. Anbar. 2014. Hypnosis in paediatric respiratory medicine. *Paediatr Respir Rev* 15 (1): 82–85. doi:10.1016/j.prrv.2013.09.002.

Naparstek, B. 1994. *Staying Well with Guided Imagery.* New York: Warner Books.

Olness, K., and G. G. Gardner. 1978. Some guidelines for uses of hypnotherapy in pediatrics. *Pediatrics* 62 (2): 228–233.

Palsson, O. S., and M. van Tilburg. 2015. Hypnosis and guided imagery treatment for gastrointestinal disorders: Experience with scripted protocols developed at the university of North Carolina. *Am J Clin Hypn* 58 (1): 5–21. doi:10.1080/00029157.2015.1012705.

Parvizi, J., V. Rangarajan, W. R. Shirer, N. Desai, and M. D. Greicius. 2013. The will to persevere induced by electrical stimulation of the human cingulate gyrus. *Neuron* 80 (6): 1359–1367. doi:10.1016/j.neuron.2013.10.057.

Pendergrast, R. A. 2017. Incorporating hypnosis into pediatric clinical encounters. *Children (Basel)* 4 (3): 18. doi:10.3390/children4030018.

Potie, A., F. Roelants, A. Pospiech, M. Momeni, and C. Watremez. 2016. Hypnosis in the perioperative management of breast cancer surgery: Clinical benefits and potential implications. *Anesthesiol Res Pract* 2016: 2942416. doi:10.1155/2016/2942416.

Reid, D. B. 2016. Hypnotic induction: Enhancing trance or mostly myth? *Am J Clin Hypn* 59 (2): 128–137. doi:10.1080/00029157.2016.1190310.

Rutten, J. M., A. M. Vlieger, C. Frankenhuis, E. K. George, M. Groeneweg, O. F. Norbruis, A. Ten. et al. 2017. Home-based hypnotherapy self-exercises vs individual hypnotherapy with a therapist for treatment of pediatric irritable bowel syndrome, functional abdominal pain, or functional abdominal pain syndrome: A randomized clinical trial. *JAMA Pediatr* 171 (5): 470–477. doi:10.1001/jamapediatrics.2017.0091.

Section on Integrative Medicine. 2016. Mind–body therapies in children and youth. *Pediatrics* 138 (3): e6–e7. doi:10.1542/peds.2016-1896.

Silove, D., V. Manicavasagar, R. Beltran, G. Le, H. Nguyen, T. Phan, and A. Blaszczynski. 1997. Satisfaction of Vietnamese patients and their families with refugee and mainstream mental health services. *Psychiatr Serv* 48 (8): 1064–1069. doi:10.1176/ps.48.8.1064.

van Tilburg, M. A., D. K. Chitkara, O. S. Palsson, M. Turner, N. Blois-Martin, M. Ulshen, and W. E. Whitehead. 2009. Audio-recorded guided imagery treatment reduces functional abdominal pain in children: A pilot study. *Pediatrics* 124 (5): e890–e897. doi:10.1542/peds.2009-0028.

Weigensberg, M. J., C. J. Lane, Q. Avila, K. Konersman, E. Ventura, T. Adam, Z. Shoar, M. I. Goran, and D. Spruijt-Metz. 2014. Imagine HEALTH: Results from a randomized pilot lifestyle intervention for obese Latino adolescents using Interactive Guided Imagery[SM]. *BMC Complement Altern Med* 14: 28. doi:10.1186/1472-6882-14-28.

8 Mindfulness

INTRODUCTION AND BACKGROUND

Mindfulness has been described by Jon Kabat-Zinn, PhD, as the cultivation of awareness in the present moment, on purpose, without judgment (Kabat-Zinn et al. 1985).

A practice with ancient roots, mindfulness has entered the mainstream medicine primarily on the strength of Kabat-Zinn's pioneering 8-week program introduced in the late 1970s originally to chronic pain patients. Now widely known as mindfulness-based stress reduction (MBSR), the program combines a variety of mind–body therapies such as breath work, progressive muscle relaxation, mindful eating, mindful movement, yoga, and meditation to introduce the concept of mindfulness in such a way as to allow people with a range of skills and awareness to access the material and learn to apply it in a wide range of clinical conditions and settings.

Although MBSR is not the only type of mindfulness training, it has gained broad acceptance in the medical community, and nearly 80% of the 140 accredited medical schools or their associated university programs in the United States have incorporated some type of mindfulness intervention into clinical treatment, educational, and or research programs (Buchholz 2015).

In part, this is due to the use of MBSR as a treatment intervention in a range of randomized controlled trials which, taken as a whole, have shown impressive benefits, including reduction of emotional reactivity, improvement in quality of life and coping capacity, reduction of anxiety and depression, decreased emotional reactivity, and modulation of inflammatory markers. Engagement of the patient in their own care and healing is another important element of mindfulness training (Rosenkranz et al. 2013).

A classic MBSR course is led by one or more trained instructors and includes an introductory session outlining the program and updating participants on the connections between emotions, stress, and overall health. A focus on patterns of habitual response to stressors is introduced early, as is an explanation of the physiologic relaxation response which underpins the mindfulness exercises. A core component of the course is a daily home practice of meditation, which is used to introduce new techniques and reinforces the course material while helping students bring a sense of discipline to their practice. The MBSR course has been offered in the classroom setting, in residential retreats, in recurring weekly sessions online, and in distance learning models where classes meet together on conference calls weekly. Guided exercises are available by CD, and a workbook often accompanies the course.

Each week, a new topic is introduced, often beginning with breath work. One of the early challenges in mindfulness is learning to focus one's attention, and breath work is often used as a focusing tool. This is important, as awareness of how and why one is focusing one's attention is a powerful tool, allowing incremental mastery of worry or chaotic thoughts, self-doubt, and suffering of all types.

In his book, *Full Catastrophe Living* (*Using the Wisdom of Your Body and Mind to Face Stress, Pain, and Illness*) (Revised Edition, 2013, Random House), Kabat-Zinn identifies seven essential attitudes for mindfulness practice. They include:

Non-judging: It is essential to bring a neutral, compassionate awareness to mindfulness practice. Many of us have long-established habits of judging and reacting to emotions or circumstance that we may not even have awareness of. This is an important element in meditation practice when thoughts arise. The goal is to acknowledge and release, without positive or negative judgment.

Patience: A sense of impatience may accompany meditation, especially early in training. When this occurs, one is encouraged to bring their attention to the sense of impatience—and to notice the sensation and how it may change as one brings their full attention to the feeling. Over time, the goal is to cultivate a feeling of spaciousness and presence in the moment and allow the feelings of impatience to pass.

Beginner's mind: This might be described as the sense of experiencing something for the first time—even if it is familiar. This is part of the exercise of maintaining one's attention in the present moment, noticing with every sense and remaining present to the full experience, moment to moment.

Trust: A focus of mindfulness training is the development of trust in oneself and one's feelings. This may build gradually and can serve as a reliable navigational tool when processing the emotional input of the day.

Non-striving: In essence, the idea is to simply bring kind awareness to the moment, with a sense of nowhere to go and nothing to do. This may be one of the most challenging elements of attention for students of mindfulness in modern society, especially for busy clinicians. This can also pose a challenge for students new to mindfulness who are hoping to *progress*, in that paradoxically, there is nowhere to go.

Acceptance: Essentially, acceptance describes the ability and willingness to see things just as they are in the present moment, rather than to resist, deny, rationalize, or deflect. This is the foundation for the ability to change. An important nuance of acceptance is that it does not imply passive acceptance or the need to like the situation or emotion—only that one is able to clearly acknowledge what is in the present moment.

Letting go: Letting go is also taught as non-attachment, which can be quite challenging if there is a goal, expectation, emotion, object, or person that one wants to hold on to. The idea is again to remain present in the moment, able to accept what is, and letting go of feelings of clinging, grasping, or need. Just letting go and allowing things to be.

One of the benefits of mindfulness training is the development of the ability to recognize experiences or emotions as they are happening, with a new sense of awareness in the present moment. Applying the principles of non-judging, patience, beginner's mind, and non-striving, one can facilitate the process of learning to trust one's insights and develop a sense of recognition without attachment. In this way, new insights and wisdom can be gained that can be reinforced by a sense of gratitude and appreciation for every experience we receive as a source of continual growth. Kabat-Zinn describes being mindful as acknowledging what is here and now and the practice of mindfulness as remaining aware of what is unfolding in the experience. The skill of mindfulness can help people face, accept, and navigate intense emotions and circumstances in a way that allows them to accept and release in a way that cultivates courage and equanimity over time. For example, emotions associated with post-traumatic stress or the challenge of dealing with a difficult diagnosis. Mindfulness practice can help people draw on deeper wells of courage, insight, discernment, and wisdom and learn to release difficult emotions rather than allowing them to define their lives.

A typical second-week lesson in MBSR includes introduction to the process of the body scan, similar to the process used in progressive muscle relaxation described in Chapter 5. Rather than a tensing and releasing, some programs use a practice of directing breath into and out of sequential areas of the body, expelling tension or unease with the outbreath. This promotes mindful awareness of the body's reactions to pleasant and stressful experiences and increases understanding of the intricate mind–body connections. A second mindfulness exercise includes mindful eating. This may involve a slow and mindful guided experience of eating a raisin or a piece of chocolate. Both of these exercises offer opportunities to practice focused attention. The body scan also helps develop early recognition of stress- or illness-related symptoms and is another approach to gathering accurate information about what is really happening in the moment. Students are encouraged to continue to practice the body scan in conjunction with their daily meditation practice and may use recorded CDs to guide the home exercise. The mindful eating exercise can be practiced at home around any meal or snack as students gradually increase awareness of feeling and emotions related to hunger and satiety.

Another important theme taught in MBSR training is the concept of impermanence— an ancient Buddhist teaching. This is reinforced in a variety of ways, including maintaining diaries of both positive and unpleasant events and emotions throughout the week. Tracking these events and feelings helps refine awareness and allows students to appreciate the ever-changing nature of life. This, in turn, promotes the strengthening of equanimity (mental calmness, composure, evenness of temper, especially in a difficult situation—Merriam-Webster derived from the Latin aequus *level* or *equal* and animus *soul* or *mind* essentially *even mind*). Ideally, these insights lead to what is referred to as a virtuous cycle (insight of impermanence, equanimity, further insight of impermanence, and so on in a positive feedback loop of personal growth).

A further exercise in MBSR is mindful movement, usually a walking exercise of 15–20 paces done very slowly and mindfully with specific attention to posture and body sensations.

One of the keys in slowing down movement and directing attention to precise physical sensations, as in the mindful eating exercise, is that this builds the ability to notice subtle physical changes. This can help act as an early warning system to symptoms of stress and thereby provides the ability to detect and redirect pre-existing habitual reactions early in the process. This can be broken down into a series of mini-steps that begin with placing kind awareness on one's reactions to help identify and name the trigger and note resulting physical and mental changes. When a situation is met in this manner, coupled with conscious breathing to balance sympathetic and parasympathetic nervous system activity, it allows a sense of discernment and insight that may help to redirect a habitual response. Although initially, this process can seem cumbersome, over time a more skillful reaction to stressors becomes automatic and becomes a buffer against the mental and physical toll of stress over-reactivity.

For example, this practice might help a student shift from an experience of feeling "I am angry" to "I am experiencing anger" or "I am in pain" to "I am experiencing a sensation of pain." Subtle shifts in perspective with important implications. One of the important concepts in this area is the development of stress hardiness, defined by Kobasa in the late 1970s (Kobasa 1979), to help identify characteristics associated with resilience in stressful situations. In a study of 86 male business executives, personality traits of:

- Commitment to self with an attitude of active involvement and curiosity
- Internal focus of control—in that one believes their actions can influence outcomes
- Attitude of vigor as opposed to passivity in response to challenge were significantly associated with lower rates of illness independent of variables such as exercise, age, education, and job level (Kobasa et al. 1985)

An introduction to yoga is another important component of MBSR. Yoga, which discussed in detail in Chapter 10, is incorporated into MBSR as a technique that reinforces the powerful interactions of mind, body, and spirit. As the MBSR course progresses, more formal types of meditation are introduced to continue cultivation of equanimity, for example, a traditional type of Buddhist Metta meditation (loving kindness meditation) that offers kind compassion to self, loved ones, neutral parties, and eventually to those with whom you perceive as difficult then to all sentient beings (Salzberg 1995).

A classic approach includes phrases such as:

- May I be happy
- May I be healthy
- May I be peaceful
- May I be safe

Offered to the self first, then to others, for example:

- May you be happy
- May you be healthy
- May you be peaceful
- May you be safe

A final part of a classic MBSR course culminates a day of silent meditation. This is often done in a group setting and includes instructors and students. A typical schedule for the retreat day includes elements learned in the course, for example, breath work, sitting meditation, walking meditation, body scan, yoga, and loving kindness meditation.

MINDFULNESS RESEARCH UPDATE

Research support for the efficacy of mindfulness and MBSR courses in adults, adolescents, and children continues to accrue. The following is a sampling of clinical studies and an overview of emerging research on the mechanisms of action of mindfulness. New imaging and measurement techniques are accelerating research in this area and helping to shed light on these complex interactions and how to most effectively harness them to improve health.

Chronic disease

A systematic review by Niazi included 18 studies examining the use of MBSR in a range of chronic medical conditions, including: cancer, hypertension, diabetes, HIV/AIDS, chronic pain, and skin disorders and found improvement across studies, although study design varied. The most significant changes were seen psychological symptoms, including anxiety, depression, and psychological distress and overall quality of life (Niazi and Niazi 2011).

Anxiety, depression, and pain

A meta-analysis of 47 actively controlled trials with 3,515 participants showed that mindfulness programs were effective in improving symptoms of self-reported anxiety, depression, and pain (Goyal et al. 2014). Reduction in rumination and improved coping ability has also been documented (Jain et al. 2007).

Pain

Several systematic review and meta-analysis have been done in pain patients and have shown varying outcomes in the effectiveness of MBSR to address pain in diverse patient populations.

One systematic review by Hilton et al. examined 38 randomized controlled trials that involved 3,536 patients. Intervention length ranged from 3 to 12 weeks, with the majority being 8 weeks long. Studies used either classic MBSR or mindfulness-based cognitive therapy (MBCT) with no significant adverse events noted. In this meta-analysis, mindfulness meditation showed a small impact on pain symptoms—although significant study heterogeneity was present. Improvements were seen in depression, physical-health-related quality of life, and mental health-related quality of life. Authors note the need for more well-designed, rigorous, randomized controlled trials of longer duration before offering definitive recommendations (Hilton et al. 2017).

An earlier systematic review included 16 paper, eight of which involved controlled trials and eight uncontrolled. Significant reduction in perception of pain intensity was seen in the mindfulness-based intervention groups across studies with sustained improvements in many of the groups (Reiner et al. 2013).

One study by Grant et al. compared pain sensitivity and tolerance in experienced meditators ($N = 17$) and 18 controls. In this study, the meditators showed significantly reduced pain sensitivity, and thicker cortex was seen on measurement with MRI in brain areas associated with pain processing and in the somatosensory cortex. A greater number of hours of meditation was positively associated with increased gray matter in specific areas related to pain processing (Grant et al. 2010).

A systematic review and meta-analysis of MBSR for low back pain evaluated seven randomized controlled studies involving 864 patients and found that MBSR was associated with short-term improvement in pain intensity in four studies but suggest longer trials are needed to more fully establish effectiveness in this study population (Anheyer et al. 2017).

Vascular disease

A systematic review and meta-analysis of the use of mindfulness (MBSR and MBCT) in 578 patients with vascular disease (hypertension, type 1 diabetes, stroke, and heart disease) included nine studies, eight of which were randomized controlled trials. Meta-analysis showed positive evidence of stress reduction (−0.36; 95% CI −0.67 to −0.09; $p = 0.01$), depression (−0.35; 95% CI −0.53 to −0.16; $p = 0.003$), and anxiety (−0.50; 95% CI −0.70 to −0.29; $p < 0.001$), although authors called for further longitudinal studies prior to making generalized recommendations (Abbott et al. 2014).

Fibromyalgia

A randomized controlled trial of MBSR in women with fibromyalgia found that women in the treatment group ($n = 51$) versus wait-listed controls ($n = 40$) had improvements in perceived stress, sleep disturbance, and overall symptom severity—but no significant changes in pain, cortisol levels, or overall physical functioning (Cash et al. 2015).

Gastrointestinal diseases

A substantial literature exists supporting the use of mind–body therapies in gastrointestinal conditions. Mindfulness is among the best studies, especially in irritable bowel syndrome (Ballou and Keefer 2017).

For example, in one prospective randomized controlled trial 75 women with IBS were assigned to an 8-week MBSR course or support group. Women in the treatment group had a statistically significant decrease in IBS symptoms immediately after completion of training (26.4% vs. 6.2% reduction) ($p = 0.006$) which increased at 3-month follow-up to (38.2% vs. 11.8% $p = 0.001$) with control group (Gaylord et al. 2011).

A study in 60 adults with inflammatory bowel disease randomized ($n = 33$) into treatment group of an 8-week MBSR course and ($n = 27$) controls into treatment as usual. Results showed significant improvement in the treatment group in a range of parameters measured, including anxiety, quality of life, mindfulness, and reduction in depression with the last three maintained at 6-month follow-up (Neilson et al. 2016).

Stress and inflammation

One of the most important areas of benefit in mindfulness training is stress reduction, especially relevant to those living with chronic inflammatory conditions. For example, a study by Rosenkranz et al. compared physiologic stress reaction and response to an inflammatory topical irritant in 31 highly experienced meditators versus control group ($n = 37$). Both groups underwent a modified Trier Social Stress Test to provoke psychological stress (impromptu, video-taped, judged, 5-minute speech, followed by 5 minutes of mental arithmetic). Capsaicin cream was applied to forearm skin to induce a neurogenic inflammatory response.

Results showed experienced meditators to have lower psychological stress response by measurement of salivary cortisol (62.62 ± 2.52 vs. 70.38 ± 2.33; $p < 0.05$) and perceived stress (4.18 ± 0.41 vs. 5.56 ± 0.30; $p < 0.01$). The meditators also had smaller flare reactions to the topical cream (81.55 ± 4.6 vs. 96.76 ± 4.26; $p < 0.05$) as compared to controls. The magnitude of inflammatory response to capsaicin was positively associated with the magnitude of the cortisol response, lending support to the theory that psychological stress is a driver of the neurogenic inflammatory response. A finding relevant to many chronic inflammatory diseases such as asthma, inflammatory bowel disease, arthritis, and other conditions. Overall, the experienced meditators also had higher levels of well-being and resilience in this study (Rosenkranz et al. 2016).

These results supported findings in a prior randomized study by Rosenkranz et al., which was designed to tease out the specific effect of an 8-week MBSR course versus a health education program designed to mirror MBSR program structure without including mindfulness. The study question was whether mindfulness could buffer the effects of physiologic stress and dermal inflammation in healthy adults and involved 49 adult men. Psychological stress was induced by the modified Trier Social Stress Test as described earlier. The inflammatory stimulus used was topical capsaicin cream at 0.1% concentration. Results showed that those in the MBSR group showed smaller flare reactions to the topical capsaicin irritant compared to controls (Rosenkranz et al. 2013).

Mechanisms of action for the influence of MBSR on the immune system remains an area of active study. A systematic review of 20 controlled trials by Black and Slavich focused on randomized controlled trials with a focus on five specific outcomes, including: circulating and stimulated inflammatory proteins, cellular transcription factors and gene expression, immune cell count, immune cell aging, and antibody response. Mean sample size of the studies was $n = 20$, and total number of participants was 1,602. Results showed mindfulness-related effects for four outcomes: reduction in transcription of cellular transcription factor NF-kB, reduction in circulating levels of C-reactive protein, increases in CD4+ T cell count in HIV-positive patients, and increases in telomerase activity. Conversely, no related effects were seen, or replicated, for IgA, IgG, or influenza antibodies; IL-1, IL-6, IL-8, IL-10, IFN, TNF interleukins; and measures of various immune cell counts. Authors conclude that, while promising connections are seen in reduction of pro-inflammatory processes, cellular-mediated immune defense, and increase in telomerase activity associated with reduction in cellular aging that more specific and larger studies are needed to deepen understanding of the potential for mindfulness to benefit immune processes (Black and Slavich 2016).

It remains unclear how meditation reduces stress sensitivity, although a body of research has demonstrated that meditation can lead to increase in areas of the brain associated with regulating cortisol to stress such as the hippocampus and amygdale (Luders et al. 2009; Luders et al. 2014).

Meditation is also under active study as an approach to mitigate age-related brain degeneration (Luders and Cherbuin 2016; Last et al. 2017).

Mindfulness and telomeres

Emerging research continues to accrue on the effect of mindfulness on telomeres and telomerase, which has been linked to longevity and improved health, an area of intense research activity (Chen et al. 2014; Goglin et al. 2016; Fair et al. 2017).

Loving kindness meditation has been shown to be associated with longer telomere length in a study comparing experienced adult meditators ($n = 15$) with control group ($n = 22$). Loving kindness meditators have longer relative telomere length than controls ($p = 0.083$), and women meditators ($n = 9$) had even more significantly longer telomere length ($p = 0.007$) in this study (Hoge et al. 2013).

A meta-analysis of the effect of mindfulness meditation on telomerase activity included four randomized controlled trials involving 190 participants found a medium-sized effect (Cohen's $d = 0.46$) (Schutte and Malouff 2014).

Mindfulness and neural connectivity

Research demonstrating how mindfulness impacts neural connectivity is on the leading edge of the field, initially reported by Gotink et al. (2016), who used fMRI study results to better understand the stress-reducing mechanism of MBSR and MBCT training. In the systematic review, 30 studies were included, 11 of which involved MBSR, 15 on certain aspects of MBSR programming, and 4 involved dispositional mindfulness. Results of the study analysis showed that prefrontal cortex, cingulate cortex, insula, and hippocampus showed increased activity, connectivity, and volume in both stressed, anxious, and healthy participants. These findings are similar to those seen in long-term meditation exercises.

The amygdala showed decreased functional activity, improved functional connectivity with the prefrontal cortex, and earlier deactivation consistent with improved emotional regulation after exposure to emotional stimuli, establishing the connection between MBSR-induced changes in behavioral and emotional states are related to both functional and structural changes in the brain (Gotink et al. 2016).

These findings are extended in work by Shao et al. in a rigorous longitudinal randomized active-controlled study design that shows the effects of an 8-week meditation program versus relaxation training on affective processing and posterior cingulate cortex connectivity. The study involved 8-week group training in either MBSR or relaxation led by an experienced instructor. Participants had 22 classes of 1.5 hours duration and had home practice assignments. Scans (MRI and fMRI) were done pre and post the last session. Results are consistent with a shift to a more non-judgmental, self-aware state.

Meditation was shown to neutralize affective processing—indicating that meditation training promotes self-referential affective regulation (enhances positive affect and reducing negative affect) and was shown to occur across resting state and during active evaluation of affective stimuli—demonstrating changes in neural functional connectivity. This is in line with the goal of equanimity in meditation wherein an even-minded appraisal of both positive and negative stimuli is achieved.

Neural connectivity from the pons to posterior cingulate cortex became more positive in the meditation group, and this enhanced connectivity has an important role in increasing self-awareness and regulating negative affective processing (Shao et al. 2016).

Mindfulness in physician wellness

Mindfulness is an active area of study in physician wellness at all stages of training and practice.

One example is seen in a randomized controlled trial in 167 Dutch medical students in their first year of clinical clerkships. Students in the treatment group ($n = 83$) undertook eight weekly, 2-hour sessions that were comprised of didactic teaching, meditation exercises, and group dialogues—similar to classic MBSR training. Parameters measured included psychological distress, positive mental health, life satisfaction, physician empathy, mindfulness skills, and dysfunctional cognitions. Assessments were done at baseline, and 3, 7, 12, 15, and 20 months. Results showed some reduction in psychological distress in the treatment group ($p = 0.03$), reduction in dysfunctional cognitions ($p = 0.05$), and improvements in positive mental health ($p = 0.002$), life satisfaction ($p = 0.01$), and mindfulness skills ($p = 0.05$) compared to a control group. No changes in empathy were seen, and no serious adverse events reported (van Dijk et al. 2017).

In a cross-sectional study in fourth year medical students in two different cohorts starting medical clerkships, group 1 ($n = 179$) and group 2 ($n = 232$) showed that 53% of group 1 and 72% of group 2 were interested in MBSR training. The study highlighted the fact that interested students showed significantly higher scores on psychological distress ($p = 0.004$) and neuroticism ($p < 0.001$) than non-interested students in group 1, and in group 2, interested students again showed significantly higher scores on psychological distress ($p = 0.001$), worrying ($p = 0.002$), problem avoidance ($p = 0.005$), and lower mindfulness skills ($p = 0.002$) than non-participants. Results of this study showed robust interest and participation in MBSR training, even in students actively on medical clerkships, and offers promise as a low-risk tool to help support students reporting higher levels of psychological distress and a relative lack of pre-existing mindfulness skills (van Dijk et al. 2015; Kraemer et al. 2016).

A systematic review of randomized and non-randomized controlled trials in a broader swath of health professional students including medical, nursing, social work, psychology, and *medical plus other* students included 19 studies and 1,815 participants and found positive results in the majority of studies, with the most common findings including decreased stress and anxiety, improved mood and mindfulness, and improved self-efficacy and empathy across student groups, adding to the literature on feasibility of introducing MBSR and related mindfulness teaching into student training (McConville et al. 2017).

Studies on the use of mindfulness in faculty physicians also show benefit. For example, a comprehensive systematic review and meta-analysis by West et al. reviewed 115 randomized controlled trials involving 716 physicians and 37 unique cohort studies including 2,914 physicians showed that the most commonly studied interventions have included mindfulness, stress management techniques, and small group discussions, although which interventions have the greatest value and impact remain unknown. Authors stress the importance of both individual and organizational approaches to addressing burnout and its comorbidities, and longitudinal studies are needed in both domains (West et al. 2016).

One study by Fortney et al. examined the question of whether an abbreviated mindfulness intervention could be effective in decreasing symptoms of burnout and increasing job satisfaction and quality of life in practicing physicians. In a single-person pre-post study design, 30 primary care physicians participated in an abbreviated mindfulness course modeled on the classic MBSR curriculum. Participants had 18 rather than approximately 30 hours of training, had 4–5 in-person training sessions beginning with a non-residential weekend immersion rather than eight weekly sessions, and were encouraged to practice at home for 10–20 minutes daily rather than 45 minutes. Results showed that extending to 9 months post-intervention, participants improved scores in emotional exhaustion ($p = 0.009$), depersonalization ($p = 0.005$), and personal accomplishment ($p < 0.001$). Improvements were also seen in anxiety ($p = 0.006$), depression ($p = 0.001$), and stress ($p = 0.002$). Classes were led by experienced mindfulness instructors and included guided sitting and walking mindfulness practices, sharing experiences in a group setting, and practicing mindfulness in the patient encounter (Fortney et al. 2013).

Another study in faculty physicians involved a series of 19 biweekly facilitated physician discussion groups that incorporated a variety of elements such as mindfulness, reflection, shared experience, and small group learning over a 9-month period. This study provided 1-hour paid protected time every other week for physicians to meet. The largest changes seen in this study were in empowerment and engagement in work ($p = 0.04$), which was sustained at 12-month follow-up, and decrease in depersonalization ($p = 0.004$), also sustained at 12 months (West et al. 2014).

CLINICAL APPLICATION MINDFULNESS

Dr. Wu is a fifth-year surgical resident who is hardworking, well respected, and known for his interest and developing skills in trauma surgery. He is single, lives alone, and has family out of the country. His residency program, similar to others in the country, is developing a wellness track for residents, and he has been nominated by his peers to lead it. He is surprised, somewhat flattered, but mainly worried because of the extra work involved. In addition, the faculty at this program, especially the department chair have expressed deep disdain for the physician wellness movement, which he views as a waste of time.

In the noon lecture where he was asked to introduce the new wellness program, Dr. Wu was met with uncomfortable silence and a derisive comment from the chair who was sitting in the front row. Afterward the residency program director approached him to offer support and suggested a way forward. The residency program director had recently been made aware of an anesthesia resident's suicide in another training program in the city which had not been widely publicized. He was committed to implementing measures to support his program's residents.

He and Dr. Wu partnered to offer a series of optional meetings on the topic for residents only to assess interest and to get ideas for what type of activities would be of greatest interest. Once word was out that the meetings were not mandatory and would not be public, residents from all years began attending. Multiple suggestions were received, including a format similar to the one used at Mayo Clinics where residents could meet for a meal and conversation about a selected topic with a facilitator versed in mind–body therapies who could help them learn and practice new skills without attaching stigma.

Based on the active research in mindfulness, it was decided that the first get together would involve a brief introductory lecture on the topic and an opportunity to experience mindfulness as a group.

Dr. Wu was filled with dread at being laughed out of the program but agreed to meet with the mindfulness teacher, an experienced child psychiatry faculty, Dr. Ellis, who reassured him all would be well. On the evening of the first group, about 10 residents gathered for dinner, supported through the departmental educational fund. They had reserved the private dining room of a nearby restaurant. The topic for the evening was *centering*, and everyone was curious. After the meal, Dr. Ellis gave a brief overview of mindfulness and invited the residents to get comfortable in their seats. He took them through a 10-minute progressive muscle relaxation exercise to highlight the discrepancy between tension and the relaxation response—then directed them to focus on their breath. They spent several minutes simply tracking the breath, in and out, and returning their attention gently to the breath if it wandered. After the exercise, they were invited to share their experiences in pairs. The residents were hesitant at first, then the groups began talking about their experience. It was eye-opening to see his colleagues so engaged with each other, and Dr. Wu felt a great sense of relief. He too had experienced just a moment of calm centering during the exercise and was eager to practice more at home.

Dr. Ellis gave the residents some resources, including recommending Dr. Kabat-Zinn's books on mindfulness, and a very simple meditation diary so they could track their practice, if they so chose, over the next 2 weeks. He suggested practicing following the breath for a few minutes a day in a quiet place.

Resident feedback on the session was very positive and a second meeting was planned. The topic of the second meeting was understanding the difference between empathy and compassion, which has been associated with decreased burnout symptoms in health care workers.

The resident wellness program continued to grow gradually, and continued to receive departmental support for its meetings. Over time, led by the residency program director, faculty organized a similar group—and the department chair gradually acknowledged the value of the work. A MBSR course was made available to the faculty and residents. Dr. Wu and the program director wrote the program up as an abstract and submitted it to one of the large academic surgical meetings—and to their surprise the abstract was accepted for oral presentation.

MINDFULNESS: PEDIATRIC RESEARCH OVERVIEW

Mindfulness has been used successfully in children with age-appropriate modifications and may be combined with breathing exercises, music, imagery, and progressive muscle relaxation depending on the setting and age group. Young children can benefit from a sensory-rich approach to mindfulness to help engage all their senses. Teaching children and adolescents mindfulness respects their capacity for coping, supports their natural ability to pay attention in the moment, and does not try to deny what is happening—for example, if a child has faced, or is facing, a challenging life event (Section on Integrative Medicine 2016).

For example, studies of mindfulness interventions in children who have faced adverse events show that mindfulness can improve mental, emotional, and physical states. Mindfulness in these circumstances have a twofold effect, first in buffering immediate stress response and second by mitigating upregulation of the physiologic hypothalamic–pituitary–adrenal (HPA) axis associated with chronic stress and its detrimental effects (Ortiz and Sibinga 2017).

Mindfulness has shown promise in a variety of pediatric conditions, including: mental health, coping skills, self-regulation, improved self-esteem, decrease in elevated blood pressure and reduction in negative school behaviors such as absenteeism (Section on Integrative Medicine 2016).

Mindfulness has also been shown to be effective in pediatric gastrointestinal conditions, especially in irritable bowel syndrome (Yeh et al. 2017).

Ideally, parents or other caretakers can serve as role models for mindful behavior and teach children to apply a mindful approach during challenging circumstances. This can be especially helpful to help children and adolescents gain perspective and reinforces their ability to learn self-regulation skills. Cultivation of a simple daily practice can help build emotional resiliency. Examples include a gratitude or appreciation practice, sending friendly wishes to self, loved ones, neutral party, and to a difficult person (if appropriate circumstances).

Mindfulness in youth has also been successfully introduced in the school setting in a variety of situations, including in inner city programs in adolescents. Outcomes in two studies by Sibinga et al. also showed significant reduction in levels of depression, somatization, negative affect, and negative coping skills, rumination, self-hostility, and post-traumatic symptom severity (all $p < 0.05$) (Sibinga et al. 2013; Sibinga et al. 2016).

Benefit of mindfulness training has also been shown in a small pilot study in children living with HIV/AIDS (Sibinga et al. 2008) and in children when parents and teachers undergo mindfulness training (Jennings et al. 2013; Gouda et al. 2016).

CLINICAL APPLICATION: MINDFULNESS IN PEDIATRICS

Ruby is a 4 year old diagnosed with acute lymphoblastic anemic (ALL). She is about halfway through her maintenance course and is spending some time in the hospital to address some cardiac symptoms. She is fearful of being back in the hospital, and her mother is simply exhausted from the strain of the last several months. Ruby's grandmother has come up to look after her younger brother, and her father is coming back and forth as able due to job demands. Ruby's mother has taken a leave of absence from her work to care for Ruby and the family.

On initial assessment, it was determined that Ruby should likely respond to treatment after stabilization and be able to go home in 5–7 days. The nurses were concerned about

Ruby's mothers stress levels and fatigue and suggested that she might be interested in attending the parent group meeting the next day. The topic was mindfulness. The children would be meeting with one of the Child Life team and were going to learn age-appropriate mindfulness skills at the same time.

Ruby's mother was skeptical but agreed to attend. Ruby expressed some separation anxiety the next day, but when she saw the playroom and a familiar Child Life worker, she agreed to go in.

The children gathered on mats or in wheelchairs, as needed, and briefly introduced themselves.

They each chose a small new stuffed animal beanbag from a basket—theirs to keep. The teacher put on some music, and they went through a 5-minute relaxation exercise. Then the teacher showed them how to balance the small beanbag on their bellies and to make it go gently up and down with their breathing. The children thought it was very funny and practiced breathing in—pushing the animal up to the sky—then exhaling and bringing the animal back down (diaphragmatic breathing). To help with exhalation, the Child Life team used bubble wands to help the children exhale completely while watching the bubbles float away.

The teacher told them they could use this whenever they wanted, for example, if they ever felt worried or scared, and encouraged them to teach their parents how to do the breathing, using bubbles as needed.

During this time, the adults were in a meeting room learning about mindfulness, breathing, and practicing *staying in the moment*. All the caretakers and parents had children who were admitted for an oncology diagnosis, but most did not know one another. The instructor taught them a progressive muscle relaxation exercise, then asked them to focus on their breathing.

She encouraged the group to allow any thoughts that arose to pass like a cloud in the sky, notice but do not react, and return their attention to their breath. Ruby's mother could feel herself relaxing for the first time in months during the muscle relaxation exercise, and she started to tear up, overwhelmed by emotion. The instructor was very calm and reassuring. She encouraged the group to simply breathe, allowing any emotion present to simply be there, acknowledged but no need to react to it, and to return to the breath. Ruby's mother allowed herself to stay in the moment and breathe. Just for an instant, she acknowledged the enormity of what had happened but did not feel the panic and fear that had been her constant companion since Ruby's diagnosis. She allowed herself to simply breathe in the moment. On conclusion of the session, the instructor asked them to bring to mind all the parents in the group and silently repeat after her:

"May you be happy.
May you be healthy.
May you be peaceful.
May you be safe and at ease."

Ruby's mother felt a deep sense of gratitude and peace and was able to go back to her daughter with an inkling of how she wanted to approach this experience with Ruby and her family going forward. She was delighted to see that Ruby had enjoyed learning about her breathing as well, and they spent time each day practicing their new skills.

MINDFULNESS RESOURCES

Centers of study

- Center for Healthy Minds at the University of Wisconsin-Madison: https://centerhealthyminds.org/join-the-movement/well-being-tips-for-children-and- their-families:
- Child Mind Institute: https://childmind.org/article/the-power-of-mindfulness/
- The Chopra Center: http://www.chopra.com/articles/4-exercises-to-teach-your-kids-about-mindfulness-and-compassion
- Center for Mindfulness University of Massachusetts Medical School, Jon Kabat-Zinn

Apps

- Stop, Breathe, Think
- Take a Chill
- Sleep Meditations for Kids
- Mindfulness for Children

Books and websites

- *Planting Seeds: Practicing Mindfulness with Children* by Thich Nhat Hanh
- *A Still Quiet Place: A Mindfulness Program for Teaching Children and Adolescents to Ease Stress and Difficult Emotions* by Amy Saltzman and Saki Santorelli
- *The Mindful Child* by Susan Kaiser Greenland
- *The Mindfulness Revolution* edited by Barry Boyce
- *Train Your Mind, Change Your Brain* by Sharon Begley
- Stressed Teens: http://stressedteens.com
- Investigating Healthy Minds: http://investigatinghealthyminds.org
- Mindful Schools: http://mindfulschools.org
- University of Massachusetts Medical School, Center for Mindfulness, MBSR Teacher Education & Certification: https://www.umassmed.edu/cfm/training/MBSR-Teacher-Education/

References

Abbott, R. A., R. Whear, L. R. Rodgers, A. Bethel, J. Thompson Coon, W. Kuyken, K. Stein, and C. Dickens. 2014. Effectiveness of mindfulness-based stress reduction and mindfulness based cognitive therapy in vascular disease: A systematic review and meta-analysis of randomised controlled trials. *J Psychosom Res* 76 (5): 341–351. doi:10.1016/j.jpsychores.2014.02.012.

Anheyer, D., H. Haller, J. Barth, R. Lauche, G. Dobos, and H. Cramer. 2017. Mindfulness-based stress reduction for treating low back pain: A systematic review and meta-analysis. *Ann Intern Med* 166 (11): 799–807. doi:10.7326/M16-1997.

Ballou, S., and L. Keefer. 2017. Psychological interventions for irritable bowel syndrome and inflammatory bowel diseases. *Clin Transl Gastroenterol* 8 (1): e214. doi:10.1038/ctg.2016.69.

Black, D. S., and G. M. Slavich. 2016. Mindfulness meditation and the immune system: A systematic review of randomized controlled trials. *Ann N Y Acad Sci* 1373 (1): 13–24. doi:10.1111/nyas.12998.

Buchholz, L. 2015. Exploring the promise of mindfulness as medicine. *JAMA* 314 (13): 1327–1329. doi:10.1001/jama.2015.7023.

Cash, E., P. Salmon, I. Weissbecker, W. N. Rebholz, R. Bayley-Veloso, L. A. Zimmaro, A. Floyd, E. Dedert, and S. E. Sephton. 2015. Mindfulness meditation alleviates fibromyalgia symptoms in women: Results of a randomized clinical trial. *Ann Behav Med* 49 (3): 319–330. doi:10.1007/s12160-014-9665-0.

Chen, S. H., E. S. Epel, S. H. Mellon, J. Lin, V. I. Reus, R. Rosser, E. Kupferman et al. 2014. Adverse childhood experiences and leukocyte telomere maintenance in depressed and healthy adults. *J Affect Disord* 169: 86–90. doi:10.1016/j.jad.2014.07.035.

Fair, B., S. H. Mellon, E. S. Epel, J. Lin, D. Revesz, J. E. Verhoeven, B. W. Penninx et al. 2017. Telomere length is inversely correlated with urinary stress hormone levels in healthy controls but not in un-medicated depressed individuals-preliminary findings. *J Psychosom Res* 99: 177–180. doi:10.1016/j.jpsychores.2017.06.009.

Fortney, L., C. Luchterhand, L. Zakletskaia, A. Zgierska, and D. Rakel. 2013. Abbreviated mindfulness intervention for job satisfaction, quality of life, and compassion in primary care clinicians: A pilot study. *Ann Fam Med* 11 (5): 412–420. doi:10.1370/afm.1511.

Gaylord, S. A., O. S. Palsson, E. L. Garland, K. R. Faurot, R. S. Coble, J. D. Mann, W. Frey, K. Leniek, and W. E. Whitehead. 2011. Mindfulness training reduces the severity of irritable bowel syndrome in women: Results of a randomized controlled trial. *Am J Gastroenterol* 106 (9): 1678–1688. doi:10.1038/ajg.2011.184.

Goglin, S. E., R. Farzaneh-Far, E. S. Epel, J. Lin, E. H. Blackburn, and M. A. Whooley. 2016. Correction: Change in leukocyte telomere length predicts mortality in patients with stable coronary heart disease from the heart and soul study. *PLoS One* 11 (12): e0168868. doi:10.1371/journal.pone.0168868.

Gotink, R. A., R. Meijboom, M. W. Vernooij, M. Smits, and M. G. Hunink. 2016. 8-week mindfulness based stress reduction induces brain changes similar to traditional long-term meditation practice: A systematic review. *Brain Cogn* 108: 32–41. doi:10.1016/j.bandc.2016.07.001.

Gouda, S., M. T. Luong, S. Schmidt, and J. Bauer. 2016. Students and teachers benefit from mindfulness-based stress reduction in a school-embedded pilot study. *Front Psychol* 7: 590. doi:10.3389/fpsyg.2016.00590.

Goyal, M., S. Singh, E. M. Sibinga, N. F. Gould, A. Rowland-Seymour, R. Sharma, Z. Berger et al. 2014. Meditation programs for psychological stress and well-being: A systematic review and meta-analysis. *JAMA Intern Med* 174 (3): 357–368. doi:10.1001/jamainternmed.2013.13018.

Grant, J. A., J. Courtemanche, E. G. Duerden, G. H. Duncan, and P. Rainville. 2010. Cortical thickness and pain sensitivity in zen meditators. *Emotion* 10 (1): 43–53. doi:10.1037/a0018334.

Hilton, L., S. Hempel, B. A. Ewing, E. Apaydin, L. Xenakis, S. Newberry, B. Colaiaco et al. 2017. Mindfulness meditation for chronic pain: Systematic review and meta-analysis. *Ann Behav Med* 51 (2): 199–213. doi:10.1007/s12160-016-9844-2.

Hoge, E. A., M. M. Chen, E. Orr, C. A. Metcalf, L. E. Fischer, M. H. Pollack, I. De Vivo, and N. M. Simon. 2013. Loving-kindness meditation practice associated with longer telomeres in women. *Brain Behav Immun* 32: 159–163. doi:10.1016/j.bbi.2013.04.005.

Jain, S., S. L. Shapiro, S. Swanick, S. C. Roesch, P. J. Mills, I. Bell, and G. E. Schwartz. 2007. A randomized controlled trial of mindfulness meditation versus relaxation training: Effects on distress, positive states of mind, rumination, and distraction. *Ann Behav Med* 33 (1): 11–21. doi:10.1207/s15324796abm3301_2.

Jennings, P. A., J. L. Frank, K. E. Snowberg, M. A. Coccia, and M. T. Greenberg. 2013. Improving classroom learning environments by Cultivating Awareness and Resilience in Education (CARE): Results of a randomized controlled trial. *Sch Psychol Q* 28 (4): 374–390. doi:10.1037/spq0000035.

Kabat-Zinn, J., L. Lipworth, and R. Burney. 1985. The clinical use of mindfulness meditation for the self-regulation of chronic pain. *J Behav Med* 8 (2): 163–190.

Kobasa, S. C. 1979. Stressful life events, personality, and health: An inquiry into hardiness. *J Pers Soc Psychol* 37 (1): 1–11.

Kobasa, S. C., S. R. Maddi, M. C. Puccetti, and M. A. Zola. 1985. Effectiveness of hardiness, exercise and social support as resources against illness. *J Psychosom Res* 29 (5): 525–533.

Kraemer, K. M., C. M. Luberto, E. M. O'Bryan, E. Mysinger, and S. Cotton. 2016. Mind-body skills training to improve distress tolerance in medical students: A pilot study. *Teach Learn Med* 28 (2): 219–228. doi:10.1080/10401334.2016.1146605.

Last, N., E. Tufts, and L. E. Auger. 2017. The effects of meditation on grey matter atrophy and neurodegeneration: A systematic review. *J Alzheimers Dis* 56 (1): 275–286. doi:10.3233/JAD-160899.

Luders, E., and N. Cherbuin. 2016. Searching for the philosopher's stone: Promising links between meditation and brain preservation. *Ann N Y Acad Sci* 1373 (1): 38–44. doi:10.1111/nyas.13082.

Luders, E., N. Cherbuin, and F. Kurth. 2014. Forever Young(er): Potential age-defying effects of long-term meditation on gray matter atrophy. *Front Psychol* 5: 1551. doi:10.3389/fpsyg.2014.01551.

Luders, E., A. W. Toga, N. Lepore, and C. Gaser. 2009. The underlying anatomical correlates of long-term meditation: Larger hippocampal and frontal volumes of gray matter. *Neuroimage* 45 (3): 672–678.

McConville, J., R. McAleer, and A. Hahne. 2017. Mindfulness training for health profession students-the effect of mindfulness training on psychological well-being, learning and clinical performance of health professional students: A systematic review of randomized and non-randomized controlled trials. *Explore (NY)* 13 (1): 26–45. doi:10.1016/j.explore.2016.10.002.

Neilson, K., M. Ftanou, K. Monshat, M. Salzberg, S. Bell, M. A. Kamm, W. Connell et al. 2016. A controlled study of a group mindfulness intervention for individuals living with inflammatory bowel disease. *Inflamm Bowel Dis* 22 (3): 694–701. doi:10.1097/MIB.0000000000000629.

Niazi, A. K., and S. K. Niazi. 2011. Mindfulness-based stress reduction: A non-pharmacological approach for chronic illnesses. *N Am J Med Sci* 3 (1): 20–23. doi:10.4297/najms.2011.320.

Ortiz, R., and E. M. Sibinga. 2017. The role of mindfulness in reducing the adverse effects of childhood stress and trauma. *Children (Basel)* 4 (3): 16. doi:10.3390/children4030016.

Reiner, K., L. Tibi, and J. D. Lipsitz. 2013. Do mindfulness-based interventions reduce pain intensity? A critical review of the literature. *Pain Med* 14 (2): 230–242. doi:10.1111/pme.12006.

Rosenkranz, M. A., R. J. Davidson, D. G. Maccoon, J. F. Sheridan, N. H. Kalin, and A. Lutz. 2013. A comparison of mindfulness-based stress reduction and an active control in modulation of neurogenic inflammation. *Brain Behav Immun* 27 (1): 174–184. doi:10.1016/j.bbi.2012.10.013.

Rosenkranz, M. A., A. Lutz, D. M. Perlman, D. R. Bachhuber, B. S. Schuyler, D. G. MacCoon, and R. J. Davidson. 2016. Reduced stress and inflammatory responsiveness in experienced meditators compared to a matched healthy control group. *Psychoneuroendocrinology* 68: 117–125. doi:10.1016/j.psyneuen.2016.02.013.

Salzberg, S. 1995. *Loving-Kindness: The Revolutionary Art of Happiness*. Boston, MA: Shambhala Publications.

Schutte, N. S., and J. M. Malouff. 2014. A meta-analytic review of the effects of mindfulness meditation on telomerase activity. *Psychoneuroendocrinology* 42: 45–48. doi:10.1016/j.psyneuen.2013.12.017.

Section on Integrative Medicine. 2016. Mind-body therapies in children and youth. *Pediatrics* 138 (3): e6–e8.doi:10.1542/peds.2016-1896.

Shao, R., K. Keuper, X. Geng, and T. M. Lee. 2016. Pons to posterior cingulate functional projections predict affective processing changes in the elderly following eight weeks of meditation training. *EBioMedicine* 10: 236–248. doi:10.1016/j.ebiom.2016.06.018.

Sibinga, E. M., C. Perry-Parrish, S. E. Chung, S. B. Johnson, M. Smith, and J. M. Ellen. 2013. School-based mindfulness instruction for urban male youth: A small randomized controlled trial. *Prev Med* 57 (6): 799–801. doi:10.1016/j.ypmed.2013.08.027.

Sibinga, E. M., M. Stewart, T. Magyari, C. K. Welsh, N. Hutton, and J. M. Ellen. 2008. Mindfulness-based stress reduction for HIV-infected youth: A pilot study. *Explore (NY)* 4 (1): 36–37. doi:10.1016/j.explore.2007.10.002.

Sibinga, E. M., L. Webb, S. R. Ghazarian, and J. M. Ellen. 2016. School-based mindfulness instruction: An RCT. *Pediatrics* 137 (1): 1–8. doi:10.1542/peds.2015-2532.

van Dijk, I., P. L. Lucassen, and A. E. Speckens. 2015. Mindfulness training for medical students in their clinical clerkships: Two cross-sectional studies exploring interest and participation. *BMC Med Educ* 15: 24. doi:10.1186/s12909-015-0302-9.

van Dijk, I., P. Lucassen, R. P. Akkermans, B. G. M. van Engelen, C. van Weel, and A. E. M. Speckens. 2017. Effects of mindfulness-based stress reduction on the mental health of clinical clerkship students: A cluster-randomized controlled trial. *Acad Med* 92 (7): 1012–1021. doi:10.1097/ACM.0000000000001546.

West, C. P., L. N. Dyrbye, P. J. Erwin, and T. D. Shanafelt. 2016. Interventions to prevent and reduce physician burnout: A systematic review and meta-analysis. *Lancet* 388 (10057): 2272–2281. doi:10.1016/S0140-6736(16)31279-X.

West, C. P., L. N. Dyrbye, J. T. Rabatin, T. G. Call, J. H. Davidson, A. Multari, S. A. Romanski, J. M. Hellyer, J. A. Sloan, and T. D. Shanafelt. 2014. Intervention to promote physician well-being, job satisfaction, and professionalism: A randomized clinical trial. *JAMA Intern Med* 174 (4): 527–533. doi:10.1001/jamainternmed.2013.14387.

Yeh, A. M., A. Wren, and B. Golianu. 2017. Mind-body interventions for pediatric inflammatory bowel disease. *Children (Basel)* 4 (4): 22. doi:10.3390/children4040022.

9 Creative arts therapies

INTRODUCTION

Use of creative arts therapies in health care taps into the important belief that our health exceeds the sum of our physiologic parts. Embracing the World Health Organization's definition of health as complete physical, mental, and social well-being rather than absence of disease or infirmity reminds us of the complex dimensions of human health and healing and the need for tools that extend the reach beyond conventional medicines. Creative arts therapies help address elements of human suffering and capacity for resilience and joy, even when the path is very challenging (Stuckey and Nobel 2010).

The creative arts therapies comprise a range of interventions that can be used successfully in both children and adults. Common examples include music therapy, visual arts therapy, movement-based creative expression, and expressive writing. Other creative arts exist and vary by location, culture, resources, and availability of trained practitioners. Creative arts can be used in a variety of venues, including home care, outpatient, inpatient, skilled care, rehabilitation, mental health and substance abuse programs, schools, and in critical care settings—and may benefit caretakers as well as patients. The use of creative arts therapies is recognized internationally and often relies up the endorsement of multiple members of the health care team, not only to facilitate scheduling and coordination of supplies but also to lend professional endorsement and belief that the interventions provide patient value and benefit. A review by Wilson et al. on health care professionals' attitudes toward creative arts therapies reviewed 27 articles written from 2004 to 2014 and suggests that the majority of those surveyed believed that creative arts interventions had positive benefit on patients' stress, mood, sleep quality, and pain. Staff also noted improved sense of communication and rapport with patients. Feelings of staff burnout were also reduced (Wilson et al. 2016).

MUSIC THERAPY

Brief background and historical perspective

Music therapy is among the creative arts therapies with the most robust supporting research and is described by the American Music Therapy Association (AMTA) as the evidence-based use of music in the clinical setting by a credentialed music therapist. It can be used to address a range of conditions with physical, psychological, and/or social implications in patients of all ages. One of the unique factors of music therapy is that it can be used to catalyze physical and emotional change that may seem unrelated to the actual musical intervention (O'Kelly et al. 2016).

A music therapy treatment consists of a detailed individualized assessment, treatment plan, and ongoing evaluation by a trained and credentialed therapist. Patient treatment goals are set and revisited regularly. Music therapy can use instrumental or voice as primary approaches and may vary from session to session based on patient need and interests. According to the AMTA, sessions might consist of music improvisation, receptive listening, therapeutic song writing, discussion of lyrics, music and imagery, performance, or movement to music. Music therapists often function as members of inter-professional teams to support the patient's overarching goals for healing.

It is important to note that many types of music are used in music therapy, and the patient does not require any sort of musical aptitude for the therapy to be successful. Specific treatment is determined by the patient's preferences, specific health circumstances, and their goals for treatment.

Historical records from the AMTA show that modern use of music in the health care setting organized around veterans of World Wars I and II when volunteers went to veterans' hospitals to play and sing for injured and traumatized soldiers and officers. As demand grew, training programs developed, eventually leading to the first music degree program internationally being offered at Michigan State University in 1944. The AMTA was founded in 1998 resulting from the joining of the National Association for Music Therapy and the American Association for Music Therapy.

Strengths

Strengths of music therapy are its ability to be tailored to the individual patient's needs and preferences. Music therapy can be thought of as an extremely rich type of sensory stimulation with potential to access complex neural pathways using non-pharmacologic and non-invasive approaches. Music therapy also has benefit of being non-threatening and may be accepted as a treatment in patients where other approaches have been unsuccessful. It may allow patients to address stress and symptoms of anxiety, pain, and may provide a safe conduit to express challenging emotions or encourage patients or caretaker to communicate more effectively.

Potential challenges

Potential challenges include the need for a trained and credentialed practitioner and the need for appropriate equipment or instruments. Further research is also needed to fully elucidate mechanisms and applications of music therapy in the clinical setting.

Proposed mechanism of action

Functional neuroimaging studies on the impact of music on emotions have demonstrated the intricate interplay of neural networks and function. Music has been widely associated with areas of the brain involved in emotional processing including: the amygdala, hippocampus, anterior cingulate cortex, nucleus accumbens, and orbitofrontal cortex (Koelsch 2014), leading researchers to question the potential of music on emotional regulation and its possible utility in patients seeking maintenance and regulation of appropriate, goal-directed emotional targets. Advanced imaging has allowed documentation of shifts in functional connectivity and hemodynamic changes associated with changes in dopaminergic activity and other neurotransmitters associated with emotional regulation. Similarly, the hippocampus is intricately connected to a range of other brain areas affected by music and emotion (Hou et al. 2017).

Amygdala

Subcortically, the amygdala receives both auditory and sensory input and processes positive and negative stimuli (Roozendaal et al. 2009).

It has been shown to have increased functional activity and connectivity when emotion is experienced originating from exposure to music, with increased connectivity seen in some studies with exposure to joyful music as opposed to fear-inducing music (Koelsch 2014).

Hippocampus

The hippocampus plays an integral role in short- and long-term memory, spatial navigation, and emotional responses to music. Functional connectivity has been shown to increase between the hippocampus and the hypothalamus during exposure to joyful music—which subsequently is associated with neuroendocrine responses that correlate with reduced emotional stress states, an area of active study (Chanda and Levitin 2013).

Interestingly, it has been shown in some people with reduced ability to experience positive emotion, that the hippocampal volume is reduced and demonstrates reduced neuronal activity in response to music (Koelsch 2014).

Nucleus accumbens

The nucleus accumbens is part of the ventral striatum and has been strongly associated with music associated feelings of pleasure and reward, which has been associated with increased dopamine in the area with exposure to enjoyable music. Again, an increase in functional connectivity of the region to other areas associated with positive emotion has been documented on exposure to pleasant music (Hou et al. 2017).

At the level of the cortex, the anterior cingulate cortex has an important role in decision making, control of impulses, and in emotional regulation, among other things. Reactions in this area of the brain have been correlated with a variety of musical variations, both positive and less so, for example, tempo, rhythm, and major or minor chords that are associated with joyful or sad emotions (Moore 2013).

The orbitofrontal cortex is another cortical structure that has been clearly associated with activation in response to music and is involved with reward valuation and emotional regulation.

The prefrontal cortex plays a central role in emotional regulation, and the left prefrontal cortex has been shown to promote positive emotional function with exposure to joyful music, while the right prefrontal cortex promotes negative emotional functions during unpleasant music exposure (Davidson et al. 2000).

RESEARCH

Research in music therapy covers a wide range of topics. In adults, particularly active areas of research include:

- Mental health
- Dementia
- Respiratory function in people with long-term neurological conditions

Conditions where music therapy has been used successfully in adults and children:

- Respiration
- Pain (acute and chronic)
- To calm or sedate
- Sleep aid
- Counteract fear
- Aid in progressive muscle relaxation
- Physical rehabilitation—used to promote movement
- Used in elderly to enhance social, emotional, and physical function
- Headache
- Diabetes
- Obstetrics–gynecology
- Cardiac conditions
- Surgery
- Stress
- Psychiatric/mental health patients
- Positive mood changes, emotional regulation, increased sense of control, and problem solving
- Decreased length of stay
- Can increase emotional connection between patient and family
- Reduce stress in family members
- Help give structure to time spent together in the medical setting
- Bring a sense of normalcy to highly stressful times
- Overall quality of life
- Used to support physical activity
- During labor and delivery
- Special Education—can be used as part of individualized education plan
- Enhance coordination and communication skills
- Autism
- Mental health
- Vets
- Trauma, depression, and substance abuse
- Williams syndrome
- Alzheimer's
- Peri-operatively

RESEARCH OVERVIEW

Mental health

Although questions remain about its mechanism of action, music therapy has been shown to be effective in reducing symptoms of depression, anxiety, and general functioning in a randomized controlled study of 79 adult patients undergoing standard care + music therapy ($n = 33$) versus standard care alone ($n = 46$). The music therapy intervention consisted of an individualized active music therapy session with a trained music therapist for a total of 20 biweekly sessions lasting 60 minutes each. Sessions involved improvisational playing of music and direct interaction with the music therapist. The number needed to treat in the study was 4, with effect size ranging from 0.65 for depression to 0.49 for anxiety. Findings were maintained at 3-month follow-up (Erkkila et al. 2011).

A meta-analysis of 12 studies evaluating the efficacy of music therapy in patients with agitation and dementia ($n = 658$) showed that music therapy helped to decrease symptoms of restlessness, wandering, and aggressive behaviors, with a medium overall effect that the authors conclude suggests robust clinical relevance. Music was used in either active (singing, dancing, instrument playing), passive (listening to live or recorded music), or in individual sessions with a trained therapist in the included studies. Both active and passive applications were seen to be beneficial (Pedersen et al. 2017).

A Cochrane Database Systematic Review of interventions for improving psychological and physical outcomes in cancer patients included 52 trials and a total of 3,731 patients in a variety of clinical settings. Analysis showed positive reduction in anxiety in cancer patients and a moderately strong, positive impact on depression. A large pain-reducing effect was seen, as was a small positive effect on fatigue. Several studies showed significant improvement in quality of life, but this was not consistent across studies (Bradt et al. 2016).

Critical care setting

A series of additional Cochrane Database Systematic Reviews evaluating the efficacy of music therapy in mechanically ventilated adult patients showed favorable impact on reduction of anxiety and reductions in respiratory rate and systolic blood pressure readings. Reductions in sedative and analgesic dosing were also noted (Bradt and Dileo 2014; Bradt et al. 2016) and for preoperative anxiety in adults in 26 trials ($n = 2,051$) with the use of pre-recorded music as compared to controls ($p < 0.00001$; 95% CI -0.90 to -0.31, $P < 0.0001$) (Bradt et al. 2013b).

Music therapy was also shown to be of benefit in patients diagnosed with myocardial infarction with reduction in anxiety being the most significant finding in this group (95% CI -7.99 to -3.75, $P < 0.00001$, $I^2 = 53\%$).

Reductions in heart rate, respiratory rate, and systolic blood pressure were seen. Despite study heterogeneity, patients given a choice of musical selection showed the greatest effects (Bradt et al. 2013a).

Music therapy was also shown to have positive impact on anxiety, pain, and insomnia in critically ill adult patients in a review by Meghani et al. (2017).

Brain injury

An additional area showing promise is the use of music therapy in individuals with acquired brain injury. A Cochrane Review including 29 trials and 775 participants showed that music was beneficial in several symptom categories, including: gait velocity, cadence, and stride length; timing of upper extremity function; and in communication in those suffering from aphasia after stroke. Naming and speech repetition was also improved. An overall large effect in improvement in quality of life was also found. Authors note that more randomized controlled trials are needed in this area before definitive recommendations can be given, although results are encouraging (Magee et al. 2017).

Labor and delivery

Music therapy has also been shown to have a significant beneficial effect during labor and delivery. A controlled study in 156 first-time mothers ($n = 77$ music group) undergoing vaginal delivery showed that women in the treatment group experienced significantly lower pain and anxiety at all stages of labor ($p < 0.001$). Improvement in fetal heart rate and maternal hemodynamics was also seen to be significant ($P < 0.01$), and need for postpartum pain medication was also fund to be significantly decreased in the music group ($p < 0.01$) (Simavli et al. 2014).

Dental anxiety

The use of music therapy has been shown to be effective in reduction of dental anxiety in both children and adults (Mejia-Rubalcava et al. 2015; Bradt and Teague 2016).

CLINICAL APPLICATION: MUSIC THERAPY IN ADULTS

Mr. Williams is a 70-year-old formerly healthy man who had an acute myocardial infarction on the golf course. He is intubated and sedated in the cardiac intensive care unit where he has had a complex post-operative course with multiple arrhythmias. On evening rounds, the family is present and upset that Mr. Williams' monitors are repeatedly alarming. His wife feels that Mr. Williams is experiencing pain and wonders else what might be done to reduce his distress. On chart review, it appears that Mr. Williams has received the maximum doses of analgesic and sedative medications. Based on the strength of research in this area, Mr. Williams may be an excellent candidate for a trial of music therapy.

The unit has a selection of MP3 players, and after some trial and error with song choice, Mr. Williams appears to relax. His heart rate slows to normal, his breathing becomes better synchronized with the ventilator, and the family around him seems to relax as well. The music is played via headphones at a low level throughout the night, with occasional breaks. In the morning, Mr. Williams is successfully extubated and relates a feeling of calm coming over him when he heard the familiar tunes, despite the fact that he was feeling pain and disorientation from the unexpected events.

MUSIC THERAPY IN PEDIATRICS

Neonatal intensive care unit (ICU)

Music therapy has become widely used in the neonatal ICU setting. Preferred types are soothing, relatively simple music such as a lullaby or soft voice or instrumental music. Music can be played through an audio recorder in or beside the incubator or can be delivered through a pacifier activated lullaby whereby sucking motion activates a recorder. Live music such as harp or guitar music has also been used.

A systematic review of 20 studies including 1,128 babies between 24 and 40 weeks gestation evaluated exposure to live or recorded music interventions. Outcomes were grouped into several overarching groups: physiologic parameters; growth and feeding; and behavioral state, relaxation outcomes, and pain. Although study heterogeneity made definitive conclusions difficult, several positive trends were noted, including improved sleep and decreased heart rate and improvement in feeding and sucking measured by feeding rate and volumes (van der Heijden et al. 2016).

Peri-operative setting

Music has also been used in the peri-operative setting in pediatrics to good effect. For example, a randomized controlled study of 42 children aged 3–14 years undergoing day surgery examined the effect of music in the immediate post-operative period. The treatment group received music exposure using a mixture of 20 minutes of recorded slow and fast classical music versus standard care in the control group. Music exposure during the awakening period was associated with less increase in systolic and diastolic blood pressure in the treatment group and improved ratings on a standardized pain scale in the older children. The music group also showed statistically lower stress-induced hyperglycemia as compared to controls ($p < 0.001$) (Calcaterra et al. 2014).

A later systematic review and meta-analysis included three randomized controlled trials that included a total of 196 pediatric patients aged 1 day to 18 years old, undergoing orthopedic, cardiac, and day surgery. A mixture of live and recorded music was used. Although study heterogeneity was present, findings showed an overall significant positive effect on pediatric post-operative pain, anxiety, and distress in this group of patients, lending further support to the use of music in the pediatric post-operative setting (van der Heijden et al. 2015).

Autism spectrum disorder

Another area of active study is the use of music therapy to improve the quality of social interaction, particularly social emotional reciprocity, in children with autism spectrum disorder.

A 2104 Cochrane Database Systematic Review that included 10 studies involving 165 children with autism found that music therapy was superior to placebo in improving social interaction, verbal communication, initiating behavior, and social-emotional reciprocity, although larger studies are needed (Geretsegger et al. 2014).

A more recent blinded, randomized clinical trial by Bieleninik et al. evaluated the impact of music therapy in children with autism spectrum disorder aged 4–7 years. The study involved children in nine countries and included ($n = 182$) controls receiving usual care plus parental counseling and ($n = 182$) receiving usual care, parental counselling, and improvisational music therapy delivered by trained music therapists over 5 months. The median number of music therapy sessions delivered was 19. In this study, no significant difference was seen in symptom severity as measured by the Autism Diagnostic Observation Schedule between the treatment group and controls (Broder-Fingert et al. 2017).

Hematology–oncology

Music therapy has also been used in critically ill pediatric patients undergoing hematopoietic stem cell transplants. A pilot study in 24 patients up to age 16 years that exposed children to both expressive and receptive music therapy in two sessions per week as compared to controls, found that children in the treatment group had significantly reduced resting heart rates in the evenings sustained from 4 to 8 hours post-intervention ($p < 0.001$) with no significant adverse effects reported (Uggla et al. 2016).

Acute care setting

In another use of music therapy in the acute care setting, a combined Child Life music therapy intervention in children aged 4–11 years undergoing placement of an intravenous line was found to enhance adaptive coping and minimize distress based on parental evaluation using a four-question pre/post test assessment ($P < 0.05$) (Ortiz et al. 2017).

Another similar randomized controlled trial using music therapy in children aged 3–11 years undergoing intravenous line placement in the pediatric emergency department showed that those in the music treatment group showed significantly less distress ($p < 0.05$), and health care providers found it was significantly easier to place the lines in children in the treatment group, and the health care providers were more satisfied with the placement in those children (86% very satisfied) compared to control (48% satisfied) ($p = 0.02$) (Hartling et al. 2013).

EMERGING AREAS OF INTEREST

Community music therapy is an emerging area of interest in that it allows opportunity for creative expression in less formal settings and increased sense of social support, connection, self-confidence, and self-esteem. Trials are underway in patients with depression (Carr et al. 2017).

CLINICAL APPLICATION: MUSIC THERAPY IN ADOLESCENTS

Robyn is a 16-year-old girl with a recent diagnosis of Crohn's disease. She failed a trial of enteral feeding and has been admitted for treatment. She and her parents are highly anxious, and she has a history of multiple difficult phlebotomy attempts in the pediatrician's office.

This is an important moment in Robyn's care and the beginning of a new chapter that requires her to focus on successful management of a chronic illness. An opportunity exists to help Robyn and her family develop effective coping strategies that will return a sense of control. Based on the strength of current pediatric research in music therapy, Robyn is offered some techniques that she might use to help reduce her pain and worry around the treatment plan.

Both Robyn and her parents express interest, and the music therapist from the Child Life Department talks with Robyn and presents a variety of options. Robyn is fortunate to work with an experienced music therapist that day who is able to provide an interactive listening experience with music she likes while the intravenous line is placed, labs are drawn, and a thin feeding tube is placed.

Ultimately, Robyn did extremely well and was proud of herself for getting through the challenges successfully. While an inpatient, Robyn used the music therapy every day for procedures and to fall asleep. Going forward, she continued to use the music therapy when she came in for infusions or lab work. Over time, Robyn's anticipatory anxiety dampened, and she was able to adapt without allowing the anxiety to dominate her life.

Robyn's parents also benefitted from her reduction in anxiety and were relieved to see their daughter's level of fear and suffering decrease significantly.

TRAINING, CREDENTIALING, AND LICENSING

AMTA is the largest professional association in the United States for music therapy and establishes criteria for education and clinical training of music therapists. It has a widely recognized Code for Ethics and Standards of Practice for the delivery of services in music therapy. Applicants must have earned bachelor's degree or higher in music therapy from an AMTA-approved program and have a minimum entry level Music Therapy–Board Certified (MT-BC) to practice.

According to the AMTA, undergraduate coursework includes a variety of topics, including music, music therapy, biology, physiology, and social and behavioral sciences in addition to general studies. There is a requirement of 1,200 hours of fieldwork and an internship in either the educational or health care setting prior to being eligible for the national certifying exam, administered by the Certification Board for Music Therapists (CBMT), an independent, nonprofit certifying agency accredited by the National Commission for Certifying Agencies at http://www.cbmt.org. Music therapists are themselves highly skilled musicians with mastery of a range of instruments.

The National Music Therapy Registry (NMTR) lists qualified music therapy professionals with the following designations:

* Registered Music Therapist
* Certified Music Therapist
* Advanced Certified Music Therapist

MEDICARE COVERAGE

Since 1994, reimbursable service under benefits for Partial Hospitalization Programs (PHP), come under Activity Therapy.

Active treatment

If prescribed by a physician

> Be reasonable and necessary for treatment of individual's illness or injury
>
> Be goal directed and based on a documented treatment plan

The goal cannot be to maintain current level of functioning; individual must exhibit some level of improvement. The most recent Healthcare Common Procedure Coding System (HCPCS*) Code for PHP is G0176 Activity Therapy (includes music, dance, art, or play therapies not for recreation, related to care and treatment of patient's disabling mental health problems, per session).

---

* HCPCS is a standardized coding system used to identify products, supplies, and services not included in the Current Procedural Terminology (CPT) codes.

Medicaid

Coverage varies from state to state.

Private insurance coverage

Current Procedural Terminology (CPT) codes for music therapy are not discipline specific and have overlap with other health care providers for example physical, occupational, speech, and recreational therapy. Individual assessments are provided for each client, and service must be reasonable and necessary and include a goal oriented treatment plan. Prior authorization is often required. There is a range of established codes applicable to different types of visits.

RESOURCES

- American Music Therapy Association—a result of merged entities in 1998. Mission is to advance public knowledge of music therapy benefits and increase access to quality music therapy services:

  American Music Therapy Association, 8455

  Colesville Road, Suite 1000, Silver Spring, MD 20910

  Phone (301) 589-3300

  Fax (301) 589-5175

  Web: www.musictherapy.org

  Email: info@musictherapy.org

- *Journal of Music Therapy*
- *Music Therapy Perspectives*
- *International Journal of Community Music*
- *International Society for Music Education*

OTHER CREATIVE ARTS THERAPIES

Visual arts

Use of the visual arts can help people express emotions that may be too difficult or painful to put into words and can help people gain insight into their illness. It may also provide an avenue for processing grief or loss. Working with textures, such as with modeling clay, or with textiles may also help reach different areas of connection or facilitate emotional release through somatic experience. Studies have shown that working with visual arts (textiles, cards, collage, pottery, watercolor, oil, acrylics, and others) can help remove the focus from the illness temporarily, may enhance sense of self worth, help maintain a sense of social identity despite even a devastating illness, and can help them express feelings in a symbolic manner (Stuckey and Nobel 2010).

An innovative artist-led creative arts program (Arts-in-Medicine) was instituted in a dialysis unit where patients, technicians, nurses, and physicians overwhelmingly reported positive impact on the unit. At 6-month follow-up, participating patients ($n = 46$) showed a significant improvement in symptom scores (including weight, serum carbon dioxide levels, phosphate levels) and a trend toward decreased depression ($p = 0.07$). Social functioning was improved, and pain scores were reduced overall ($p = 0.04$) (Ross et al. 2006).

Creative arts programs have also benefitted caregivers of adult cancer patients. Forty caregivers participated in a variety of creative arts activities designed to be completed at the patient bedside. Measurements of stress, anxiety, and positive-negative affect showed improvements in short-term well-being and increases in positive communications with the cancer patients and with the health care teams (Walsh et al. 2004).

Creative movement can be used as a therapy intervention in both children and adults. For example, a dance and movement class was shown to benefit breast cancer survivors ($n = 35$) who completed a 12-week randomized control trial with wait-list intervention focused on healing and dance movements. Quality of life, shoulder range of motion, and body image all showed significant improvement in group members (Sandel et al. 2005).

Emerging research in movement therapy in children involves testing of computer game-based movement to encourage balance, mobility, problem solving, and gross and fine motor control (Kanitkar et al. 2017).

Expressive writing

Expressive writing has been used in medicine in a variety of ways, including the use of focused writing on an important emotional issue which has been shown in a number of studies to improve immune function and decrease blood pressure and other stress-related markers (Campbell and Pennebaker 2003).

Other examples of creative writing include the use of directed writing to express anger in the face of chronic illness. In a group of 102 chronic pain patients ($n = 51$ anger expression group), patients in a 9-week writing program showed greater improvements in pain control and depressed mood than the control group and found greater meaning in their symptoms over time (Graham et al. 2008).

Expressive writing has also been used in adult HIV-infected patients and has been shown to reduce HIV viral loads in small studies as compared to controls (Petrie et al. 2004).

Poetry and journaling are other forms of written expression that have been shown to be healing, for health care providers as well as for patients (Coulehan and Clary 2005).

Journaling has been used in the senior population and in survivors of childhood sexual abuse as a way to help patients identify feelings, and use creative approaches to describe and process abusive and traumatic experiences (Stuckey and Nobel 2010).

Creative play

Creative play therapy can be instrumental in reduction of uncertainly, anxiety, and fear in pediatrics. It can incorporate movement and allow children a chance to practice procedures, such as venipuncture, using puppets or dolls (Li et al. 2016). Some hospitals incorporate play interventions to help prepare children for surgery or other procedures (William Li et al. 2007; He et al. 2015).

Animal-assisted therapy

The benefits of animal companionship are widely recognized and include reduction in loneliness and increased regular physical activity. One survey study in 643 children, mean age 6.7 years, in a primary pediatric care setting found that the presence of a pet dog in the home was associated with statistically decreased probability of pediatric anxiety ($p = 0.01$). Animal-assisted therapy is also used frequently in the pediatric population to reduce feelings of stress, pain, and fear as well as to facilitate positive communication between patient, family, and the health care team (Goddard and Gilmer 2015).

Equine therapy is an approach finding wide acceptance in the autistic population where it has been found to benefit children in a variety of ways, including improved social functioning and improved problem-solving skills (Borgi et al. 2016).

For example, in one randomized controlled trial of 116 children with autism ($n = 58$ treatment group), those participating in a 10-week equine therapy program were found to have significant improvements in irritability ($p = 0.02$), social cognition ($p = 0.05$), and social communication ($p = 0.003$). The total number of words and total number of new words spoken were also significant ($p = 0.01$ each) (Gabriels et al. 2015).

Animal-assisted therapy is also used in adult inpatient and palliative care settings and has been shown to have a beneficial effect on mood and stress reduction, enhancement of socialization, decreased loneliness, and overall improvement in sense of well-being (Munoz Lasa et al. 2011; MacDonald and Barrett 2016).

Clinical application: Equine therapy

Jason is a 7-year-old boy with a diagnosis of autism spectrum disorder who has been having a particularly hard time in school this year. He was placed in a part-time mainstream class but experienced repeated bullying and difficulty connecting with classmates. Over the course of the year, he appears to have lost ground verbally and is beginning to exhibit increasing school resistance. Multiple parent teacher conferences have shown the parents that Jason's teacher feels overwhelmed and unsure of how best to accommodate Jason in class. The parents are concerned.

Based on the emerging body of evidence supporting equine therapy in autism, a trial is suggested, and Jason expresses interest. The following week, parents report that the first session went well, and Jason was able to mount the pony with help from the highly experienced staff. He watched the other children take their lessons and expressed a desire to return for another ride. Over the course of the summer, Jason went weekly and regained vocabulary he had extinguished and learned several new words related to control of the pony such as "go," "whoa," and "walk." In addition, he very gradually established a trusting relationship with the lead teacher/therapist who was able to encourage Jason to speak up for himself when the pony was not following his command and to praise the pony when it did as it was asked. One of the most significant benefits parents reported was the bond that developed between Jason and the pony. They said they had never seen Jason spontaneously hug another person or animal, and now he ended every lesson by giving the pony a hug—and a carrot.

Based on conversations with the medical team, parents, and the lead therapist, it was decided that Jason would be better served in a different school placement in the upcoming school year and that he would greatly benefit from ongoing equine therapy.

RESOURCES

• National Coalition of Creative Arts Therapies Associations: http://www.nccata.org

Founded in 1979, represents 15,000 individual members of seven creative arts therapies associations in the United States:

• American Music Therapy Association: https://www.musictherapy.org/
• American Dance Therapy Association: https://adta.org/

- American Art Therapy Association: https://arttherapy.org/
- North American Drama Therapy Association: http://www.nadta.org/
- National Association of Poetry Therapy: http://poetrytherapy.org/
- American Society for Group Psychotherapy and Psychodrama: http://www.asgpp.org/
- University of Florida General Arts in Medicine Program: http://arts.ufl.edu/academics/center-for-arts-in-medicine/

References

American Music Therapy Association. Retrieved from https://www.musictherapy.org/.

Borgi, M., D. Loliva, S. Cerino, F. Chiarotti, A. Venerosi, M. Bramini, E. Nonnis et al. 2016. Effectiveness of a standardized equine-assisted therapy program for children with autism spectrum disorder. *J Autism Dev Disord* 46 (1): 1–9. doi:10.1007/s10803-015-2530-6.

Bradt, J., and C. Dileo. 2014. Music interventions for mechanically ventilated patients. *Cochrane Database Syst Rev* (12): CD006902. doi:10.1002/14651858.CD006902.pub3.

Bradt, J., C. Dileo, L. Magill, and A. Teague. 2016. Music interventions for improving psychological and physical outcomes in cancer patients. *Cochrane Database Syst Rev* (8): CD006911. doi:10.1002/14651858.CD006911.pub3.

Bradt, J., C. Dileo, and N. Potvin. 2013a. Music for stress and anxiety reduction in coronary heart disease patients. *Cochrane Database Syst Rev* (12): CD006577. doi:10.1002/14651858.CD006577.pub3.

Bradt, J., C. Dileo, and M. Shim. 2013b. Music interventions for preoperative anxiety. *Cochrane Database Syst Rev* (6): CD006908. doi:10.1002/14651858.CD006908.pub2.

Bradt, J., and A. Teague. 2016. Music interventions for dental anxiety. *Oral Dis*. doi:10.1111/odi.12615.

Broder-Fingert, S., E. Feinberg, and M. Silverstein. 2017. Music therapy for children with autism spectrum disorder. *JAMA* 318 (6): 523–524. doi:10.1001/jama.2017.9477. Oral Dis. Apr 24 (3): 300–306.

Calcaterra, V., S. Ostuni, I. Bonomelli, S. Mencherini, M. Brunero, E. Zambaiti, S. Mannarino et al. 2014. Music benefits on postoperative distress and pain in pediatric day care surgery. *Pediatr Rep* 6 (3): 5534. doi:10.4081/pr.2014.5534.

Campbell, R. S., and J. W. Pennebaker. 2003. The secret life of pronouns: Flexibility in writing style and physical health. *Psychol Sci* 14 (1): 60–65. doi:10.1111/1467-9280.01419.

Carr, C. E., J. O'Kelly, S. Sandford, and S. Priebe. 2017. Feasibility and acceptability of group music therapy vs. wait-list control for treatment of patients with long-term depression (the SYNCHRONY trial): Study protocol for a randomised controlled trial. *Trials* 18 (1): 149. doi:10.1186/s13063-017-1893-8.

Chanda, M. L., and D. J. Levitin. 2013. The neurochemistry of music. *Trends Cogn Sci* 17 (4): 179–193. doi:10.1016/j.tics.2013.02.007.

Coulehan, J., and P. Clary. 2005. Healing the healer: Poetry in palliative care. *J Palliat Med* 8 (2): 382–389. doi:10.1089/jpm.2005.8.382.

Davidson, R. J., D. C. Jackson, and N. H. Kalin. 2000. Emotion, plasticity, context, and regulation: Perspectives from affective neuroscience. *Psychol Bull* 126 (6): 890–909.

Erkkila, J., M. Punkanen, J. Fachner, E. Ala-Ruona, I. Pontio, M. Tervaniemi, M. Vanhala, and C. Gold. 2011. Individual music therapy for depression: Randomised controlled trial. *Br J Psychiatry* 199 (2): 132–139. doi:10.1192/bjp.bp.110.085431.

Gabriels, R. L., Z. Pan, B. Dechant, J. A. Agnew, N. Brim, and G. Mesibov. 2015. Randomized controlled trial of therapeutic horseback riding in children and adolescents with autism spectrum disorder. *J Am Acad Child Adolesc Psychiatry* 54 (7): 541–549. doi:10.1016/j.jaac.2015.04.007.

Geretsegger, M., C. Elefant, K. A. Mossler, and C. Gold. 2014. Music therapy for people with autism spectrum disorder. *Cochrane Database Syst Rev* (6): CD004381. doi:10.1002/14651858.CD004381.pub3.

Goddard, A. T., and M. J. Gilmer. 2015. The role and impact of animals with pediatric patients. *Pediatr Nurs* 41 (2): 65–71.

Graham, J. E., M. Lobel, P. Glass, and I. Lokshina. 2008. Effects of written anger expression in chronic pain patients: Making meaning from pain. *J Behav Med* 31 (3): 201–212. doi:10.1007/s10865-008-9149-4.

Hartling, L., A. S. Newton, Y. Liang, H. Jou, K. Hewson, T. P. Klassen, and S. Curtis. 2013. Music to reduce pain and distress in the pediatric emergency department: A randomized clinical trial. *JAMA Pediatr* 167 (9): 826–835. doi:10.1001/jamapediatrics.2013.200.

He, H. G., L. Zhu, S. W. Chan, P. Klainin-Yobas, and W. Wang. 2015. The effectiveness of therapeutic play intervention in reducing perioperative anxiety, negative behaviors, and postoperative pain in children undergoing elective surgery: A systematic review. *Pain Manag Nurs* 16 (3): 425–439. doi:10.1016/j.pmn.2014.08.011.

Hou, J., B. Song, A. C. N. Chen, C. Sun, J. Zhou, H. Zhu, and T. P. Beauchaine. 2017. Review on neural correlates of emotion regulation and music: Implications for emotion dysregulation. *Front Psychol* 8: 501. doi:10.3389/fpsyg.2017.00501.

Kanitkar, A., T. Szturm, S. Parmar, D. B. Gandhi, G. R. Rempel, G. Restall, M. Sharma et al. 2017. The effectiveness of a computer game-based rehabilitation platform for children with cerebral palsy: Protocol for a randomized clinical trial. *JMIR Res Protoc* 6 (5): e93. doi:10.2196/resprot.6846.

Koelsch, S. 2014. Brain correlates of music-evoked emotions. *Nat Rev Neurosci* 15 (3): 170–180. doi:10.1038/nrn3666.

Li, W. H., J. O. Chung, K. Y. Ho, and B. M. Kwok. 2016. Play interventions to reduce anxiety and negative emotions in hospitalized children. *BMC Pediatr* 16: 36. doi:10.1186/s12887-016-0570-5.

MacDonald, J. M., and D. Barrett. 2016. Companion animals and well-being in palliative care nursing: A literature review. *J Clin Nurs* 25 (3–4): 300–310. doi:10.1111/jocn.13022.

Magee, W. L., I. Clark, J. Tamplin, and J. Bradt. 2017. Music interventions for acquired brain injury. *Cochrane Database Syst Rev* 1: CD006787. doi:10.1002/14651858.CD006787.pub3.

Meghani, N., M. F. Tracy, N. N. Hadidi, and R. Lindquist. 2017. Part I: The effects of music for the symptom management of anxiety, pain, and insomnia in critically ill patients: An integrative review of current literature. *Dimens Crit Care Nurs* 36 (4): 234–243. doi:10.1097/DCC.0000000000000254.

Mejia-Rubalcava, C., J. Alanis-Tavira, H. Mendieta-Zeron, and L. Sanchez-Perez. 2015. Changes induced by music therapy to physiologic parameters in patients with dental anxiety. *Complement Ther Clin Pract* 21 (4): 282–286. doi:10.1016/j.ctcp.2015.10.005.

Moore, K. S. 2013. A systematic review on the neural effects of music on emotion regulation: Implications for music therapy practice. *J Music Ther* 50 (3): 198–242.

Munoz Lasa, S., G. Ferriero, E. Brigatti, R. Valero, and F. Franchignoni. 2011. Animal-assisted interventions in internal and rehabilitation medicine: A review of the recent literature. *Panminerva Med* 53 (2): 129–136.

O'Kelly, J., J. C. Fachner, and M. Tervaniemi. 2016. Editorial: Dialogues in music therapy and music neuroscience: Collaborative understanding driving clinical advances. *Front Hum Neurosci* 10: 585. doi:10.3389/fnhum.2016.00585.

Ortiz, G. S., T. O'Connor, J. Carey, A. Vella, A. Paul, D. Rode, and A. Weinberg. 2017. Impact of a child life and music therapy procedural support intervention on parental perception of their child's distress during intravenous placement. *Pediatr Emerg Care*. pp. 1–8. doi:10.1097/PEC.0000000000001065.

Pedersen, S. K. A., P. N. Andersen, R. G. Lugo, M. Andreassen, and S. Sutterlin. 2017. Effects of music on agitation in dementia: A meta-analysis. *Front Psychol* 8: 742. doi:10.3389/fpsyg.2017.00742.

Petrie, K. J., I. Fontanilla, M. G. Thomas, R. J. Booth, and J. W. Pennebaker. 2004. Effect of written emotional expression on immune function in patients with human immunodeficiency virus infection: A randomized trial. *Psychosom Med* 66 (2): 272–275.

Roozendaal, B., B. S. McEwen, and S. Chattarji. 2009. Stress, memory and the amygdala. *Nat Rev Neurosci* 10 (6): 423–433. doi:10.1038/nrn2651.

Ross, E. A., T. L. Hollen, and B. M. Fitzgerald. 2006. Observational study of an arts-in-medicine program in an outpatient hemodialysis unit. *Am J Kidney Dis* 47 (3): 462–468. doi:10.1053/j.ajkd.2005.11.030.

Sandel, S. L., J. O. Judge, N. Landry, L. Faria, R. Ouellette, and M. Majczak. 2005. Dance and movement program improves quality-of-life measures in breast cancer survivors. *Cancer Nurs* 28 (4): 301–309.

Simavli, S., I. Gumus, I. Kaygusuz, M. Yildirim, B. Usluogullari, and H. Kafali. 2014. Effect of music on labor pain relief, anxiety level and postpartum analgesic requirement: A randomized controlled clinical trial. *Gynecol Obstet Invest* 78 (4): 244–250. doi:10.1159/000365085.

Stuckey, H. L., and J. Nobel. 2010. The connection between art, healing, and public health: A review of current literature. *Am J Public Health* 100 (2): 254–263. doi:10.2105/AJPH.2008.156497.

Uggla, L., L. O. Bonde, B. M. Svahn, M. Remberger, B. Wrangsjo, and B. Gustafsson. 2016. Music therapy can lower the heart rates of severely sick children. *Acta Paediatr* 105 (10): 1225–1230. doi:10.1111/apa.13452.

van der Heijden, M. J., S. Oliai Araghi, J. Jeekel, I. K. Reiss, M. G. Hunink, and M. van Dijk. 2016. Do hospitalized premature infants benefit from music interventions? A systematic review of randomized controlled trials. *PLoS One* 11 (9): e0161848. doi:10.1371/journal.pone.0161848.

van der Heijden, M. J., S. Oliai Araghi, M. van Dijk, J. Jeekel, and M. G. Hunink. 2015. The effects of perioperative music interventions in pediatric surgery: A systematic review and meta-analysis of randomized controlled trials. *PLoS One* 10 (8): e0133608. doi:10.1371/journal.pone.0133608.

Walsh, S. M., S. C. Martin, and L. A. Schmidt. 2004. Testing the efficacy of a creative-arts intervention with family caregivers of patients with cancer. *J Nurs Scholarsh* 36 (3): 214–219.

William Li, H. C., V. Lopez, and T. L. Lee. 2007. Effects of preoperative therapeutic play on outcomes of school-age children undergoing day surgery. *Res Nurs Health* 30 (3): 320–332. doi:10.1002/nur.20191.

Wilson, C., H. Bungay, C. Munn-Giddings, and M. Boyce. 2016. Healthcare professionals' perceptions of the value and impact of the arts in healthcare settings: A critical review of the literature. *Int J Nurs Stud* 56: 90–101. doi:10.1016/j.ijnurstu.2015.11.003.

10 Movement therapies

INTRODUCTION: A FOCUS ON YOGA

This chapter on movement therapies emphasizes yoga as it currently has the most compelling evidence. Other movement therapies such as dance therapy are mentioned in Chapter 9—"Creative Arts Therapies."

Yoga is an ancient practice with a rapidly growing body of supporting research for efficacy in modern medicine. Traditionally viewed in the realm of the East, yoga practice is becoming more mainstream as its beneficial physiologic effects are recognized. Descriptions of yoga often include translation from Sanskrit which is said to be "union" from the Sanskrit root "yuj" which translates roughly as "to unite" and is thought to capture the full dimension of yoga practice which encompasses physical, mental, and spiritual components working together to promote optimal health. This combination gives yoga unique potential to address complex illnesses such as chronic pain using a multidimensional approach to healing by decreasing sympathetic nervous system activation, improving tissue perfusion and physical flexibility, and facilitating positive emotions, heightened self-awareness, and improved sense of self-efficacy (Posadzki et al. 2011).

One of most widely recognized classic texts on yoga is called the *Yoga Sutras of Patanjali*, written by a second century Indian sage who recorded a pattern of ideas and practices that are still used today (Rosen et al. 2015).

In Patanjali's work, eight paths are outlined that are used to prepare the practitioner. The first two paths are used to outline and reinforce moral guidelines and principles for healthy living; the next two introduce the physical practice of asana (postures) and pranayama (breathing). These first four paths are considered preparation for more advanced meditation techniques discussed in the final four paths which focus on attention and awakening of consciousness through concentration and practice until enlightenment occurs. Although there are many variations of yoga practices, for example, kundalini, tantra, and others, the traditional yogic practices have a common theme of breath control (pranayama), meditation (dharana and dhyana), use of specific body postures (asana), and self-reflective practices (Stephens 2017).

In the United States, data from the 2012 National Health Interview Survey ($n = 34{,}525$) showed that approximately 31 million adults had ever used yoga, and approximately 21 million had practiced yoga in the prior year. Reasons given for its use included general wellness and disease prevention (78.4%), to improve energy (66.1%), or to improve immune function

(49.7%). The primary medical conditions identified for yoga use included back pain (19.7%), stress (6.4%), and arthritis (6.4%) (Cramer et al. 2016).

In modern practice, medical yoga can be prescribed by clinicians and is used to promote well-being and to address specific physical, mental, or emotional challenges. Similar to the vast majority of complementary and integrative practices, yoga in the medical setting is used to enhance rather than compete with conventional therapies and emphasizes a proactive approach to healthy living. This might include mindful eating, restful sleep, healthy social interactions, and consistent self-care of mind, body, and spirit. It is important to note that medical yoga differs from a typical community yoga class. A trained yoga therapist has undergone specific training in order to introduce yoga in the clinical setting.

The benefits of individualized yoga therapy include the practitioner's ability to tailor treatments and address weakness, imbalance, or gaps in the patient's care. Early intervention may help prevent injury and enhance the patient's sense of self efficacy and self-control. Other overarching benefits of yoga include a low prevalence of adverse effects in most age groups. A longitudinal survey of yoga-associated injuries in adults in the United States based on data from the National Electronic Injury Surveillance System from 2001 to 2014 showed that 29,590 yoga-related injuries were evaluated in emergency departments, with adults over 65 years recording the highest prevalence (57.9/100,000) as compared to those 18–44 years (11.9/100,000). Most injuries were recorded as strain or sprain, with the trunk being the primary location of injury (Swain and McGwin 2016).

Minimal equipment requirements, relative cost effectiveness, and flexibility of use are other strengths.

Breath: An important healing component of yoga

One of the particular strengths of yoga is the focus on breath (pranayama). Emerging research has emphasized this as one of only two physiologic conduits to both the voluntary and involuntary nervous systems. Eye blink is the other. Most patients, regardless of the medical condition, can learn breath work exercises. Mastery of the breath brings the patient a lever of control over the parasympathetic nervous system and allows them a non-pharmacologic option to reduce stress by triggering the physiologic relaxation response, decreasing blood pressure, heart rate, respiratory rate, and stress hormones. A small controlled study by Twal et al. in 20 adults ($n = 10$ treatment group) showed a significant decrease in levels of inflammatory interleukin cytokines ($p < 0.05$) in the treatment group who engaged in two types of yogic breathing for 10 minutes each. Salivary samples were collected pre, during, and after completion of the exercises (Twal et al. 2016).

One hypothesis suggests that voluntary long, slow, deep breaths activate stretch-induced inhibitory signals in the lungs which trigger modulation of the nervous system, stimulating the parasympathetic nervous system and slowing respiratory and heart rate (Jerath et al. 2006).

A review by Nivethitha et al. on the physiologic effects of a variety of breath exercises found overall positive findings on both cardiovascular and autonomic measurements, including improved heart rate variability, decreased blood pressure, and decreased sympathetic tone. Studies examining the specific breathing exercises, such as alternating nostril yogic breathing, were too small and heterogeneous to allow definitive condition-specific recommendations. Positive physiologic findings were recorded for slow pranayama practices but were less favorable for rapid or bellows breathing techniques. These are discussed in more detail in Chapter 5 (Nivethitha et al. 2016).

Challenges

Yoga therapy may be unfamiliar to some and perceived as outside the normal practice of medicine. Medical yoga requires a trained teacher which may not be available or feasible depending on local resources. Some people may be uncomfortable or self-conscious about the idea of movement therapies or experience worsening of their pain, stiffness, or discomfort related to their medical condition or to trying a new exercise.

Yoga and stress

A growing number of studies support the use of yoga in addressing stress, although many questions remain, and the mechanism is highly likely to be multifactorial. A systematic review of the literature by Riley and Park (2015) identified a variety of psychological and biological factors that have been examined as potential contributing factors. Those with some evidence for enhancing stress reduction in this review included: improvement in the positive effect, presence of mindfulness and self-compassion, inhibition of activity in the posterior hypothalamus associated with decreased blood pressure, and reduction in biomarkers such as salivary cortisol, interleukin-6, and C-reactive protein. The authors stress that larger and more rigorous studies are needed to determine specific mechanisms.

An important component of yoga is meditation, which has itself been shown to have an important range of physiologic benefits, including increased telomerase activity associated with increased telomere length. This was demonstrated in a seminal study by Ornish et al. in which a program of comprehensive lifestyle changes that included yoga, meditation, and a plant-based diet. In this pilot study, 24 men with low-risk prostate cancer were followed to see if a 3-month program of intensive lifestyle change resulted in increased telomerase activity. Participants showed increased peripheral blood mononuclear cell telomerase activity ($p = 0.031$), as well as a decrease in psychological distress ($p = 0.047$), and a decrease in LDL-cholesterol ($p = 0.041$) (Ornish et al. 2008).

A 5-year follow-up study of these participants showed the persistence of increased telomerase activity and telomere length over age-matched controls (Ornish et al. 2013).

Another small randomized controlled trial in 25 university students ($n = 13$ treatment group) examined the effect of yoga on markers of physiologic stress. Students in the yoga group practiced with an instructor for 90 minutes weekly for 12 weeks and were asked to do daily home practice for 40 minutes with the aid of a DVD. The practices consisted of the three typical arms of yogic practice (pranayama, asanas, meditation). Fasting blood samples were taken at 0 and 12 weeks to compare levels of immune-related cytokines, stress hormones, and antioxidants. Results showed a significant reduction in serum levels of nitric oxide, F2-isoprostane, and lipid peroxide ($p < 0.05$ or $p = 0.01$) and a significant increase in immune-related cytokines interleukin-12, and interferon-γ, in serum ($p < 0.05$ or $p = 0.01$). Yoga practice also significantly reduced the plasma levels of adrenalin ($p < 0.05$) and increased plasma levels of serotonin compared with the control group ($p < 0.05$) (Lim and Cheong 2015).

A more recent, open label, prospective study in 96 healthy adults examined the impact of a 12-week yoga- and meditation-based lifestyle intervention on cellular aging. Measurements included telomerase activity, telomerase length, oxidative stress markers, total antioxidant capacity, and evidence of DNA damage through 8-hydroxy-2'-deoxyguanosine. Other endpoints measured included beta-endorphin, interleukin-6, and brain-derived neurotrophic factor (BDNF). Participants had an initial 2-week onsite training consisting of an integrated yoga and meditation based lifestyle intervention program delivered on 5 days per week, the remaining 10 weeks of the program were home-based practice, 90 minutes per day. Elements included asanas (physical postures or poses), pranayama (breathing exercises), and meditation. Home practice was monitored through a diary and phone monitoring. Blood biomarkers were checked on day 0 and at 12 weeks. Ninety-four subjects completed the study. Results showed statistically significant increase in telomerase activity and total antioxidant capacity and lowering of oxidative stress markers, all $p < 0.05$. Mean levels of cortisol and interleukin-6 were significantly lower ($p < 0.05$), and beta-endorphin and BDNF were also significantly increased ($p < 0.05$). Body mass index was also significantly decreased in the group ($P < 0.01$) (Tolahunase et al. 2017).

The effects of yoga have also been evaluated in an extended retreat setting in a study by Cahn et al. in 38 adults. The retreat included daily meditation and yoga practice, vegetarian diet, and participation in community projects around the retreat center. Daily activities included 2 hours of sitting meditation, 1–2 hours of yoga practice which had a meditation component, and 1 hour of chanting. Subjects had increases in self-reported mindfulness ($p < 0.0001$) and decreases in reported anxiety ($p < 0.0001$) and depression ($p < 0.01$). Measures of BDNF (associated with enhanced neurogenesis/neuroplasticity) increased by threefold ($p < 0.001$) and were inversely associated with anxiety scores in pre-retreat ($p < 0.05$, $r = 0.40$) and post-retreat ($p < 0.005$, $r = 0.52$) samples. Body mass index decreased in the group ($p < 0.0001$). Changes in pro-inflammatory markers were mixed, with some decreasing significantly, such as the pro-inflammatory IL-12 ($p < 0.05$) whereas other such as IL-6 increased. Significant increases in cortisol awakening response were seen, reflecting the improved rhythm of adrenocortical activity which is related to enhanced levels of alertness and physiologic arousal, considered a positive marker of stress resilience (Cahn et al. 2017).

The length of optimal treatment for stress using yoga is an unanswered question. One study by Yadav et al. in 86 patients with chronic inflammatory diseases included only 2 hours of yoga, theory, and practice, on each of 10 days. Significant reductions were seen in plasma cortisol ($p = 0.001$) and in interleukin-6 ($p = 0.36$), with an increase in beta-endorphin from baseline to day 10 ($p = 0.024$). The program consisted of asanas, pranayama, stress management, discussions, lectures, and individualized health advice (Yadav et al. 2012).

RESEARCH OVERVIEW

Pain

Over the past decade, yoga has been evaluated by a number of investigators for its efficacy in pain management. A 2011 systematic review evaluated 10 randomized clinical trials evaluating the use of yoga for pain in 492 patients (adults and adolescents) with a range of pain symptoms. Authors found high study heterogeneity in length of treatment, type of yoga used, and duration and frequency of interventions. Common factors included specific stretching exercises, breath work, relaxation exercises, and specific postures to align the body (asanas). No serious adverse events were reported. Overall, authors found a promising suggestion for the use of yoga in pain but fell short of specific recommendations due to a lack of compelling evidence and called for further work in this area (Posadzki et al. 2011).

A more recent comprehensive review of recent literature on the use of yoga in the medical setting by Field included a wide range of psychiatric and medical conditions (pregnancy, pre- and postnatal depression, stress, post-traumatic stress disorder, anxiety, obesity, cardiovascular disease, hypertension, arthritis, headache, low back pain, asthma, type 2 diabetes, HIV, breast cancer, balance, osteoporosis, and Parkinson's disease). While benefit was seen in most conditions, again, small sample size, lack of active control groups, and heterogeneity of types of yoga practice limited definitive conclusions in many studies (Field 2016).

One area showing greater promise is in the use of yoga in low back pain in adults. Clinical guidelines for treatment of low back pain by the American College of Physicians recommend a variety of non-pharmacologic approaches, including yoga (Qaseem et al. 2017).

A randomized trial of yoga for adults with chronic low back pain ($n = 156$ treatment group) versus usual care ($n = 157$) found that those in the treatment group who undertook a 12-class, 3-month program in yoga reported better back function at 3, 6, and 12 months compared to the control group.

Those in the yoga group also reported an increased sense of self-efficacy at months 3 and 6, although not at month 12. Twelve of the 156 patients in the yoga group experienced an adverse event (increased pain) in this study group versus 2 of 157 in the control group (Tilbrook et al. 2011).

A systematic review by Cramer et al. evaluated 10 randomized controlled trials with a total of 967 patients with a history of chronic low back pain found strong evidence for short-term effectiveness and moderate supporting evidence for the use of yoga in these patients when used as an additional therapy in their treatment. No studies reported serious adverse events (Cramer et al. 2013).

Other conditions where yoga has been shown to be useful in the clinical setting are discussed below.

Depression

A systematic review of the role of yoga as an add-on therapy in the treatment of major depressive disorder offered some insight into potential mechanisms of action. Authors found supporting evidence in five studies to support links between increased mindfulness and decreased rumination. Three studies correlated yoga therapy with alterations in cortisol, increase in BDNF, and improved heart rate variability. Authors note the need for larger studies with rigorous designs to gain further understanding of the involved mechanisms (Meister and Juckel 2017).

Another randomized controlled trial compared a series of 10 weekly yoga classes ($n = 63$) to healthy living education classes ($n = 59$) in adults with a history of depression and antidepressant medication use. Follow-up of depressive symptoms was done at week 10 and 3 and 6 months post intervention. No change was seen in the first evaluation at 10 weeks, but at 6-month follow-up, 51% of the yoga treatment group showed a 50% reduction in depressive symptoms as compared to 31% of the control group. (odds ratio = 2.31; $p = 0.04$). Additional benefits in the yoga group included improved social functioning and more positive general health perceptions consistent with accumulating benefits over time (Uebelacker et al. 2017).

And a prospective randomized pilot study of 38 adults with a diagnosis of major depression was randomized to 90-minute hatha yoga twice weekly for 8 weeks ($n = 18$) versus education groups as a control. Classes were led by certified yoga instructors at a university-based clinic. At the 8-week endpoint, those in the yoga group had a significant improvement in Beck Depression Inventory-II scores as compared to controls ($p = 0.034$) and were more likely to achieve remission; effect size was large per Cohen's $d = -0.96$ (95% CI, -1.81 to -0.12) (Prathikanti et al. 2017).

A further randomized controlled study in adults with depression examined the most effective *dose* of yoga and coherent breathing, comparing effects of two 90-minute yoga classes ($n = 15$ low dose) versus three weekly classes ($n = 15$ high dose). In the study, a significant reduction in depressive symptoms was seen in both groups, with a slightly higher percentage in the high dose group exhibiting Beck Depression Inventory–II scores at or below 10 at week 12 (Streeter et al. 2017).

Breast cancer

A small randomized study in breast cancer survivors with persistent fatigue evaluated the effect of a 12-week Iyengar yoga program on inflammation-related gene expression and inflammatory cytokines. The treatment group ($n = 16$) showed a reduction in the pro-inflammatory transcription factor nuclear factor kappa B (NF-kB) and in markers of tumor necrosis factor, both ($p < 0.05$). No changes in IL-6, C reactive protein, or diurnal cortisol were seen. A significant increase in the expression of genes associated with glucocorticoid responsiveness was seen—authors hypothesized that glucocorticoid receptors may become more sensitive to the anti-inflammatory effects of cortisol, subsequently leading to decreased inflammatory signaling, rather than decreased in cortisol levels. Results in this study also showed down-regulation of genes involved in interferon-related transcription factors which may be related to fatigue in cancer treatment (Bower et al. 2014).

A 2017 Cochrane Database Systematic Review involving 23 studies and 2,166 participants with breast cancer found benefit of yoga for improving health-related quality of life, reduction of fatigue, and improved sleep, as well as reducing symptoms of depression, fatigue, and anxiety as compared to educational or psychosocial interventions (Cramer et al. 2017).

A small study ($n = 17$) examining the benefit of yoga in adults with rheumatoid arthritis in the community setting identified several positive themes, including improvement in physical and psychologic symptoms related to the diagnosis of rheumatoid arthritis, including stretching, strengthening, stress management, and positive support from instructors (Greysen et al. 2017).

Another survey study examining the types of complementary movement therapies used by 2,140 adults with arthritis found that 19% ($n = 398$) were using some type of movement therapy, and 89.2% of those reported use of yoga (Mielenz et al. 2016).

Prenatal yoga

A range of studies have been done examining the safety and efficacy of prenatal yoga. Reviews have shown prenatal yoga to be safe and efficacious when taught by an experienced instructor and to be more beneficial than walking or standard prenatal exercise (Polis et al. 2015).

A randomized trial of 59 high risk pregnant women were randomized to yoga ($n = 27$) or control. The yoga group received standard care plus 1-hour yoga sessions three times per week from the 12th to the 28th week of gestation. Findings in the yoga group showed significantly better growth measures for the fetus of women in the yoga group, including parietal diameter ($p = 0.001$), femur length ($p = 0.005$), head circumference ($p = 0.002$), and fetal weight ($p = 0.019$). Uterine artery resistance was also noted to be significantly lower in the yoga group in this study ($p = 0.048$), suggesting improved fetal circulation (Rakhshani et al. 2015). Yoga has also been shown to have a beneficial effect on perinatal depression and anxiety (Gong et al. 2015; Sheffield and Woods-Giscombe 2016).

YOGA AND TELEHEALTH

Many questions remain about the feasibility or effectiveness of implementing yoga in health care settings. A study evaluating the efficacy of yoga implemented via telehealth through a Veterans Affairs Medical Center showed promising results. Courses taught in person at a central health clinic were telecast in real time to groups at outlying community centers. The instructor was able to see students in the outlying centers on the screen. In the study by Schultz-Heik et al., 64 veterans who completed the course evaluation of yoga classes administered by certified teachers showed that 82% rated the classes as excellent, 96% reported symptom improvement after class, and 98% indicated enjoyment of the class. Only 13% of students reported no symptom improvement, with 62% reporting partial improvement and 26% reporting full improvement of symptoms. There were no statistically significant differences between students attending class in person versus via a telehealth class. Patients experienced symptom improvement in many areas, including pain, fatigue, and psychological distress. Students reported high levels of satisfaction with the course. No adverse events were reported. Authors concluded that the program was feasible, acceptable to students, and effective at addressing a range of physical and psychological issues in a group setting (Schulz-Heik et al. 2017).

This study raises interesting ideas about other routes of distribution of yoga and other movement therapies to homebound patients, those in rehabilitation centers, or those confined in the hospital setting.

TAI CHI

Tai chi is another movement therapy that shows some promising research. It is an ancient Chinese practice that combines slow gentle movement, relaxation, and controlled breathing exercises. It has been shown to be beneficial in promoting functional capacity and reducing falls in a study in patients with Parkinson's disease (Li et al. 2012) and in improving balance in Parkinson's patients (Tsang 2013). Another area where tai chi has shown benefit is in patients with knee osteoarthritis. A small study by Ghandali et al. (2017) showed that an 8-week course (2 × 60-minute classes per week) in tai chi improved balance and stability in a group of 20 patients >60 years of age in a physical therapy rehabilitation program.

CLINICAL APPLICATION: YOGA

Diana is a 42-year-old mother of three who is 2 years post diagnosis of breast cancer, stage III. She has experienced significant anxiety over the past year and is now having an acute increase in anxiety symptoms before her next follow-up appointment. She is finding it nearly impossible to get through her normal activities, sleep at night, or to maintain her work schedule. She had tried benzodiazepines for anxiety in the past but did not tolerate them, and she is now interested in exploring non-pharmacologic options for anxiety. Given the accruing research on the use of yoga in breast cancer survivors, it is mentioned as a possible option.

Diane is not very familiar with yoga and would like to know more. She is surprised it is being mentioned in a medical visit. In this scenario, how might one introduce the practice of yoga?

- First, it will be important to use language that is easily understandable and that ties in the evidence-based mental and physiologic benefits without insulting Diana or minimizing her symptoms as *just stress*. In this case, an emphasis could be placed on the important physiologic benefits of each of the three components of yoga, controlled breathing (pranayama) which serves to balance the sympathetic and parasympathetic nervous systems, mindfulness which has been linked with decreased perceived stress and improvement in inflammatory markers, and gentle movement (asanas) which can lend increased flexibility and improved balance.
- It may be reassuring to suggest to her that the three-pronged approach used in yoga, (breath, mindfulness, and movement) offers a non-pharmacologic approach that is greater than the sum of its parts with significant potential to help with stress, sleep, and overall coping with her diagnosis and is becoming widely accepted in the medical community for patients with a range of conditions.
- Another potential benefit to mention might be the social connection and support of a class if there is a patient program or a community-based program available. Connecting with others who are outside her family, or sharing a cancer diagnosis, may offer a chance to process stress in a healthy way. Alternatively, if no clinic or community-based resources are available, Diana could investigate the wide variety of online or CD/DVD resources available for home practice.

Diana was curious and interested to try yoga, especially due to her motivation to avoid prescription drugs for anxiety. She was able to find a 90-minute weekly class through the university nursing school and began attending the beginner sessions in addition to adding short sessions of nightly mindfulness meditation. She reported that initially the meditation component was challenging, but over time she mastered several breathing exercises that made a significant difference in her baseline anxiety, and gradually the evening *homework* meditation became easier and more enjoyable.

Diana found connecting with other patients in this way very helpful, and this prompted her to reach out to her nurse case coordinator to lay groundwork for a breast cancer support group in her community. Her goal was to start a beginner's yoga course.

Ultimately, Diana was able to avoid the use of pharmaceuticals for the treatment of her anxiety, and at her last follow-up reported an increase in overall quality of life which she, in part, attributed to the yoga practice.

YOGA IN PEDIATRICS

Yoga can be used successfully in the pediatric population and had been studied in a variety of settings. Results from the 2012 National Health Interview Survey showed that the use of yoga and yoga therapy had increased in children since the 2007 survey from 2.5% to 3.2% which correlates to more than 400,000 children (Rosen et al. 2015).

A review of yoga in the pediatric population by Rosen et al. included 15 studies, although authors note small sample size, absence of systematic randomization, and high variability between interventions. Pediatric conditions in which yoga was found to be beneficial included: irritable bowel syndrome, polycystic ovarian disease, eating disorders, obesity, anxiety, ADHD (hyperactivity, impulsiveness), psychological well-being in the school setting, mood, perceived stress and resilience, anger, and fatigue. One of the most encouraging conclusions from this review was the successful use of yoga in a variety of school settings and age groups. Due to methodological limitations, small sample sizes, lack of randomization, and variability of interventions, the need for larger, well-designed trials was emphasized (Rosen et al. 2015).

Yoga has also been studied in pediatric inpatients. A randomized trial in 73 pediatric inpatients with sickle cell disease vaso-occlusive crisis compared yoga with attention control on pain. The yoga was delivered to children while in the hospital bed ($n = 35$). The intervention consisted of mindfulness and mindful breathing, asanas, and pranayama and guided relaxation led by an experienced yoga instructor. Compared to control, the yoga group had significantly greater reduction in mean pain score after only one session (-0.6 ± 0.96 vs. 0.0 ± 1.37; $P = 0.029$). This was the first randomized controlled trial of yoga for children in acute pain and showed benefit as well as feasibility in the inpatient setting. To increase familiarity and acceptance of the yoga intervention, educational material and experiential sessions were offered to nurses and other caregivers on the unit (Moody et al. 2017).

CLINICAL APPLICATION: PEDIATRIC YOGA

Maya is a 12 year old admitted to the hospital for work up of weight loss and recurrent abdominal pain. She is scheduled to undergo a variety of tests, including endoscopy, over the next few days. Child Life Services are called on because Maya is experiencing anticipatory anxiety about the endoscopy and is also worried about having an IV placed. While meeting with Maya and the family, the Child Life Specialist mentions the yoga class that is held every afternoon in the activity room. The younger kids have a class in the morning. Maya is curious and agrees to walk down the hall that afternoon to see the class.

What she saw surprised her in that there were adolescents from different units of the hospital, many on IV's and in wheelchairs gathering to participate in the yoga class. There was one instructor and a handful of aides and nurses who stayed to monitor the children. Some patients were new to the class, but others had been inpatient for weeks and attended regularly. The instructor started with a simple guided meditation and breath work exercise. She then added progressive muscle relaxation that lasted about 10 minutes.

The instructor then led a gentle series of asanas with easy to follow instructions. Each of the children did what they were able to do comfortably. The session ended with a short meditation encouraging the children to send themselves good thoughts and to send good thoughts to all in the room. Maya could feel herself relaxing simply watching the class and decided she wanted to participate the next day.

As it turned out, Maya ended up requiring a longer than anticipated stay and needed nasogastric feeds. The placement of the nasogastric tube was challenging, and she was very upset about the way she looked, the discomfort, and her inability to eat. Once again, the Child Life Specialist was able to speak with her and encourage Maya to attend the afternoon yoga sessions if she felt up to it. Maya initially resisted, and the yoga instructor was able to come to her hospital room for several private sessions. Eventually, Maya agreed to join the group, and during the classes the instructor worked with the adolescents on accepting themselves as they were and gaining strength every day. Maya found the breathing exercises especially helpful to reduce her sense of anger and anxiety about her situation.

She found herself more and more able to remain in the moment and accept the treatment that was helping her to heal.

On discharge, the yoga instructor made sure Maya had recordings and some high-quality CD/DVDs to follow at home. Maya's family intended to speak with her pediatrician about local yoga classes for children or explore starting a group through the pediatric practice.

RESOURCES

In the United States, Yoga Alliance is a nonprofit 501(c)(6) membership professional and trade association. It serves as an association for yoga teachers, schools, and yoga studios. Yoga Alliance Registry is a nonprofit 501(c)(3) public charity. As of 2017, the group estimates they serve 9,700 Registered Yoga Teachers and 380 Registered Yoga Schools. To register with Yoga Alliance, you must complete either a 200- or a 500-hour teacher training program at a Registered Yoga School. There is no standard credentialing for teaching yoga to children. A minimum of 200 hours is recognized by the U.S. Yoga Alliance (www.yogaalliance.org), but this applies for adult teaching only.

PEDIATRIC YOGA RESOURCES

- International Association of Yoga Therapists: http://iayt.org/
- Kripalu Yoga in the Schools: http://kripalu.org/be_a_part_of_kripalu/812
- NCCAM Yoga for Health: http://nccam.nih.gov/health/yoga
- Yoga Alliance: http://www.yogaalliance.org/
- Yoga in Schools: http://yogainschools.org
- YogaKids: http://yogakids.com/
- Yoga for the Special Child: http://www.specialyoga.com/

References

Bower, J. E., G. Greendale, A. D. Crosswell, D. Garet, B. Sternlieb, P. A. Ganz, M. R. Irwin, R. Olmstead, J. Arevalo, and S. W. Cole. 2014. Yoga reduces inflammatory signaling in fatigued breast cancer survivors: A randomized controlled trial. *Psychoneuroendocrinology* 43: 20–29. doi:10.1016/j.psyneuen.2014.01.019.

Cahn, B. R., M. S. Goodman, C. T. Peterson, R. Maturi, and P. J. Mills. 2017. Yoga, meditation and mind-body health: Increased BDNF, cortisol awakening response, and altered inflammatory marker expression after a 3-month yoga and meditation retreat. *Front Hum Neurosci* 11: 315. doi:10.3389/fnhum.2017.00315.

Cramer, H., R. Lauche, H. Haller, and G. Dobos. 2013. A systematic review and meta-analysis of yoga for low back pain. *Clin J Pain* 29 (5): 450–460. doi:10.1097/AJP.0b013e31825e1492.

Cramer, H., R. Lauche, P. Klose, S. Lange, J. Langhorst, and G. J. Dobos. 2017. Yoga for improving health-related quality of life, mental health and cancer-related symptoms in women diagnosed with breast cancer. *Cochrane Database Syst Rev* 1: CD010802. doi:10.1002/14651858.CD010802.pub2.

Cramer, H., L. Ward, A. Steel, R. Lauche, G. Dobos, and Y. Zhang. 2016. Prevalence, patterns, and predictors of yoga use: Results of a U.S. nationally representative survey. *Am J Prev Med* 50 (2): 230–235. doi:10.1016/j.amepre.2015.07.037.

Field, T. 2016. Yoga research review. *Complement Ther Clin Pract* 24: 145–161. doi:10.1016/j.ctcp.2016.06.005.

Ghandali, E., S. T. Moghadam, M. R. Hadian, G. Olyaei, S. Jalaie, and E. Sajjadi. 2017. The effect of Tai Chi exercises on postural stability and control in older patients with knee osteoarthritis. *J Bodyw Mov Ther* 21 (3): 594–598. doi:10.1016/j.jbmt.2016.09.001.

Gong, H., C. Ni, X. Shen, T. Wu, and C. Jiang. 2015. Yoga for prenatal depression: A systematic review and meta-analysis. *BMC Psychiatry* 15: 14. doi:10.1186/s12888-015-0393-1.

Greysen, H. M., S. R. Greysen, K. A. Lee, O. S. Hong, P. Katz, and H. Leutwyler. 2017. A qualitative study exploring community yoga practice in adults with rheumatoid arthritis. *J Altern Complement Med* 23 (6): 487–493. doi:10.1089/acm.2016.0156.

Jerath, R., J. W. Edry, V. A. Barnes, and V. Jerath. 2006. Physiology of long pranayamic breathing: Neural respiratory elements may provide a mechanism that explains how slow deep breathing shifts the autonomic nervous system. *Med Hypotheses* 67 (3): 566–571. doi:10.1016/j.mehy.2006.02.042.

Li, F., P. Harmer, K. Fitzgerald, E. Eckstrom, R. Stock, J. Galver, G. Maddalozzo, and S. S. Batya. 2012. Tai chi and postural stability in patients with Parkinson's disease. *N Engl J Med* 366 (6): 511–519. doi:10.1056/NEJMoa1107911.

Lim, S. A., and K. J. Cheong. 2015. Regular yoga practice improves antioxidant status, immune function, and stress hormone releases in young healthy people: A randomized, double-blind, controlled pilot study. *J Altern Complement Med* 21 (9): 530–538. doi:10.1089/acm.2014.0044.

Meister, K., and G. Juckel. 2017. A systematic review of mechanisms of change in body-oriented yoga in major depressive disorders. *Pharmacopsychiatry*. doi:10.1055/s-0043-111013.

Mielenz, T. J., C. Xiao, and L. F. Callahan. 2016. Self-management of arthritis symptoms by complementary and alternative medicine movement therapies. *J Altern Complement Med* 22 (5): 404–407. doi:10.1089/acm.2015.0222.

Moody, K., B. Abrahams, R. Baker, R. Santizo, D. Manwani, V. Carullo, D. Eugenio, and A. Carroll. 2017. A randomized trial of yoga for children hospitalized with sickle cell vaso-occlusive crisis. *J Pain Symptom Manage* 53 (6): 1026–1034. doi:10.1016/j.jpainsymman.2016.12.351.

Nivethitha, L., A. Mooventhan, and N. K. Manjunath. 2016. Effects of various pranayama on cardiovascular and autonomic variables. *Anc Sci Life* 36 (2): 72–77. doi:10.4103/asl.ASL_178_16.

Ornish, D., J. Lin, J. M. Chan, E. Epel, C. Kemp, G. Weidner, R. Marlin et al. 2013. Effect of comprehensive lifestyle changes on telomerase activity and telomere length in men with biopsy-proven low-risk prostate cancer: 5-year follow-up of a descriptive pilot study. *Lancet Oncol* 14 (11): 1112–1120. doi:10.1016/S1470-2045(13)70366-8.

Ornish, D., J. Lin, J. Daubenmier, G. Weidner, E. Epel, C. Kemp, M. J. Magbanua et al. 2008. Increased telomerase activity and comprehensive lifestyle changes: A pilot study. *Lancet Oncol* 9 (11): 1048–1057. doi:10.1016/S1470-2045(08)70234-1.

Polis, R. L., D. Gussman, Y. H. and Kuo. 2015. Yoga in pregnancy: An examination and fetal responses to 26 yoga postures. *Obstet Gynecol* 126: 1237–1241.

Posadzki, P., E. Ernst, R. Terry, and M. S. Lee. 2011. Is yoga effective for pain? A systematic review of randomized clinical trials. *Complement Ther Med* 19 (5): 281–287. doi:10.1016/j.ctim.2011.07.004.

Prathikanti, S., R. Rivera, A. Cochran, J. G. Tungol, N. Fayazmanesh, and E. Weinmann. 2017. Treating major depression with yoga: A prospective, randomized, controlled pilot trial. *PLoS One* 12 (3): e0173869. doi:10.1371/journal.pone.0173869.

Qaseem, A., T. J. Wilt, R. M. McLean, M. A. Forciea, for the Clinical Guidelines Committee of the American College of Physicians. 2017. Noninvasive treatments for acute, subacute, and chronic low back pain: A clinical practice guideline from the American college of physicians. *Ann Intern Med* 166 (7): 514–530. doi:10.7326/M16-2367.

Rakhshani, A., R. Nagarathna, R. Mhaskar, A. Mhaskar, A. Thomas, and S. Gunasheela. 2015. Effects of yoga on utero-fetal-placental circulation in high-risk pregnancy: A randomized controlled trial. *Adv Prev Med* 2015: 373041. doi:10.1155/2015/373041.

Riley, K. E., and C. L. Park. 2015. How does yoga reduce stress? A systematic review of mechanisms of change and guide to future inquiry. *Health Psychol Rev* 9 (3): 379–396. doi:10.1080/17437199.2014.981778.

Rosen, L., A. French, and G. Sullivan. 2015. Complementary, holistic, and integrative medicine: Yoga. *Pediatr Rev* 36 (10): 468–474. doi:10.1542/pir.36-10-468.

Schulz-Heik, R. J., H. Meyer, L. Mahoney, M. V. Stanton, R. H. Cho, D. P. Moore-Downing, T. J. Avery et al. 2017. Results from a clinical yoga program for veterans: Yoga via telehealth provides comparable satisfaction and health improvements to in-person yoga. *BMC Complement Altern Med* 17 (1): 198. doi:10.1186/s12906-017-1705-4.

Sheffield, K. M., and C. L. Woods-Giscombe. 2016. Efficacy, feasibility, and acceptability of perinatal yoga on women's mental health and well-being: A systematic literature review. *J Holist Nurs* 34 (1): 64–79. doi:10.1177/0898010115577976.

Stephens, I. 2017. Medical yoga therapy. *Children (Basel)* 4 (2). doi:10.3390/children4020012.

Streeter, C. C., P. L. Gerbarg, T. H. Whitfield, L. Owen, J. Johnston, M. M. Silveri, M. Gensler et al. 2017. Treatment of major depressive disorder with iyengar yoga and coherent breathing: A randomized controlled dosing study. *J Altern Complement Med* 23 (3): 201–207. doi:10.1089/acm.2016.0140.

Swain, T. A., and G. McGwin. 2016. Yoga-related injuries in the United States from 2001 to 2014. *Orthop J Sports Med* 4 (11): 2325967116671703. doi:10.1177/2325967116671703.

Tilbrook, H. E., H. Cox, C. E. Hewitt, A. R. Kang'ombe, L. H. Chuang, S. Jayakody, J. D. Aplin et al. 2011. Yoga for chronic low back pain: A randomized trial. *Ann Intern Med* 155 (9): 569–578. doi:10.7326/0003-4819-155-9-201111010-00003.

Tolahunase, M., R. Sagar, and R. Dada. 2017. Impact of yoga and meditation on cellular aging in apparently healthy individuals: A prospective, open-label single-arm exploratory study. *Oxid Med Cell Longev* 2017: 7928981. doi:10.1155/2017/7928981.

Tsang, W. W. 2013. Tai Chi training is effective in reducing balance impairments and falls in patients with Parkinson's disease. *J Physiother* 59 (1): 55. doi:10.1016/S1836-9553(13)70148-6.

Twal, W. O., A. E. Wahlquist, and S. Balasubramanian. 2016. Yogic breathing when compared to attention control reduces the levels of pro-inflammatory biomarkers in saliva: A pilot randomized controlled trial. *BMC Complement Altern Med* 16: 294. doi:10.1186/s12906-016-1286-7.

Uebelacker, L. A., G. Tremont, L. T. Gillette, G. Epstein-Lubow, D. R. Strong, A. M. Abrantes, A. R. Tyrka, T. Tran, B. A. Gaudiano, and I. W. Miller. 2017. Adjunctive yoga v. health education for persistent major depression: a randomized controlled trial. *Psychol Med* 47 (12): 2130–2142. doi:10.1017/S0033291717000575.

Yadav, R. K., D. Magan, N. Mehta, R. Sharma, and S. C. Mahapatra. 2012. Efficacy of a short-term yoga-based lifestyle intervention in reducing stress and inflammation: Preliminary results. *J Altern Complement Med* 18 (7): 662–667. doi:10.1089/acm.2011.0265.

Yoga Alliance. Retrieved from https://www.yogaalliance.org/Credentialing.

Part III

Clinical Application

Part III builds on the material presented in Part I (introduction, stress physiology, self-care, language, and mind–body interview) and Part II (review of selected mind–body therapies) and explores the use of mind–body therapies in a group of common conditions where research on their use in the clinical setting shows promise. These selected conditions include anxiety and depression; oncologic and surgical diagnosis; gastroenterologic conditions, including GERD, IBD, IBS, and pediatric functional abdominal pain disorders; and pain—including low back pain, headache, fibromyalgia, arthritis, and pediatric chronic pain.

Overlap of the use of mind–body therapies is common, and although accruing research can be used to guide choices, in reality there are no hard and fast rules for their application. Clinicians are encouraged to exercise curiosity and creativity in partnership with the patient to find the best therapeutic fit. The wide margin of safety of the mind–body therapies in most patients allows room for trial with little downside.

A typical approach would include review of relevant research, inquiry about a patient's prior experience with mind–body therapies, special interests or reservations, assessment or identification of available resources, selection of a trained provider if needed, trial, follow-up, and reassessment.

For some clinicians, even consideration of the potential use of the mind–body therapies will require a shift in perspective. Some may be skeptical, others worried about colleague's perceptions or doubtful their patients will accept their recommendations. Probably the most important elements in successful introduction of the mind–body therapies are gaining familiarity with the depth of supporting research and adoption of an open-minded approach toward their use. Understanding that some reassessment and fine tuning is common should reassure practitioners and patients and may even encourage a sense of partnership and shared learning if the therapy is unfamiliar to either party.

Hopefully, the patient cases woven through Part III accurately convey the curiosity, creativity, flexibility, and motivation to feel better that these patients brought to their care. Each benefited from the confidence of their medical team that they could improve and the encouragement to try something new. Resources mentioned in Part III are aggregated at the end of the book for convenience.

11 Anxiety and depression

INTRODUCTION

Mental illness affects millions of adults, adolescents, and children in the United States, taking a significant toll on quality of life, work productivity, academic advancement, and family life (Lipari et al. 2013). Many affected individuals lack access to treatment, and an estimated 50% have symptoms that limit life activity. In the range of mental illness, anxiety and depression are two of the most common diagnoses reported, often overlapping in the same individual (McCall-Hosenfeld et al. 2014).

Pharmaceutical treatment can be confounded by unwanted side effects, leading to discontinuation of medications (Gartlehner et al. 2008). Some individuals may avoid prescriptions altogether due to stigma, price, or a desire to avoid long-term medication exposure or due to a preference for more natural treatments, especially in children.

The etiologies of many mental illnesses are complex and remain under active study. Emerging research focusing on the interplay of microbiome-derived peptides in the bidirectional regulation of gut–brain signaling has opened exciting new frontiers of research and treatment interventions (Lach et al. 2017).

Stress-related mental health disorders are common and cover a wide range of diagnoses, comprehensively described within the International Classification of Diseases, 10th Edition (ICD-10) and the *Diagnostic and Statistical Manual for Mental Disorders* (DSM-V), the primary diagnostic guide used for mental health classification in the United States. Diagnostic categories include acute stress disorder, post-traumatic stress disorder, adjustment disorder, and unspecified stress reactions. Comorbid health conditions are often associated with stress disorders, and conversely, living with chronic health conditions can drive symptoms of anxiety and depression (Gradus 2017).

Of concern, stress disorders have consistently been found to have a strong epidemiological association with completed suicide, highlighting the urgency of early referral to a mental health consultant if the patient verbalizes any type of suicidal ideation or if the clinician feels the patient's symptoms warrant additional consultation at any time. A patient with post-traumatic stress disorder (PTSD) should ideally be cleared by a mental health specialist before use of any type of mind–body therapy, especially imagery or hypnosis to avoid inadvertently provoking symptoms (Gradus 2017).

ANXIETY IN THE GENERAL POPULATION

A large population study estimates lifetime prevalence of anxiety disorder in the United States at near 40% (McCall-Hosenfeld et al. 2014), with an estimated prevalence of 15%–20% in children and adolescents (which includes categories of separation anxiety disorder, social phobia, specific phobia, agoraphobia, panic disorder, and generalized anxiety disorder) (Beesdo et al. 2009).

Anxiety can be experienced as a variety of sensations, including nervousness, apprehension, worry, palpitations, increased perspiration, tremors, hypervigilance, feeling overwhelmed, uncertainty, agitation, difficulty concentrating, and increased fearfulness. These feelings of discomfort can appear in any sector of life, impacting school, work, social activities, relationships, and travel. Insomnia is a recognized comorbidity, and somatic complaints are commonly seen, for example, gastrointestinal symptoms, headache, or dermatologic conditions.

An estimated 5%–8% of primary care visits are associated with anxiety, making it important for clinicians to have a range of therapeutic options (Kessler et al. 2012; McPherson and McGraw 2013).

SCREENING FOR EXACERBATING FACTORS

In any patient with anxiety, it is important to consider and rule out clinical conditions that can present with features of anxiety such as thyroid disorders, pheochromocytoma (adrenal gland tumor that produces adrenaline), and the use of any exacerbating food, caffeinated beverages, sympathomimetics, beta-agonists, corticosteroids, thyroid supplements, stimulant medications, drugs of abuse, or over-the-counter products with caffeine or other stimulant ingredients. Certain dietary supplements such as S-adenosylmethionine (SAM-e) typically used for osteoarthritis pain and depression can cause anxiety in some individuals. Yerba mate is another popular natural product high in caffeine, typically prepared as a tea.

ANXIETY AS A COMORBID CONDITION

Anxiety can be diagnosed as a primary condition, for example, Generalized Anxiety Disorder (ICD-10 F41.1), or can present as a comorbidity in nearly any medical condition experienced by children and adults. The non-pharmacologic nature of mind–body therapies is especially valuable in this patient population to help reduce the risk of potential drug interactions.

Examples of conditions where anxiety is a frequently seen comorbidity

Type 1 and type 2 diabetes (T1DM, T2DM)

There is a well-recognized association between diabetes, anxiety, and depression with an estimated lifetime prevalence of any anxiety disorder for all types of diabetes of 19.5% (Li et al. 2008).

Anxiety is also prevalent in pediatric patients with diabetes, especially adolescent females (Rechenberg et al. 2017). Anxiety and depression often occur together in individuals with diabetes and have a significant impact on quality of life and illness management (Purewal and Fisher 2017). For example, higher levels of anxiety in diabetic patients have been associated with suboptimal glycemic control related to less frequent glucose monitoring (Herzer and Hood 2010). In addition to the internal effects of HPA axis dysregulation, impacted by glucose fluctuation, patients with diabetes may have symptoms of anxiety related to needle sticks, frequent clinic visits, financial burden, and worry about adherence to diet, medication regimens, monitoring needs, fear of hyper- or hypoglycemic episodes, complications, and body image issues (Tareen and Tareen 2017).

Metabolic syndrome and obesity

A survey of 2,111 adults ($n = 1,155$ female and 956 male) found that both depression and anxiety were statistically higher in female participants and increased with age. Depression and anxiety were higher in both females and males with metabolic syndrome ($p < 0.001$ for both), as well as in those with diabetes ($p < 0.001$ both sexes) (Shinkov et al. 2017). In addition to impacting the quality of life, anxiety can interfere with the patient's ability to pursue healthy lifestyle measures such as exercise and restorative sleep and may significantly increase health care costs.

Cardiovascular disease

Large population studies in adults have suggested a correlation between anxiety and coronary heart disease, although a causal relationship has not been established (Janszky et al. 2010; Nabi et al. 2010; Roest et al. 2010; Altino et al. 2017). One theory of interaction proposed is the accumulated physiologic toll anxiety takes on the autonomic and cardiac systems due to excessive activation of the HPA axis with subsequent release of pro-inflammatory cytokines and catecholamines that can damage endothelial tissue, catalyzing atherosclerotic changes that precede cardiovascular disease. Some studies have also shown a significant correlation between anxiety in the 2-hour time frame preceding acute myocardial infarction, suggestive of vasoconstrictive coronary artery effects (Mittleman et al. 1995). European guidelines on cardiovascular disease prevention list depression and anxiety as well as psychosocial stressors such as work stress, lack of social support, and other social stressors as risk factors for cardiac events and as predictors of poorer outcomes in those with cardiovascular disease (Cohen et al. 2015).

Cancer

Anxiety has been widely reported to be prevalent in both adult and pediatric cancer patients, potentially affecting every part of the patient's journey, including diagnosis, pre-treatment consultation, during treatment, recovery, survival and ongoing surveillance, and palliative care if needed. Compounding factors include loss of control, uncertainty about the future, complex treatment options, fear of recurrence, pain, fatigue, financial stressors, and school, family, and work disruption (Carlson et al. 2017).

A sub-study of a large randomized controlled trial evaluating the effect of mindfulness-based stress reduction (MBSR) breast cancer (BC) compared to standard care on pro-inflammatory cytokines in breast cancer survivors showed that those in the MBSR BC group were able to normalize pro-inflammatory cytokine levels after cancer treatment. Results suggested that B cell modulation may be involved in the recovery of the immune system after breast cancer treatment and that the changes were seen in TNF alpha and IL-6 in this study group may be markers for immune system normalization (Reich et al. 2017).

Polycystic ovarian disease

Anxiety in patients with polycystic ovarian disease (PCOS) may be related to physical changes such as hirsutism, acne, and weight gain, and also associated with quality of life issues such as stress due to infertility or the need to manage heavy irregular menstrual bleeding (Cooney and Dokras 2017; Cooney et al. 2017).

Dermatological conditions

The connection between emotion and skin disorders is a topic of active research interest.

A systematic review on the prevalence of mental disorders in patients with psoriasis included 34 papers and found that anxiety affected 30% of participants and depression affected 27.6% of participants (Ferreira et al. 2017). Patients with dermatologic conditions can also experience significant social anxiety, which in turn can aggravate skin symptoms through flushing and perspiration as well as upregulation of the inflammatory response (Dixon et al. 2017b).

Lupus

Mindfulness can play a part in symptom relief for anxiety in individuals living with autoimmune illnesses such as lupus (Solati et al. 2017).

Sleep disorders

Anxiety can be a significant driver of sleep disorders, and sleep disorders themselves can worsen anxiety in a challenging negative feedback loop (Dixon et al. 2017a; Short et al. 2017).

Psychosis

Anxiety can foreshadow the development of psychosis in some individuals. A small study in 20 adults with anxiety and depression underwent 4 weeks of training in heart rate variability biofeedback and showed improvement in the ability to tolerate normal stressors ($P < 0.001$) and improvement in dysphoric mood ($p < 0.001$), although no changes in anxiety scores were seen in the initial evaluation; feedback and adherence to the intervention was positive, and further studies are planned (McAusland and Addington 2016).

INTEGRATIVE MEDICINE APPROACHES TO ANXIETY

An integrative medicine approach to anxiety would typically include a comprehensive evaluation of lifestyle, including nutrition, physical activity, sleep, supplements, environmental factors, potential whole systems approaches such as traditional Chinese medicine or Ayurveda, and evaluation of the need or potential benefit of conventional treatments (e.g., pharmaceuticals) in addition to the range of mind–body therapies. A large survey by Bystritsky et al. (2012) showed that the most commonly used complementary therapies for anxiety include: relaxation, imagery, meditation, botanicals, yoga, acupuncture, massage, and spiritual approaches to healing.

Encouraging the patient to initiate or continue healthy lifestyle choices can add to their feeling of self-efficacy and is generally approached as a foundational part of any integrative treatment plan.

MIND–BODY THERAPIES IN ANXIETY

Some of the better studied mind–body therapies for anxiety include yoga, biofeedback, and mindfulness—both MBSR and MBCT.

MINDFULNESS AND ANXIETY

Components of mindfulness include learning to focus attention on a moment-by-moment approach, on purpose, with an attitude of detachment, curiosity, and acceptance (Marchand 2012).

Intention, attention, and attitude

Shapiro et al. (2006) have distilled the mindfulness components into three main facets: intention, attention, and attitude. When considered as components, a patient with anxiety might form the *intention* to use mindfulness to decrease their experience of suffering or pain associated with their medical condition or to decrease worry about possible side effects of treatment. Further consideration might lead to an intention to explore the root of the symptom of anxiety and to cultivate the intention to increase their self-regulation skills, which have been associated with improved outcomes.

Attention in mindfulness allows moment-to-moment awareness, paying attention in the moment rather than dwelling in the past or projecting thoughts into the future. This again has obvious utility in the clinical approach to anxiety by limiting the scope of thoughts to what is actually happening in the present moment.

The aspect of *attitude* in the application of mindfulness in anxiety is important in that one is encouraged to bring a sense of self-compassion to the practice, to give oneself a break from worry and fearfulness, to recognize one's discomfort but not to indulge or magnify it. To simply accept what is happening and to be curious, without judgment or blame.

The conscious focuses of attention in mindfulness practice demonstrates the usefulness of this practice in anxiety, where thoughts may be scattered, racing, or ruminative. In MBSR, attention is also given to sensory input, again with a sense of curiosity, in an observational manner. The focus is on the moment, and the steady stream of thoughts, emotions, and comfortable or uncomfortable sensations are allowed to pass through the mind without the need to engage or react. The idea is to bring the mental processes under voluntary control and to quiet the mind. The skills of mindfulness can be cultivated from formal learning and practice into day-to-day life over time, making them extremely useful for those living with anxiety.

Emerging research on mindfulness in children has shown that more mindful children and adolescents report lower anxiety symptoms (Greco et al. 2011).

There are many types of mindfulness practices, several of which are described in Chapter 8. Rather than an extensive review, common themes will be explored here for their potential benefit to patients living with anxiety. Although interest is high, study size and heterogeneity have been limiting factors. For example, a meta-analysis of eight randomized controlled trials that evaluated MBSR and MBCT on anxiety showed moderate benefit—but high study heterogeneity and mixed quality of study design (Strauss et al. 2014).

An early study of MBSR in anxiety disorder examined its efficacy in 53 patients with social anxiety disorder using a classic 8-week MBSR course versus 12 weeks of CBGT (cognitive behavioral group therapy). In this trial, patients in the CBGT had significantly greater improvements in anxiety measures, although those in the MBSR group reported improvement in mood, functionality, and quality of life (Koszycki et al. 2007).

Another study on mindfulness in social anxiety disorder examined 16 patients who underwent fMRI scanning while reacting to and experiencing negative beliefs and then while regulating negative emotions. After MBSR training, 14 of 16 patients underwent neuroimaging. Post-MBSR training, participants showed improvement in both anxiety and depression and showed increased activity in areas of the brain associated with enhanced emotional regulation (Goldin and Gross 2010).

A further study on mindfulness tested for effectiveness in generalized anxiety disorder in 76 adult patients randomized to MBSR course or wait-list control. Those in the treatment group who completed the program had medium to large effect sizes of improvement in anxiety and large effect sizes in improvement in depressive symptoms, with improvements persisting to 6-month follow-up (Vollestad et al. 2011).

A 2017 review of mindfulness-based interventions for anxiety and depression finds that MBSR and MBCT are superior in the reduction of anxiety symptoms compared to most control arms in a range of studies and work comparably to CBT (Hofmann and Gomez 2017).

MINDFULNESS IN PEDIATRIC ANXIETY

A review of mindfulness-based interventions in adolescents with chronic illness included eight papers, all of which were quite small—most had fewer than 20 participants. Outcomes were positive for acceptance of the training, although studies were underpowered to make definitive conclusions regarding efficacy, and larger studies are needed (Ahola Kohut et al. 2017).

A randomized controlled trial of MBSR versus health education by Sibinga et al. in 300 fifth to eighth graders in an urban school found significantly lower levels of somatization, depression, negative effect, rumination, and self-hostility and post-traumatic stress symptom severity (all $p < 0.05$) in the MBSR group (Sibinga et al. 2016).

Another example of research on the use of mindfulness in the pediatric population is found in a small feasibility study by Freedenberg et al. in 10 teens with cardiac illnesses who showed a significant decrease in mean anxiety scores and frequency of anxiety symptoms after undertaking MBSR training ($p < 0.01$). Coping strategies improved ($p = 0.04$) and levels of depression also decreased ($p = 0.001$) (Freedenberg et al. 2015).

In a follow-up to this study, the group compared MBSR to a video online support group in 46 teens with a cardiac diagnosis (congenital heart disease, cardiac device, postural orthostatic tachycardia syndrome) conditions associated with high psychosocial stress.

Results showed that both a 6-week MBSR and six weekly video online group interactions had significant benefit to participants and were well tolerated. Interestingly, in addition to serving as a control group, the video group also experienced reduced stress and increased coping skills, pointing to the unique benefit of group connection in this patient population (Freedenberg et al. 2017).

Mindfulness has also been evaluated in adolescents with cancer to address symptoms of psychological distress, anxiety, pain, and the full range of disruption to day-to-day life due to cancer diagnosis. Results in small studies are promising, although further studies are needed (Jones et al. 2013).

CLINICAL APPLICATION: PEDIATRIC ANXIETY

Quinn is a high-performing student in a magnet high school known for her 4.0 GPA and disciplined study habits. In her freshman year, she began experiencing intermittent symptoms of extreme anxiety before test days with racing thoughts, palpitations, inability to sleep, and progressive exhaustion. She began missing days of school, which added to her academic stress. She found ways to accommodate for the anxiety by limiting most social activities and using weekends for studying. Her family also hired a tutor in an attempt to reduce her stress. Some of the measures helped, but at the start of her senior year, she was finding it difficult to leave the house to go to school and becoming fearful of peer ridicule if she received anything less than 100% on her assignments. Her general health was good, and she was seen by her primary care clinician who discussed treatment options with the family who were very reluctant to place her on short- or long-term medication.

In this case, in addition to balancing her school work load, screening for external drivers of anxiety (e.g., in off-use prescriptions such as Adderall, over-the-counter products or dietary supplements, foods, or beverages) and encouraging regular enjoyable physical activity, MBSR was proposed to introduce Quinn to a range of mindfulness practices that included education about stress as well as specific coping skills. These included: sitting meditation, body scan to encourage awareness of bodily sensations, yoga, breath exercises, and walking meditation. Other skills covered included learning to observe thoughts rather than being controlled by them, accepting the present moment, and practicing non-judging.

Over the course of 8 weeks, Quinn practiced in the class and applied herself to the *homework*, which included guided meditation, progressive muscle relaxation, breath work, and reflective questions. Over time, she became able to recognize feelings of anxiety at the earliest stages, and rather than allowing the sensation to accelerate, she trained herself to become a curious observer, letting the feelings pass without reacting. It took months, but eventually, she was able to trigger a state of calm awareness simply using her breath and was then able to use mindfulness in any situation, including at school and before and during test taking.

One of the key concepts Quinn learned is that "the anxiety is not me," she was able to fundamentally shift her perspective so that non-judgmental attention took the place of being swept away by the sensation of anxiety so the sensation gradually lost its power over her. In addition, although she was relatively young, Quinn was gradually able to appreciate the unrealistic pressure she was placing on herself to be *perfect* and how counterproductive this was to sustain. She recognized the mental and physical toll the anxiety was taking and was able to bring a sense of self-compassion to bear that significantly helped her change her perspective.

The intervention served as a wake-up call to her parents and resulted in them slowing the overall pace of the family's activities and recognition of the pressure to excel that had been building in their daughter. The family was able to work together to identify trouble spots, and over time, they all made several adjustments to rebalance work–school–life integration. Quinn was able to complete her senior year—earning a B in honor's physics, which she was able to accept with equanimity. For her, a victory.

MUSIC THERAPY FOR ANXIETY

Music therapy has been evaluated to address anxiety in medically acute patients, such as in post-operative patients, those who have had coronary events, or undergoing treatment for cancer. The overall risk of music therapy is low, although more studies are needed before conclusive recommendations are given. Lack of access to a trained music therapist can be a limiting factor (Bradt et al. 2016).

A review on psychosocial interventions included 12 randomized controlled trials involving 1,393 pediatric oncology patients (Coughtrey et al. 2017), two of the studies included music therapy in which the adolescents produced music videos, including song selection, lyric writing, photo and artwork selection, video design, and digitally recording songs in an inpatient setting. Benefit was seen in the significant reduction of anxiety and depression in the majority of participants (Robb et al. 2014).

YOGA FOR ANXIETY

Small studies on yoga for anxiety have shown benefit (Reddy and Vijay 2016). Yoga can be used alone or in conjunction with conventional treatments. The combination of movement, breath work, and meditation address both psychological stress and physiologic inflammation.

A 2015 review by Pascoe and Bauer includes 25 studies and examined changes in physiologic parameters related to yoga practice. Although larger studies are needed, overall benefits were seen in blood pressure, heart rate, cortisol and peripheral cytokine expression, and in structural and functional brain measures in areas related to emotional regulation and stress. The authors concluded that yoga has the potential to improve sympathetic regulation and decrease symptoms of anxiety and depression in the studies population (Pascoe and Bauer 2015).

Yoga practice has also been shown to improve measures of survivorship in women with breast cancer. One case control study in early breast cancer survivors compared those with prior yoga experience ($n = 27$) to no yoga experience ($N = 25$). The comparison showed that women in the yoga group had significantly lower stress, anxiety, and depression scores and improved quality of life measures ($p < 0.001$). Global quality of life and trait anxiety were significantly associated with yoga practice (Amritanshu et al. 2017).

A review of 16 studies on the use of yoga in children found six randomized controlled trials, two pre–post non-randomized control group design studies, seven uncontrolled prep–post intervention studies, and one case study. Collectively, the studies showed improvement in anxiety measures in participants, but variation in study design and small numbers precluded definitive recommendations (Weaver and Darragh 2015).

A 2016 pre-post study examining the benefit of yoga in 20 children (aged 7–20 years) with cystic fibrosis found that six one-on-one sessions over a 10-week study period with a certified yoga instructor showed improvement in mean immediate anxiety scores ($P < 0.001$) and improvement in joint pain ($p = 0.028$) and found the intervention to be acceptable with no adverse related events (McNamara et al. 2016).

CLINICAL HYPNOSIS FOR ANXIETY IN ONCOLOGY PATIENTS

A review by Carlson et al. found that clinical hypnosis has good supporting evidence for decreasing symptoms of anxiety without the need for anxiolytic medication in both adult and pediatric oncology patient populations. Depending on the study participants, both therapist-guided and self-hypnosis were found to be effective in moderating pain, reducing overall emotional distress, sleep disturbance, and overall health-related quality of life (Carlson et al. 2017).

A meta-analysis by Chen et al. (2017) of 20 studies found that hypnosis had an immediate and significant effect on anxiety in the cancer patients studied ($p < 0.01$), with therapist-directed hypnosis being significantly more effective in these subjects than self-directed hypnosis. The highest effects were seen in pediatric studies and in studies with procedure-related stressors.

PLAY THERAPY FOR ANXIETY IN CHILDREN

A study by Al-Yateem and Rossiter (2017) in 165 hospitalized children ages 4–7 years old found that those in the treatment group ($n = 81$) evaluated the impact of unstructured age-appropriate play sessions of 30 minutes twice daily for 3 days showed a statistically significant decrease in anxiety scores on days 2 and 3 of hospitalization ($p < 0.001$, day 3).

Therapeutic clowning is another approach under study in the acute pediatric care setting as a way to address anxiety but must be approached with training and sensitivity to the specific environment to avoid striking the wrong tone with both families and clinicians (Mortamet et al. 2017a,b; van Venrooij and Barnhoorn 2017).

ONLINE MINDFULNESS-BASED STRESS REDUCTION AND DISTANCE LEARNING PROGRAMS

A review and meta-analysis of 15 randomized controlled trials evaluating the efficacy of online mindfulness training showed that online mindfulness interventions had a small but significant positive effect on anxiety, depression, and overall well-being with the highest effect seen for a reduction in stress. This is an area of active research with the potential to be tailored to specific patient populations (Spijkerman et al. 2016).

DEPRESSION

Depression is characterized by persistent low mood, sadness, hopelessness, amotivation, (dysthymia), and loss of ability to enjoy formerly enjoyable activities (anhedonia). Its global disease burden is substantial, and in the 2010 World Health Organization ranking of years lived with disability (YLD), depressive disorders were ranked second overall. Higher prevalence is seen in females and adults of working age. Major depressive disorder (experiencing depressed mood almost all day, every day for at least 2 weeks) is also associated with significant disease burden from related ischemic heart disease and suicide (Ferrari et al. 2013).

Depression impacts individuals from all socioeconomic layers and is also found in the pediatric population. National Institute of Mental Health 2015 statistics report an increase of 12% in the prevalence of major depressive disorder among U.S. adolescents aged 12–17 years, weighted toward females (36.1%) over males (13.6%). Depression prevalence has also increased in young adults, with an estimated 8.8%–9.6% in the 18- to 25-year-old group (Mojtabai et al. 2016).

This is especially concerning in part because suicide is the second-leading cause of death in adolescents. Depression in adolescence has also been shown to predispose to depressive symptoms in adulthood (Bhatta et al. 2017).

In addition to the inflammatory and cardiovascular comorbidities mentioned in the following with respect to depression, adolescents and children with depression face academic pressures and interruption with social relationships of peer groups and family. Somatic symptoms such as headaches, abdominal pain, and musculoskeletal pain can be markers of depression in the pediatric population. Sleep disruption and irritability are also common. As in adults, the prevalence of depression increases significantly in the presence of chronic illness (Bhatta et al. 2017). The use of digital media and associated light at night exposures are additional factors of consequence in depression prevalence, in both adults and youth (LeBourgeois et al. 2017).

Depression has been associated with chronic stress and is considered a neurochemical disorder involving, in part, alteration of neurotransmitters, especially serotonin and dopamine (Blier 2013; Montoya et al. 2016; Jeon and Kim 2017).

Commonly recognized comorbidities of depression include obesity, cardiovascular disease, metabolic syndrome, pain, anxiety, irritability, and substance abuse. Sleep disorders are also frequently seen in depression, for example, sleep latency, insomnia, frequent nocturnal awakenings, and early morning waking (Zhang et al. 2017).

Depression screening should be done with a high index of suspicion in those living with chronic illness and with family history of depression.

TREATMENT

Compounding factors in depression treatment include inhibition of motivation for healthy lifestyle behaviors such as exercise and difficulty adhering to regular medical treatment.

Emerging research demonstrates that chronic treatment with antidepressants has a positive effect on neuroplasticity through increases in dendritic density and synaptic plasticity possibly related to brain-derived neurotrophic factor, among other factors. This may in part account for the delay in treatment effect that can be seen when some depression medications are started and raises an interesting and important question about the use of mindfulness and other mind–body therapies that have been shown to positively impact neuroplasticity in this time period (Zhang et al. 2017).

LIFTING THE STIGMA OF DEPRESSION

It is important for clinicians to continue to destigmatize depression and to be able to offer more options to patients in the treatment of this serious condition and to feel confident in recommending mind–body therapies when appropriate—either as a sole therapy or as a complementary approach when appropriate. In any depressed patient, close monitoring is needed along with a low threshold for referral to a trained mental health provider for screening and ongoing treatment and monitoring for worsening of symptoms.

CHRONIC ILLNESSES ASSOCIATED WITH DEPRESSION

Diabetes

An estimated 415 million people globally suffer from diabetes, and approximately 20% of those with type 1 diabetes have a comorbid diagnosis of depression (Fisher et al. 2012; Li et al. 2017). Studies in adults in the primary care setting have shown slightly higher prevalence (25%) of recurrent depression in adults with type 2 diabetes (Nefs et al. 2012).

Depression in diabetes patients has been associated with decreased adherence to treatment and self-care regimens, higher HbA1c and fasting blood glucose levels, and increased microvascular and macrovascular complications. Higher rates of heath care expenditures are also a significant factor (de Groot et al. 2001; Bhattacharya et al. 2016; Bogner and McClintock 2016).

Cardiovascular disease

A review by Cohen et al. reports that one in five patients with cardiovascular disease suffers from depression, which is associated with poorer outcomes, higher health care costs, and reduced quality of life. Prevalence of depression is estimated to effect one in three stroke patients and is similarly correlated with worse outcomes. In addition to impacting adherence to self-care activities and medication regimens, depression in cardiovascular patients is associated with upregulation of inflammatory markers, impairment of autonomic nervous system function, and increased risk of myocardial ischemia (Cohen et al. 2015).

The American Heart Association recognizes depression as a risk factor for poor outcomes in patients who have had acute coronary events (Lichtman et al. 2014), as do the European guidelines on cardiovascular disease prevention (Perk et al. 2012).

CANCER

Similar to anxiety, depression has been widely reported to be prevalent in cancer patients and can affect every aspect of care, including: diagnosis, pre-treatment, during treatment, recovery, survival and ongoing surveillance, or need for palliative care. Depression can be compounded by the loss of control or loss of body function, uncertainty about the future, burden of deciding best treatment options, fear of recurrence, fatigue, financial stressors, and disruption of work and family routines and relationships. Small studies exist on the use of a variety of mind–body therapies, including relaxation and imagery, hypnosis, yoga, meditation, tai chi and qi gong, and creative arts therapies. The mind–body therapies have been used to address the full range of symptoms, including nausea and vomiting, pain, fatigue, and overall quality of life. Some of the challenges identified include standardizing treatments in diverse patient populations, and the variation in training of providers. Overall results are encouraging with few adverse events reported (Carlson 2017).

MINDFULNESS IN DEPRESSION

The most common form of mindfulness studied in depression to date is MBCT, which can be used as a sole treatment or as an augmentation therapy to conventional treatment (Strauss et al. 2014; Khusid and Vythilingam 2016).

Data for the use of mindfulness as a maintenance treatment to prevent relapse of depression are encouraging. A systematic review and meta-analysis by Clark et al. involving 2,742 participants showed a 21% reduction in average risk of recurrence with the use of MBCT, although, because it was tested after medication use, results must be interpreted accordingly (Clarke et al. 2015).

Additional trials comparing the use of MBCT as sole therapy (Segal et al. 2010) and as compared to standard CBT showed equally encouraging results (Kuyken et al. 2015). The Canadian Network for Mood and Anxiety Disorders identifies MBCT as a second-line therapy for major depressive disorder and a first-line therapy for prevention of recurrence (Parikh et al. 2016).

Mindfulness in oncology and depression

Mindfulness has been shown to be of benefit in cancer patients with depression at various stages of treatment.

Small studies have examined the use of mindfulness in cancer patients to address both depression and anxiety. While effects on anxiety have been stronger than in depression, positive effects have been documented (Zhang et al. 2015; Carlson 2017; Carlson et al. 2017).

Medication adherence

A paper on the use of mindfulness to increase adherence to medical therapy highlights another benefit of this approach in chronic illnesses such as heart failure and HIV where depression affects a significant number of patients (Salmoirago-Blotcher and Carey 2017).

Mindfulness for caretakers

Mindfulness has also been studied in caretakers where in one small study in 40 wives of men confined to rehabilitation centers for schizophrenia found that those in the treatment group ($n = 10$) who underwent training in MBCT, one 1.5-hour session weekly for 8 weeks, had statistically significant improvement in resilience scores (Solati 2017).

Light therapy

Phototherapy has shown promise in addressing seasonal affective disorder and depression (Freeman et al. 2010; Ravindran et al. 2016), although a 2015 Cochrane Database review states that more information is needed for definitive recommendations to be made (Nussbaumer et al. 2015). The recommended time in front of the light box (20–60 minutes of exposure to 10,000 lux of cool-white fluorescent light with the average recommendation of 30 minutes daily in the early morning for up to 6 weeks) presents an excellent opportunity for the use of mind–body therapies as a complementary treatment. For example, consider the addition of a selected guided imagery, self-hypnosis, or mindfulness practice to address depression symptoms during that time frame for those who may be interested in combining therapies.

MUSIC THERAPY IN DEPRESSION

A 2017 Cochrane Database review of the use of music therapy in depression included nine studies and a total of 421 participants primarily evaluating the short-term benefits of music therapy in depression. The reviewers concluded that music therapy had moderate quality of evidence in favor as compared to treatment as usual for depression and was not associated with adverse effects. In addition, music therapy added to *treatment as usual* improved symptoms more than just *treatment as usual*. Anxiety levels were also improved, as was the level of functioning. Studies in children and adolescents are currently lacking in this area, and more and larger studies are needed overall to support the development of broader usage of music therapy in depression (Aalbers et al. 2017).

YOGA IN DEPRESSION

Reviews on the use of yoga for depression are promising, although small and with variable study design (Louie 2014; Uebelacker et al. 2017b).

A study by Uebelacker et al. (2017b) randomized adults with continued depressive symptoms on antidepressive treatment ($n = 63$) to weekly yoga class versus ($n = 59$) in a Healthy Living health education class. The intervention was 10 weeks, followed by 3- and 6-month post follow-ups. Initially, there was not a significant difference in depressive symptoms noted ($p = 0.36$), but at 6-month follow-up, 51% of those in the yoga group showed a greater than 50% reduction in depressive symptoms compared to 31% in health education class ($p = 0.04$) and had a significantly better social functioning and general perception of improved health over time.

After the earlier study, participants were asked to comment on their participation in the sessions. Positive findings that increased acceptability in depressed participants included the non-competitive and non-judgmental culture of the classes, knowledgeable instructors who were caring and kind, the inclusion of depression-themed skill building, and guidance in translating class to home teaching. Some students felt their physical limitations were a factor in fully benefitting from the classes—although no adverse events were reported (Uebelacker et al. 2017a).

POST-TRAUMATIC STRESS DISORDER (PTSD)

Mind–body therapies have shown some benefit for PTSD, although pre-screening and awareness of the potential to precipitate adverse events are important. Multiple small trials have been published which have demonstrated small to moderate benefits—but no definitive recommendations currently exist for depression related to PTSD (Asher et al. 2017).

CLINICAL APPLICATION: DEPRESSION

Suni is a 47-year-old woman who is in the maintenance phase of chemotherapy for ovarian cancer. She is experiencing a significant amount of stress and fatigue due to the disruptions in her family and professional life and does not have a robust support system to help her meet all her responsibilities. She is sleeping poorly and eating more fast food than usual. It was recommended to her that she participate in the MBSR program through the oncology clinic to address her increasing anxiety and growing sense of hopelessness over her situation. She has no background in mind–body medicine but trusts the nurse who made the recommendation so decided to give it a try.

After attending the first class, Suni felt more irritated than calm. She felt the pace of the class was very slow and repetitive, and the other students seemed to have a grasp on the skills already. She found the teaching on diaphragmatic breathing especially irritating, and almost got up to leave midway through the class. She stayed and took the CD home for daily practice which was on progressive muscle relaxation (PMR). Throughout the first week, she was only able to get through 5 minutes of the PMR before experiencing an overwhelming feeling of anxiety and internal discomfort. On arrival in the second class, she was glad to see a walking meditation on the schedule; however, when the time came to practice, the instructor insisted that the movements be extremely slow and methodical. Suni tried to accommodate the instructions but felt as though she was going to burst with irritation and struggled to complete the class.

On follow-up with her clinician, she was asked how she was enjoying the mindfulness class and in a moment of candor told the clinician that she hated it. She said that the excruciatingly slow pace made her more anxious, and she felt defeated because she could not even *do relaxing well*. She asked about medication to calm her anxiety and to lift her spirits. The clinician took some time to explore her stressors and was able to connect Suni to the social worker and to the financial advisor to help problem solve. She was also assigned a patient navigator to help manage the complex logistics of her upcoming treatments. The clinician mentioned a new research study starting up that involved the home use of yoga videos in women in treatment. One in-person class was needed, then the sessions were delivered at home with weekly check-in by phone with the study nurse.

Suni agreed to hold off on adding medication for anxiety and depression to her treatment and decided to give the yoga a try. The first class was attended by a group of women who were interested in maintaining as much activity and function as possible during their treatment. The instructor was enthusiastic and highly skilled. She met with each woman individually to understand her goals and potential limitations. Suni learned that the study group was part of an eight-center study designed to gather enough data to make a meaningful contribution to the ovarian cancer research, a fact she found very appealing.

The yoga class started with a warm-up that was active and enjoyable. Suni found to her surprise that she was able to do all the movements and enjoyed learning the meanings behind the postures and breathing exercises. She found the home videos easy to follow, with enough activity to keep her mind engaged and with enough slow time to help her progressively relax. Overall, she found the yoga a much better fit than the MBSR, and she loved the idea of helping out other women, despite her very limited personal resources. Suni was able to move through the middle section of her treatment regimen without starting an antidepressant medication and found herself sleeping more restfully after she committed to doing the yoga home videos five evenings a week. On follow-up with the study nurse during her weekly check-in calls, Suni reported a significant reduction in her feelings of hopelessness and depression and a desire to continue with yoga after her treatment course ended.

References

Aalbers, S., L. Fusar-Poli, R. E. Freeman, M. Spreen, J. C. Ket, A. C. Vink, A. Maratos, M. Crawford, X. J. Chen, and C. Gold. 2017. Music therapy for depression. *Cochrane Database Syst Rev* 11: CD004517. doi:10.1002/14651858.CD004517.pub3.

Ahola Kohut, S., J. Stinson, C. Davies-Chalmers, D. Ruskin, and M. van Wyk. 2017. Mindfulness-based interventions in clinical samples of adolescents with chronic illness: A systematic review. *J Altern Complement Med* 23 (8): 581–589. doi:10.1089/acm.2016.0316.

Al-Yateem, N., and R. C. Rossiter. 2017. Unstructured play for anxiety in pediatric inpatient care. *J Spec Pediatr Nurs* 22 (1): e12166. doi:10.1111/jspn.12166.

Altino, D. M., L. A. Nogueira-Martins, A. L. B. L. de Barros, and J. L. Lopes. 2017. Predictive factors of anxiety and depression in patients with acute coronary syndrome. *Arch Psychiatr Nurs* 31 (6): 549–552. doi:10.1016/j.apnu.2017.07.004.

Amritanshu, R. R., R. M. Rao, R. Nagaratna, V. H. Veldore, M. U. Usha Rani, K. S. Gopinath, and B. S. Ajaikumar. 2017. Effect of long-term yoga practice on psychological outcomes in breast cancer survivors. *Indian J Palliat Care* 23 (3): 231–236. doi:10.4103/IJPC.IJPC_93_17.

Asher, G. N., J. Gerkin, and B. N. Gaynes. 2017. Complementary therapies for mental health disorders. *Med Clin North Am* 101 (5): 847–864. doi:10.1016/j.mcna.2017.04.004.

Beesdo, K., S. Knappe, and D. S. Pine. 2009. Anxiety and anxiety disorders in children and adolescents: Developmental issues and implications for DSM-V. *Psychiatr Clin North Am* 32 (3): 483–524. doi:10.1016/j.psc.2009.06.002.

Bhatta, S., J. D. Champion, C. Young, and E. Loika. 2017. Outcomes of depression screening among adolescents accessing school-based pediatric primary care clinic services. *J Pediatr Nurs* 38: 8–14. doi:10.1016/j.pedn.2017.10.001.

Bhattacharya, R., C. Shen, A. B. Wachholtz, N. Dwibedi, and U. Sambamoorthi. 2016. Depression treatment decreases healthcare expenditures among working age patients with comorbid conditions and type 2 diabetes mellitus along with newly-diagnosed depression. *BMC Psychiatry* 16: 247. doi:10.1186/s12888-016-0964-9.

Blier, P. 2013. Neurotransmitter targeting in the treatment of depression. *J Clin Psychiatry* 74 (Suppl 2): 19–24. doi:10.4088/JCP.12084su1c.04.

Bogner, H. R., and H. F. McClintock. 2016. Costs of coexisting depression and diabetes. *J Gen Intern Med* 31 (6): 594–595. doi:10.1007/s11606-016-3675-5.

Bradt, J., C. Dileo, L. Magill, and A. Teague. 2016. Music interventions for improving psychological and physical outcomes in cancer patients. *Cochrane Database Syst Rev* (8): CD006911. doi:10.1002/14651858.CD006911.pub3.

Bystritsky, A., S. Hovav, C. Sherbourne, M. B. Stein, R. D. Rose, L. Campbell-Sills, D. Golinelli, G. Sullivan, M. G. Craske, and P. P. Roy-Byrne. 2012. Use of complementary and alternative medicine in a large sample of anxiety patients. *Psychosomatics* 53 (3): 266–272. doi:10.1016/j.psym.2011.11.009.

Carlson, L. E. 2017. Distress management through mind-body therapies in oncology. *J Natl Cancer Inst Monogr* 2017 (52). doi:10.1093/jncimonographs/lgx009.

Carlson, L. E., E. Zelinski, K. Toivonen, M. Flynn, M. Qureshi, K. A. Piedalue, and R. Grant. 2017. Mind-body therapies in cancer: What is the latest evidence? *Curr Oncol Rep* 19 (10): 67. doi:10.1007/s11912-017-0626-1.

Chen, P. Y., Y. M. Liu, and M. L. Chen. 2017. The effect of hypnosis on anxiety in patients with cancer: A meta-analysis. *Worldviews Evid Based Nurs* 14 (3): 223–236. doi:10.1111/wvn.12215.

Clarke, K., E. Mayo-Wilson, J. Kenny, and S. Pilling. 2015. Can non-pharmacological interventions prevent relapse in adults who have recovered from depression? A systematic review and meta-analysis of randomised controlled trials. *Clin Psychol Rev* 39: 58–70. doi:10.1016/j.cpr.2015.04.002.

Cohen, B. E., D. Edmondson, and I. M. Kronish. 2015. State of the art review: Depression, stress, anxiety, and cardiovascular disease. *Am J Hypertens* 28 (11): 1295–1302. doi:10.1093/ajh/hpv047.

Cooney, L. G., and A. Dokras. 2017. Depression and anxiety in polycystic ovary syndrome: Etiology and treatment. *Curr Psychiatry Rep* 19 (11): 83. doi:10.1007/s11920-017-0834-2.

Cooney, L. G., I. Lee, M. D. Sammel, and A. Dokras. 2017. High prevalence of moderate and severe depressive and anxiety symptoms in polycystic ovary syndrome: A systematic review and meta-analysis. *Hum Reprod* 32 (5): 1075–1091. doi:10.1093/humrep/dex044.

Coughtrey, A., A. Millington, S. Bennett, D. Christie, R. Hough, M. Su, M. Constantinou, and R. Shafran. 2017. The effectiveness of psychosocial interventions for psychological outcomes in paediatric oncology: A systematic review. *J Pain Symptom Manage.* doi:10.1016/j.jpainsymman.2017.09.022.

de Groot, M., R. Anderson, K. E. Freedland, R. E. Clouse, and P. J. Lustman. 2001. Association of depression and diabetes complications: A meta-analysis. *Psychosom Med* 63 (4): 619–630.

Dixon, L. J., A. A. Lee, K. L. Gratz, and M. T. Tull. 2017a. Anxiety sensitivity and sleep disturbance: Investigating associations among patients with co-occurring anxiety and substance use disorders. *J Anxiety Disord* 53: 9–15. doi:10.1016/j.janxdis.2017.10.009.

Dixon, L. J., S. M. Witcraft, N. K. McCowan, and R. T. Brodell. 2017b. Stress and skin disease quality of life: The moderating role of anxiety sensitivity social concerns. *Br J Dermatol.* doi:10.1111/bjd.16082.

Ferrari, A. J., F. J. Charlson, R. E. Norman, S. B. Patten, G. Freedman, C. J. Murray, T. Vos, and H. A. Whiteford. 2013. Burden of depressive disorders by country, sex, age, and year: Findings from the global burden of disease study 2010. *PLoS Med* 10 (11): e1001547. doi:10.1371/journal.pmed.1001547.

Ferreira, B. R., J. L. Pio-Abreu, J. P. Reis, and A. Figueiredo. 2017. Analysis of the prevalence of mental disorders in psoriasis: The relevance of psychiatric assessment in dermatology. *Psychiatr Danub* 29 (4): 401–406. doi:10.24869/psyd.2017.401.

Fisher, E. B., J. C. Chan, H. Nan, N. Sartorius, and B. Oldenburg. 2012. Co-occurrence of diabetes and depression: Conceptual considerations for an emerging global health challenge. *J Affect Disord* 142 Suppl: S56–S66. doi:10.1016/S0165-0327(12)70009-5.

Freedenberg, V. A., P. S. Hinds, and E. Friedmann. 2017. Mindfulness-based stress reduction and group support decrease stress in adolescents with cardiac diagnoses: A randomized two-group study. *Pediatr Cardiol* 38 (7): 1415–1425. doi:10.1007/s00246-017-1679-5.

Freedenberg, V. A., S. A. Thomas, and E. Friedmann. 2015. A pilot study of a mindfulness based stress reduction program in adolescents with implantable cardioverter defibrillators or pacemakers. *Pediatr Cardiol* 36 (4): 786–795. doi:10.1007/s00246-014-1081-5.

Freeman, M. P., M. Fava, J. Lake, M. H. Trivedi, K. L. Wisner, and D. Mischoulon. 2010. Complementary and alternative medicine in major depressive disorder: The American Psychiatric Association Task Force report. *J Clin Psychiatry* 71 (6): 669–681. doi:10.4088/JCP.10cs05959blu.

Gartlehner, G., P. Thieda, R. A. Hansen, B. N. Gaynes, A. Deveaugh-Geiss, E. E. Krebs, and K. N. Lohr. 2008. Comparative risk for harms of second-generation antidepressants: A systematic review and meta-analysis. *Drug Saf* 31 (10): 851–865.

Goldin, P. R., and J. J. Gross. 2010. Effects of mindfulness-based stress reduction (MBSR) on emotion regulation in social anxiety disorder. *Emotion* 10 (1): 83–91. doi:10.1037/a0018441.

Gradus, J. L. 2017. Prevalence and prognosis of stress disorders: A review of the epidemiologic literature. *Clin Epidemiol* 9: 251–260. doi:10.2147/CLEP.S106250.

Greco, L. A., R. A. Baer, and G. T. Smith. 2011. Assessing mindfulness in children and adolescents: Development and validation of the child and adolescent mindfulness measure (CAMM). *Psychol Assess* 23 (3): 606–614. doi:10.1037/a0022819.

Herzer, M., and K. K. Hood. 2010. Anxiety symptoms in adolescents with type 1 diabetes: Association with blood glucose monitoring and glycemic control. *J Pediatr Psychol* 35 (4): 415–425. doi:10.1093/jpepsy/jsp063.

Hofmann, S. G., and A. F. Gomez. 2017. Mindfulness-based interventions for anxiety and depression. *Psychiatr Clin North Am* 40 (4): 739–749. doi:10.1016/j.psc.2017.08.008.

Janszky, I., S. Ahnve, I. Lundberg, and T. Hemmingsson. 2010. Early-onset depression, anxiety, and risk of subsequent coronary heart disease: 37-year follow-up of 49,321 young Swedish men. *J Am Coll Cardiol* 56 (1): 31–37. doi:10.1016/j.jacc.2010.03.033.

Jeon, S. W., and Y. K. Kim. 2017. Inflammation-induced depression: Its pathophysiology and therapeutic implications. *J Neuroimmunol* 313: 92–98. doi:10.1016/j.jneuroim.2017.10.016.

Jones, P., M. Blunda, G. Biegel, L. E. Carlson, M. Biel, and L. Wiener. 2013. Can mindfulness-based interventions help adolescents with cancer? *Psychooncology* 22 (9): 2148–2151. doi:10.1002/pon.3251.

Kessler, R. C., M. Petukhova, N. A. Sampson, A. M. Zaslavsky, and H. U. Wittchen. 2012. Twelve-month and lifetime prevalence and lifetime morbid risk of anxiety and mood disorders in the United States. *Int J Methods Psychiatr Res* 21 (3): 169–184. doi:10.1002/mpr.1359.

Khusid, M. A., and M. Vythilingam. 2016. The emerging role of mindfulness meditation as effective self-management strategy, Part I: Clinical implications for depression, post-traumatic stress disorder, and anxiety. *Mil Med* 181 (9): 961–968. doi:10.7205/MILMED-D-14-00677.

Koszycki, D., M. Benger, J. Shlik, and J. Bradwejn. 2007. Randomized trial of a meditation-based stress reduction program and cognitive behavior therapy in generalized social anxiety disorder. *Behav Res Ther* 45 (10): 2518–2526. doi:10.1016/j.brat.2007.04.011.

Kuyken, W., R. Hayes, B. Barrett, R. Byng, T. Dalgleish, D. Kessler, G. Lewis et al. 2015. The effectiveness and cost-effectiveness of mindfulness-based cognitive therapy compared with maintenance antidepressant treatment in the prevention of depressive relapse/recurrence: Results of a randomised controlled trial (the PREVENT study). *Health Technol Assess* 19 (73): 1–124. doi:10.3310/hta19730.

Lach, G., H. Schellekens, T. G. Dinan, and J. F. Cryan. 2017. Anxiety, depression, and the microbiome: A role for gut peptides. *Neurotherapeutics* 15 (1): 36–59. doi:10.1007/s13311-017-0585-0.

LeBourgeois, M. K., L. Hale, A. M. Chang, L. D. Akacem, H. E. Montgomery-Downs, and O. M. Buxton. 2017. Digital media and sleep in childhood and adolescence. *Pediatrics* 140 (Suppl 2): S92–S96. doi:10.1542/peds.2016-1758J.

Li, C., L. Barker, E. S. Ford, X. Zhang, T. W. Strine, and A. H. Mokdad. 2008. Diabetes and anxiety in US adults: Findings from the 2006 behavioral risk factor surveillance system. *Diabet Med* 25 (7): 878–881. doi:10.1111/j.1464-5491.2008.02477.x.

Li, C., D. Xu, M. Hu, Y. Tan, P. Zhang, G. Li, and L. Chen. 2017. A systematic review and meta-analysis of randomized controlled trials of cognitive behavior therapy for patients with diabetes and depression. *J Psychosom Res* 95: 44–54. doi:10.1016/j.jpsychores.2017.02.006.

Lichtman, J. H., E. S. Froelicher, J. A. Blumenthal, R. M. Carney, L. V. Doering, N. Frasure-Smith, K. E. Freedland et al. 2014. Depression as a risk factor for poor prognosis among patients with acute coronary syndrome: Systematic review and recommendations: A scientific statement from the American Heart Association. *Circulation* 129 (12): 1350–1369. doi:10.1161/CIR.0000000000000019.

Lipari, R. N., S. L. Van Horn, A. Hughes, and M. Williams. 2013. State and substate estimates of serious mental illness from the 2012–2014 national surveys on drug use and health. In The CBHSQ Report, pp. 1–19, Rockville, MD.

Louie, L. 2014. The effectiveness of yoga for depression: A critical literature review. *Issues Ment Health Nurs* 35 (4): 265–276. doi:10.3109/01612840.2013.874062.

Marchand, W. R. 2012. Mindfulness-based stress reduction, mindfulness-based cognitive therapy, and zen meditation for depression, anxiety, pain, and psychological distress. *J Psychiatr Pract* 18 (4): 233–252. doi:10.1097/01.pra.0000416014.53215.86.

McAusland, L., and J. Addington. 2016. Biofeedback to treat anxiety in young people at clinical high risk for developing psychosis. *Early Interv Psychiatry*. doi:10.1111/eip.12368.

McCall-Hosenfeld, J. S., S. Mukherjee, and E. B. Lehman. 2014. The prevalence and correlates of lifetime psychiatric disorders and trauma exposures in urban and rural settings: Results from the national comorbidity survey replication (NCS-R). *PLoS One* 9 (11): e112416. doi:10.1371/journal. pone.0112416.

McNamara, C., M. Johnson, L. Read, H. Vander Velden, M. Thygeson, M. Liu, L. Gandrud, and J. McNamara. 2016. Yoga therapy in children with cystic fibrosis decreases immediate anxiety and joint pain. *Evid Based Complement Alternat Med* 2016: 9429504. doi:10.1155/2016/9429504.

McPherson, F., and L. McGraw. 2013. Treating generalized anxiety disorder using complementary and alternative medicine. *Altern Ther Health Med* 19 (5): 45–50.

Mittleman, M. A., M. Maclure, J. B. Sherwood, R. P. Mulry, G. H. Tofler, S. C. Jacobs, R. Friedman, H. Benson, and J. E. Muller. 1995. Triggering of acute myocardial infarction onset by episodes of anger. Determinants of myocardial infarction onset study investigators. *Circulation* 92 (7): 1720–1725.

Mojtabai, R., M. Olfson, and B. Han. 2016. National trends in the prevalence and treatment of depression in adolescents and young adults. *Pediatrics* 138 (6). doi:10.1542/peds.2016-1878.

Montoya, A., R. Bruins, M. A. Katzman, and P. Blier. 2016. The noradrenergic paradox: Implications in the management of depression and anxiety. *Neuropsychiatr Dis Treat* 12: 541–557. doi:10.2147/ NDT.S91311.

Mortamet, G., A. Merckx, N. Roumeliotis, C. Simonds, S. Renolleau, and P. Hubert. 2017a. Parental perceptions of clown care in paediatric intensive care units. *J Paediatr Child Health* 53 (5): 485–487. doi:10.1111/jpc.13448.

Mortamet, G., N. Roumeliotis, F. Vinit, C. Simonds, L. Dupic, and P. Hubert. 2017b. Is there a role for clowns in paediatric intensive care units? *Arch Dis Child* 102 (7): 617–620. doi:10.1136/ archdischild-2016-311583.

Nabi, H., M. Hall, M. Koskenvuo, A. Singh-Manoux, T. Oksanen, S. Suominen, M. Kivimaki, and J. Vahtera. 2010. Psychological and somatic symptoms of anxiety and risk of coronary heart disease: The health and social support prospective cohort study. *Biol Psychiatry* 67 (4): 378–385. doi:10.1016/j.biopsych.2009.07.040.

Nefs, G., F. Pouwer, J. Denollet, and V. Pop. 2012. The course of depressive symptoms in primary care patients with type 2 diabetes: Results from the diabetes, depression, type D personality Zuidoost-Brabant (DiaDDZoB) study. *Diabetologia* 55 (3): 608–616. doi:10.1007/s00125-011-2411-2.

Nussbaumer, B., A. Kaminski-Hartenthaler, C. A. Forneris, L. C. Morgan, J. H. Sonis, B. N. Gaynes, A. Greenblatt et al. 2015. Light therapy for preventing seasonal affective disorder. *Cochrane Database Syst Rev* (11): CD011269. doi:10.1002/14651858.CD011269.pub2.

Parikh, S. V., L. C. Quilty, P. Ravitz, M. Rosenbluth, B. Pavlova, S. Grigoriadis, V. Velyvis et al. 2016. Canadian network for mood and anxiety treatments (CANMAT) 2016 clinical guidelines for the management of adults with major depressive disorder: Section 2. Psychological treatments. *Can J Psychiatry* 61 (9): 524–539. doi:10.1177/0706743716659418.

Pascoe, M. C., and I. E. Bauer. 2015. A systematic review of randomised control trials on the effects of yoga on stress measures and mood. *J Psychiatr Res* 68: 270–282. doi:10.1016/j. jpsychires.2015.07.013.

Perk, J., G. De Backer, H. Gohlke, I. Graham, Z. Reiner, M. Verschuren, C. Albus et al. 2012. European Guidelines on cardiovascular disease prevention in clinical practice (version 2012). The Fifth Joint Task Force of the European Society of Cardiology and Other societies on cardiovascular disease prevention in clinical practice (constituted by representatives of nine societies and by invited experts). *Eur Heart J* 33 (13): 1635–1701. doi:10.1093/eurheartj/ehs092.

Purewal, R., and P. L. Fisher. 2017. The contribution of illness perceptions and metacognitive beliefs to anxiety and depression in adults with diabetes. *Diabetes Res Clin Pract*. doi:10.1016/j. diabres.2017.11.029.

Ravindran, A. V., L. G. Balneaves, G. Faulkner, A. Ortiz, D. McIntosh, R. L. Morehouse, L. Ravindran et al. 2016. Canadian network for mood and anxiety treatments (CANMAT) 2016 clinical guidelines for the management of adults with major depressive disorder: Section 5. Complementary and alternative medicine treatments. *Can J Psychiatry* 61 (9): 576–587. doi:10.1177/0706743716660290.

Rechenberg, K., R. Whittemore, and M. Grey. 2017. Anxiety in youth with type 1 diabetes. *J Pediatr Nurs* 32: 64–71. doi:10.1016/j.pedn.2016.08.007.

Reddy, M. S., and M. S. Vijay. 2016. Yoga in psychiatry: An examination of concept, efficacy, and safety. *Indian J Psychol Med* 38 (4): 275–278. doi:10.4103/0253-7176.185948.

Reich, R. R., C. A. Lengacher, T. W. Klein, C. Newton, S. Shivers, S. Ramesar, C. B. Alinat et al. 2017. A randomized controlled trial of the effects of mindfulness-based stress reduction (MBSR[BC]) on levels of inflammatory biomarkers among recovering breast cancer survivors. *Biol Res Nurs* 19 (4): 456–464. doi:10.1177/1099800417707268.

Robb, S. L., D. S. Burns, K. A. Stegenga, P. R. Haut, P. O. Monahan, J. Meza, T. E. Stump et al. 2014. Randomized clinical trial of therapeutic music video intervention for resilience outcomes in adolescents/young adults undergoing hematopoietic stem cell transplant: A report from the children's oncology group. *Cancer* 120 (6): 909–917. doi:10.1002/cncr.28355.

Roest, A. M., E. J. Martens, P. de Jonge, and J. Denollet. 2010. Anxiety and risk of incident coronary heart disease: A meta-analysis. *J Am Coll Cardiol* 56 (1): 38–46. doi:10.1016/j.jacc.2010.03.034.

Salmoirago-Blotcher, E., and M. P. Carey. 2017. Can mindfulness training improve medication adherence? integrative review of the current evidence and proposed conceptual model. *Explore (NY)*. doi:10.1016/j.explore.2017.09.010.

Segal, Z. V., P. Bieling, T. Young, G. MacQueen, R. Cooke, L. Martin, R. Bloch, and R. D. Levitan. 2010. Antidepressant monotherapy vs sequential pharmacotherapy and mindfulness-based cognitive therapy, or placebo, for relapse prophylaxis in recurrent depression. *Arch Gen Psychiatry* 67 (12): 1256–1264. doi:10.1001/archgenpsychiatry.2010.168.

Shapiro, S. L., L. E. Carlson, J. A. Astin, and B. Freedman. 2006. Mechanisms of mindfulness. *J Clin Psychol* 62 (3): 373–386. doi:10.1002/jclp.20237.

Shinkov, A., A. M. Borissova, R. Kovatcheva, J. Vlahov, L. Dakovska, I. Atanassova, and P. Petkova. 2017. Increased prevalence of depression and anxiety among subjects with metabolic syndrome and known type 2 diabetes mellitus—A population-based study. *Postgrad Med* 1–7. doi:10.1080/00325481.2018.1410054.

Short, N. A., J. W. Boffa, S. King, B. J. Albanese, N. P. Allan, and N. B. Schmidt. 2017. A randomized clinical trial examining the effects of an anxiety sensitivity intervention on insomnia symptoms: Replication and extension. *Behav Res Ther* 99: 108–116. doi:10.1016/j.brat.2017.09.013.

Sibinga, E. M., L. Webb, S. R. Ghazarian, and J. M. Ellen. 2016. School-based mindfulness instruction: An RCT. *Pediatrics* 137 (1). doi:10.1542/peds.2015-2532.

Solati, K. 2017. The efficacy of mindfulness-based cognitive therapy on resilience among the wives of patients with schizophrenia. *J Clin Diagn Res* 11 (4): VC01–VC03. doi:10.7860/JCDR/2017/23101.9514.

Solati, K., M. Mousavi, S. Kheiri, and A. Hasanpour-Dehkordi. 2017. The effectiveness of mindfulness-based cognitive therapy on psychological symptoms and quality of life in systemic lupus erythematosus patients: A randomized controlled trial. *Oman Med J* 32 (5): 378–385. doi:10.5001/omj.2017.73.

Spijkerman, M. P., W. T. Pots, and E. T. Bohlmeijer. 2016. Effectiveness of online mindfulness-based interventions in improving mental health: A review and meta-analysis of randomised controlled trials. *Clin Psychol Rev* 45: 102–114. doi:10.1016/j.cpr.2016.03.009.

Strauss, C., K. Cavanagh, A. Oliver, and D. Pettman. 2014. Mindfulness-based interventions for people diagnosed with a current episode of an anxiety or depressive disorder: A meta-analysis of randomised controlled trials. *PLoS One* 9 (4): e96110. doi:10.1371/journal.pone.0096110.

Tareen, R. S., and K. Tareen. 2017. Psychosocial aspects of diabetes management: Dilemma of diabetes distress. *Transl Pediatr* 6 (4): 383–396. doi:10.21037/tp.2017.10.04.

Uebelacker, L. A., M. Kraines, M. K. Broughton, G. Tremont, L. T. Gillette, G. Epstein-Lubow, A. M. Abrantes, C. Battle, and I. W. Miller. 2017a. Perceptions of hatha yoga amongst persistently depressed individuals enrolled in a trial of yoga for depression. *Complement Ther Med* 34: 149–155. doi:10.1016/j.ctim.2017.06.008.

Uebelacker, L. A., G. Tremont, L. T. Gillette, G. Epstein-Lubow, D. R. Strong, A. M. Abrantes, A. R. Tyrka, T. Tran, B. A. Gaudiano, and I. W. Miller. 2017b. Adjunctive yoga v. health education for persistent major depression: A randomized controlled trial. *Psychol Med* 47 (12): 2130–2142. doi:10.1017/S0033291717000575.

van Venrooij, L. T., and P. C. Barnhoorn. 2017. Hospital clowning: A paediatrician's view. *Eur J Pediatr* 176 (2): 191–197. doi:10.1007/s00431-016-2821-8.

Vollestad, J., B. Sivertsen, and G. H. Nielsen. 2011. Mindfulness-based stress reduction for patients with anxiety disorders: Evaluation in a randomized controlled trial. *Behav Res Ther* 49 (4): 281–288. doi:10.1016/j.brat.2011.01.007.

Weaver, L. L., and A. R. Darragh. 2015. Systematic review of yoga interventions for anxiety reduction among children and adolescents. *Am J Occup Ther* 69 (6): 6906180070p1–6906180070p9. doi:10.5014/ajot.2015.020115.

Zhang, M. Q., R. Li, Y. Q. Wang, and Z. L. Huang. 2017. Neural plasticity is involved in physiological sleep, depressive sleep disturbances, and antidepressant treatments. *Neural Plast* 2017: 5870735. doi:10.1155/2017/5870735.

Zhang, M. F., Y. S. Wen, W. Y. Liu, L. F. Peng, X. D. Wu, and Q. W. Liu. 2015. Effectiveness of mindfulness-based therapy for reducing anxiety and depression in patients with cancer: A meta-analysis. *Medicine (Baltimore)* 94 (45): e0897. doi:10.1097/MD.0000000000000897.

12 Oncology and surgery

INTRODUCTION

Due to the multiple stages of cancer diagnosis and treatment and the long-term approach necessary in the treatment of many cancers, the clinician has repeated potential opportunities to introduce of mind–body therapies into the treatment plan in both adult and pediatric patients.

Studies have shown that cancer patients of all ages use complementary and integrative therapies, with mind–body therapies being among the most popular. Their use can help both children and adults improve communication and engagement in their treatment and help buffer the many stressors inherent in treatment (Ndao et al. 2013; Jacobs 2014; King et al. 2015).

In addition to providing increasing self-regulation skills and providing emotional support, use of the mind–body therapies in oncology has been shown to strengthen the immune system and offer relief from a variety of distressing treatment side effects, including nausea and vomiting, pain, anxiety, depression, fatigue, and sleep disruption (Kanitz et al. 2013; Carlson et al. 2017).

Some of the best researched mind–body therapies in oncology include guided imagery, mindfulness, clinical hypnosis, yoga, tai chi and qigong, and creative arts therapies.

The strength of research varies by therapy, and overlapping use is common, for example combining relaxation practices and guided imagery. Despite inherent research challenges, the Society for Integrative Oncology has documented good supporting evidence for the joint use of imagery and relaxation practices in depression and other mood disturbance and some supporting evidence for their use in anxiety, symptoms of nausea and vomiting, and for overall quality of life (Greenlee et al. 2014).

Other supporting examples of combined therapies include a randomized control trial in 208 patients with breast or prostate cancer that found a combination of guided imagery and progressive muscle relaxation had statistically significant benefit in reduction of a variety of symptoms on patients undergoing chemotherapy, including nausea, vomiting, retching, pain, and perceived fatigue. The treatment group received four weekly supervised and daily unsupervised sessions of scripted guided imagery and progressive muscle relaxation augmented with music inclusive of auditory, tactile and olfactory images. The make-up of the sessions included 2 minutes of breathing exercises, a 10-minute progressive muscle relaxation exercise, and a 15-minute guided imagery session. The control group received standard symptom specific care for side effects (Charalambous et al. 2016).

PEDIATRIC ONCOLOGY

Cancer continues to be the leading cause of disease-related death in children and adolescents in the United States (Siegel et al. 2014). National survey data show that from 2001 to 2009 there were 120,137 child and adolescent cancer diagnoses, and according to the National Cancer Institute, nearly half of these patients are under 10 years of age.

Pediatric oncology patients face similar stressors as those in adult oncology patients, along with additional stressors in the form of absences from school routines, loss of independence, and emotional availability of parents and other caretakers during treatment.

Mind–body therapies in pediatric oncology are sometimes directed at parental stress, which has been shown to significantly impact perceived child stress. For example, in a group survey of 125 families whose child was undergoing treatment for cancer, more than 95% of parents reported post-traumatic stress symptoms (Kazak and Baxt 2007). And a study by Klassen et al. (2008) demonstrated the significant impact of caring for a child diagnosed with cancer on parents' health-related quality of life. One study on the use of combined mind–body therapies examined the effectiveness of guided imagery and progressive muscle relaxation (PMR) as a tool to reduce stress and improve mood in parents of children hospitalized for malignancies. The treatment group ($n = 29$ parents, control $n = 25$ parents) received individualized 25-minute sessions once weekly for 3 weeks using PMR and guided imagery scripts tailored to the intervention. Recordings in CD form were also given to the parents for continued use. Results showed a statistically significant improvement in anxiety ($p = 0.008$), a and reduction in tension ($p = 0.027$), and a decrease in sadness ($p = 0.001$) versus the control group (Tsitsi et al. 2017).

SELECTION OF A MIND–BODY THERAPY IN ONCOLOGY PATIENTS

Determining interest in mind–body therapies and feasibility for their use in oncology patients can follow the same steps as used in other patients. Ideally, one would be able to offer adults, children, and families a wide range of tools and options to best manage their symptoms and stress. First steps would include determining interest, establishing prior experience with mind–body therapies (positive or negative), and aligning interest with available resources. Qualified practitioners are needed, and patients should be encouraged to try new therapies if they are curious. Therapies can be considered for both short- and long-term use and ideally be available to the patient in both the inpatient and outpatient setting. If possible, use of mind–body therapies should be offered early in the treatment course to allow time for skill building. Different therapies may be appropriate at different times in the course of an individual's treatment.

HYPNOSIS IN ONCOLOGY

A collection of studies reviewed by Carlson et al. (2017) demonstrates strong support for the use of clinical hypnosis to address anxiety in both pediatric and adult cancer patients.

A review by Chen et al. also documents the positive impact of hypnosis on anxiety in adult and pediatric cancer patients and found more benefit in therapist-directed versus self-directed sessions (self-hypnosis) in their study population (Chen et al. 2017), although other studies have shown benefit in self-hypnosis in cancer patients for a range of treatment side effects (Bragard et al. 2017).

Clinical hypnosis has shown good efficacy in pediatric oncology patients undergoing bone marrow aspiration and lumbar puncture. One of the earliest studies in this area by Zeltzer and LeBaron (1982) found statistically significant pain reduction with hypnosis in 27 children undergoing bone marrow aspiration and in 22 undergoing lumbar puncture.

A range of other studies examining the effectiveness of the use of hypnosis in lumbar puncture, bone marrow aspiration, venepuncture, and other painful procedures support its benefit in reduction of pre-procedural anxiety and pain (Liossi and Hatira 1999, 2003; Wild and Espie 2004; Liossi et al. 2006, 2009).

A systematic review and meta-analysis of studies examining pain and needle procedures in children by Birnie et al. (2014) included 26 studies using distraction and 7 using hypnosis. Results showed strong support for efficacy in pain reduction for both techniques, although study size and design were limiting factors in both modalities.

Hypnosis has also been shown to be helpful in surgical oncology. For example, a 15-minute psychologist-guided, pre-surgery hypnosis session was found to be very effective in the management of surgical pain both intraoperatively and post-operatively in a randomized trial of 200 women undergoing excisional breast biopsy or lumpectomy in a study by Montgomery et al. Decreased nausea, emotional distress, and overall cost per patient was also seen (Montgomery et al. 2007).

Clinical hypnosis should be carried out by a trained practitioner under guidelines established by a national certifying body such as the American Society for Clinical Hypnosis. Clinicians working with children should have specialty training in both areas, pediatrics and child-directed hypnosis. Patients with any history of trauma or PTSD should be cleared by a mental health consultant to avoid precipitating setbacks or new symptoms.

CLINICAL APPLICATION: HYPNOSIS IN ONCOLOGY

May is a 43-year-old patient with a new diagnosis of breast cancer preparing to undergo lumpectomy. She had become highly anxious in the weeks preceding her procedure and wondered if there was something that could help her. She is deeply religious and prefers to avoid prescription medication. May is a single mother and needs to be able to drive and continue working. She had heard about clinical hypnosis from another patient in the clinic and is curious.

Question: Does her religious affiliation preclude the use of hypnosis?

Hypnosis is secular. It can be described as a form of focused attention or trance, where an individual is deeply relaxed yet always in control of their own faculties. In May's case, the use of hypnosis has several potential benefits, including being non-pharmaceutical and portable. Additionally, May could tailor the hypnosis to help address pre-procedural anxiety and intra-procedure self-regulation. This might include therapeutic suggestions for decreasing blood loss and reducing post-procedure pain.

A particular benefit for May would be the ability to master the skill of self-hypnosis so she could use the therapy any time she needed it, (other than while driving or doing other tasks that required her full attention for safety). People with specific belief systems can incorporate desired images or phrases into any hypnotic therapy session to help augment their strengths, confidence, sense of security, or faith.

CLINICAL APPLICATION: PATIENT FOLLOW-UP

May decided to try an introductory hypnosis session and met with a community-based certified clinical hypnosis practitioner. She remained open minded and learned self-hypnosis in the first session. The practitioner spoke with her about her upcoming procedure and recorded a 15-minute hypnosis session with her that addressed her fear of losing control under sedation, adverse outcomes, worrying about her children, and post-procedural pain. The recording started with a focused breathing exercise followed by several minutes of guided relaxation to deepen trance. This was followed by therapeutic suggestions related to her body's ability to function exactly as needed while she allowed the team to perform the needed procedure. It reviewed how her healthy heart and respiratory system are designed to take care of her and that she could rest and allow her body and health care team to work together to get the procedure done smoothly, with a minimum amount of discomfort or blood loss. It reinforced how, as she was gently waking up from the procedure, she would know that her body would only signal pain if needed to alert the team of important information, nothing in excess. The recording reviewed how her friends and family members would be caring for her children throughout the day, so she could focus on herself and her care. No need for undue anxiety. She could allow trusted others to help her.

May spoke with her patient care coordinator and received assurance that she could listen to the recording before, during, and after the procedure using headphones. She listened to the recording several times daily in the week prior to the procedure and was able to move through the procedure calmly and with confidence. Afterward, her breast surgeon remarked at her rapid recovery and shift in sense of self-confidence. May told her about the recording and was subsequently asked to come to a patient support group meeting to share her experience.

CLINICAL APPLICATION: PEDIATRIC ONCOLOGY

Sean is a 13-year-old boy with a diagnosis of soft tissue sarcoma. He has undergone multiple invasive therapies and repeated rounds of chemotherapy and radiation. The last time he was in the MRI scanner, he had a bad reaction to the sedative used. Sean and his family would like to avoid sedation for his upcoming scan, but it requires sustained time without motion, and the team is concerned about his ability to remain both comfortable and still during the scan. Sean spoke with the Child Life Specialist who suggested exploring clinical hypnosis.

The anesthesiologist lead on the sedation team was very skeptical but willing to explore the option with the family. A pediatric psychologist in the community with training was approached and agreed to work with Sean to prepare him for the scan.

Over the course of three sessions, they reviewed the basics of hypnosis, and Sean quickly mastered self-hypnosis. An approach was used that emphasized Sean's strengths and resilience as a veteran of all the challenges and procedures he has already successfully completed. The sessions emphasized the importance of Sean being motionless and reinforced that this could come easily and naturally to him during the scan. His body already knew what to do. This was simply an opportunity to rest and relax while the scanner did the work.

Sean developed a simple cue for entering into self-hypnosis and practiced so he could drop into a trance using a breath. He could not rely on headphones in the scanner, so he decided to develop a self-directed script with the psychologist that he could use in any future clinical setting. Sean wrote out the script and mentally created a safe and enjoyable sanctuary. He used an image of hibernation to help him assume a completely still position, allowing his body to take care of all necessary needs without moving a muscle. With practice, he memorized the script, which was then reinforced with the psychologist. On the day of the scan, he entered with anticipation and was able to easily trigger his self-hypnotic trance. The scan was completed without difficulty, and he emerged feeling rested and refreshed as he had practiced. Going forward, he used self-hypnosis with each subsequent procedure and hospitalization, which relieved significant anticipatory stress for both Sean and his family members.

MINDFULNESS IN ONCOLOGY

The use of mindfulness in oncology has a robust supporting literature and has been shown to improve quality of life, pain scores, stress symptoms, sense of social support, and to decrease cancer-related anxiety and depression. For example, clinical practice guidelines on the evidence-based use of integrative therapies during and after breast cancer treatment identifies meditation as having the highest grade of evidence for treatment of depression, anxiety, and overall quality of life in survivors of breast cancer (Greenlee et al. 2017).

Mindfulness-based stress reduction has also been shown to be effective in women with metastatic breast cancer by improvement in general activity, sleep, and enjoyment of life. A small wait-list control study ($n = 18$ patients, 9 in the study group) participated in an 8-week classic MBSR program with 2 hours of instruction weekly and daily home practice. Mood disturbance showed a statistically significant improvement, and improvement in pain showed a positive trend. Anxiety and depression were not impacted in this study. Members of the study reported benefit from the peer group support (Lee et al. 2017).

And in a randomized controlled study of 57 colorectal cancer patients, those in the mindfulness group ($n = 17$) who undertook a 32-minute mindfulness practice in the form of body scan during chemotherapy showed that these patients had significantly greater cortisol activity, recorded by salivary cortisol. In this study, more than twice as many patients in the mindfulness group experienced a cortisol rise from baseline in the first 20 minutes of the infusion, which reflects cortisol reactivity rather than the blunting often seen in cancer patients and survivors that is associated with hypothalamic–pituitary–adrenal (HPA) axis dysregulation seen in the chronically stressed. The study is the first to explore this physiologic reaction during chemotherapy infusion and is important because blunting of cortisol expression in cancer patients is associated with poorer health outcomes and reduced survival (Black et al. 2017).

MINDFULNESS IN PEDIATRIC ONCOLOGY

Smaller studies support the use of mindfulness to decrease psychosocial distress in adolescent and young adult cancer survivors who completed an 8-week mindfulness-based intervention. In addition to decreasing feelings of distress, a study by Van der Gucht showed participants ($n = 16$) had a significant decrease in negative self-perception and vulnerability and improvement in quality of life (Van der Gucht et al. 2017).

Meditation has also been shown to reduce pain associated with infusion of a monoclonal antibody (anti-ganglioside GD2), the standard treatment for high-risk neuroblastoma which is known for causing pain as a primary side effect. A small study by Ahmed et al. (2014) showed that children in the treatment group who participated in guided meditation ($n = 24$) required significantly fewer doses of pain medication during treatment ($p < 0.01$).

Mindfulness can be taught in a variety of ways, often as the classic 8-week Mindfulness-Based Stress Reduction course pioneered by Kabat-Zinn (described in detail in Chapter 8) (Carlson et al. 2017). Online delivery of a mindfulness curriculum has also been shown to be effective in adults (Zernicke et al. 2014) and is being piloted with parents of pediatric oncology survivors (Wakefield et al. 2015).

Marusak and colleagues have shown that martial arts therapy that incorporates mindfulness (Kids Kicking Cancer, KKC, www.kidskickingcancer.org) has a very good efficacy in reduction of pediatric cancer pain, with more than 85% of children reporting improvement in pain with an average decrease of 40% (Bluth 2016).

Mindfulness has also been used in the form of a self-compassion videoconference series designed for young adult cancer survivors to help address feelings of social isolation, distress, and body image stress. An 8-week telehealth videoconference intervention for a nationally distributed group of cancer survivors age 18–29 was piloted as a feasibility study using group-based 90-minute videoconference sessions supplemented by home practice. It was shown to be well accepted in the group of 25 attendees. Six of eight sessions were attended by 84% of the participants, and all measures except resilience (body image, anxiety, depression, social isolation, posttraumatic growth, self-compassion, and mindfulness) had significant changes ($P < 0.002$) (Campo et al. 2017).

The forward edge of mindfulness research in children reinforces the fact that it is a trainable skill that can be strengthened over time and can lead to improvement in cognitive performance, regulation of emotion, increased resilience, and improvement in symptoms of anxiety and depression. Advances in neuroimaging techniques area are being used to examine how mindfulness in children influences neural networks and functional connectivity to help determine how best to harness this powerful mind–body tool in pediatric patients (Marusak et al. 2018).

YOGA IN ONCOLOGY

Yoga is another mind–body modality with a substantial supporting literature in oncology patients. Benefits have been especially strong in addressing psychosocial aspects such as depression, anxiety, and overall distress (Danhauer et al. 2017).

The 2017 review by Danhauer et al. (2017) also reports that yoga has also been shown to improve cancer-related fatigue and is correlated with significant improvement in sleep quality in several studies. One randomized controlled study in patients with breast cancer explored the utility of yoga ($n = 53$) in improving physical functioning and physical quality of life compared to stretching ($n = 56$) or wait-list control group ($n = 54$). In this study, the yoga group experienced significantly improved physical quality of life compared to other groups, with improvements continuing at 3-month post-radiation therapy follow-up.

Another study by Bower et al. (2014) in breast cancer survivors with persistent cancer-related fatigue found that those randomized to 12-week Iyengar yoga intervention ($n = 16$) had significantly decreased activity of proinflammatory-related gene expression ($p < 0.05$) compared to the control group ($n = 15$) who received health education only.

A small feasibility study on the use of yoga in the outpatient setting in eight pediatric cancer patients found that a 12-week community-based course that included twice weekly supervised yoga sessions resulted in significant improvements in health-related quality of life ($p = 0.02$), functional mobility ($p = 0.01$), flexibility ($p = 0.02$), and total physical activity levels ($p = 0.02$) pre-post intervention (Wurz et al. 2014).

BIOFEEDBACK IN ONCOLOGY

Adult and pediatric oncology patients face a daunting gamut of procedures beginning from diagnosis through survivorship, including lumbar punctures, intravenous ports and lines, bone marrow aspirations, intramuscular injections, biopsies, possible surgeries, and more. Understandably these are accompanied by high levels of anticipatory and intra- and post-procedure anxiety on the part of patients and caretakers.

A feasibility study by Shockey et al. (2013) evaluated the use of relaxation techniques paired with biofeedback as a scheduled part of invasive procedures to evaluate benefit and efficacy. Participants included 11 children, mean age 11 years, the majority of whom were being treated for leukemia or soft tissue sarcoma. Variables measured included anticipatory fear, anxiety, heart rate and heart rate variability, and satisfaction with the study intervention. Patients received four sessions of the intervention prior to four scheduled procedures. Each relaxation session was 60 minutes long and was built into the child's waiting time in clinic. Breath work (belly breathing) was covered in session 1, biofeedback using em Wave lap top heart rate variability measurement technology at session 2; thereafter each session used a combination of breath and biofeedback. Patient response to the intervention was positive, and most were able to demonstrate improvement in coherence associated with relaxation, although study numbers were too small to establish significance. Use of the belly breathing alone was found to reduce fear in 63% (7/11 patients). Biofeedback alone reduced fear in 45% (5/11), and breath combined with biofeedback resulted in 81% (9/11) feeling more in charge of their bodies pre-procedure. The authors conclude that this combination of skills offered a feasible approach to the management of fear and pre-procedural stress in this clinical setting and served as a useful tool to increase participants' self-regulation skills.

CREATIVE ARTS THERAPIES IN ONCOLOGY

A 2013 review of the potential benefit of creative arts therapies in adult cancer patients that included 27 studies involving 1,576 patients found that participation in creative arts therapies reduced symptoms of anxiety, depression, and pain and improved overall quality of life after treatment. Although immediate results were promising, in most studies, effects were not sustained. Variation in study design, interventions, and duration of trials was high (Puetz et al. 2013).

More recently, a range of small studies using creative art therapies were reviewed by Carlson et al. (2017), and overall encouraging results were shown in coping and communication ability, especially in groups where language or cultural barriers were present, although significant variation in study design and quality was noted. Adverse events were absent, and the creative arts allowed for significant individualization to meet patients' needs.

A study on music therapy in 83 pediatric cancer patients ages 4–7 years compared active music engagement ($n = 27$) versus music listening ($n = 28$) versus audio books ($n = 28$) and found that children involved in active music engagement exhibited significantly higher coping behaviors ($p < 0.0001$). Active engagement is defined as using age-appropriate live music and providing the child multiple opportunities to choose the material and interact in a way of their choosing, guided by a certified music therapist who maintains the child's decision making as a primary focus of the session. The idea is to support the child's autonomy and encourage opportunities to self-regulate during the session (Robb et al. 2008).

Another randomized study evaluating the impact of music therapy was done in 100 patients undergoing stem cell transplantation to measure the impact on overall distress, pain, anxiety, and depression. The treatment group ($n = 50$) received live music therapy sessions twice a week for 30 minutes per session. Results showed a statistical significance for improvement of mood, reduction of anxiety, and improvement of pain ($p < 0.05$) (Doro et al. 2017).

Creative arts therapies along with other integrative therapies are often used in pediatric cancer patients in the form of art, music, play therapy, animal therapy, and other individualized therapies (Thrane 2013).

TAI CHI/QIGONG IN ONCOLOGY

Smaller studies exist supporting the use of these movement therapies in oncology patients, primarily in the elderly. In one of the larger studies, 162 participants participated in a 10-week program that combined a 90-minute weekly class in medical qigong with the assignment of 30 minutes of daily home practice ($n = 79$) versus the control group ($n = 83$). Those in the treatment group had significantly improved the overall quality of life ($p < 0.001$), improvement in fatigue ($p < 0.001$), and a decrease in C-reactive protein ($p < 0.044$) compared to controls (Oh et al. 2010).

A second study by Oh and colleagues in 81 adult cancer patients found that those who participated in a 10-week medical qigong program ($n = 37$) experienced significant improvement in perceived cognitive impairment over the control group ($p = 0.029$) and improved quality of life ($p < 0.001$) compared to controls (Oh et al. 2012).

MIND–BODY THERAPIES IN SURGERY

Given the prevalence of anxiety associated with surgery and the predictable stages involved: pre-, intra-, and post-surgical, multiple opportunities exist to introduce mind–body therapies to interested patients, although large high-quality studies are lacking. A systematic review by Nelson et al. (2013) involved 20 studies and 1,297 patients with the goal of evaluating the efficacy of pre-operative mind–body interventions on post-operative outcomes found wide variability in study design and quality. Guided imagery, relaxation, and hypnosis were the primary interventions used.

Of the studies reviewed, guided imagery was used in eight and was shown in the majority to have moderate evidence for efficacy in reduction of pain medication and strong evidence for improving psychological well-being.

Studies evaluating relaxation lacked evidence to support efficacy in reduction of pain medication and showed some support for improvement in psychological well-being measures. Hypnosis was used in four studies and showed some efficacy in improvement in psychological well-being (Nelson et al. 2013).

A more recent study evaluating the use of guided imagery on functional outcomes of total knee replacement included 58 participants ($n = 29$ treatment group, $n = 29$ controls).

The intervention included listening to a professionally produced pre-recorded 19–21-minute CDs daily for 2 weeks prior and 3 weeks after surgery. The main outcome measured was function and gait velocity. In addition to serum measures of T-cell activation and monocyte function (IL-6, IL-IS, TNF, CD69), hair cortisol concentration in the time frame reflecting 3 months before intervention and 6 months after the intervention was measured. Study results showed that guided imagery pre-post surgical intervention was superior over a placebo for gait velocity, particularly in those with highest imaging ability. Hair cortisol analysis also supported a reduction in HPA activation in the study group. The intervention was found to be feasible in this study group with no adverse events reported (Jacobson et al. 2016).

MUSIC THERAPY IN SURGERY

Music therapy has a growing body of supporting research in surgical patients in both adult and pediatric patients and has been used pre-operatively, intraoperatively, and post-operatively to help reduce anxiety and pain and decrease medication exposure (Mondanaro et al. 2017; Nelson et al. 2017).

Mind–body approaches in surgery can be tailored to the pediatric population. For example, an observational study in 78 children aged 3–11 years scheduled for general anesthesia prior to surgical procedure used an intervention of integrated art therapy with clown visits from the child's arrival at the hospital through the preoperative room. Children in the intervention group had a significant reduction in preoperative anxiety measured on a validated scale ($p < 0.001$) compared to the control group (Dionigi and Gremigni 2017).

SUMMARY

A wealth of data supports the use of mind–body therapies in both adult and pediatric oncology patients, with few adverse effects reported in the literature. Overlap of therapies is common, and the strength of the research varies by therapy, with some of the strongest supporting the use of clinical hypnosis for pain and anxiety in a variety of settings. One of the most important points is to individualize the treatment to the patient's needs and to remember that different therapies may be preferred at various stages of treatment. Ideally, a patient facing a challenging treatment course would be introduced to the mind–body therapies early to provide time for skill building before reaching highly stressful or painful stages of treatment. Mind–body therapies are adaptable to adult and pediatric oncology and surgery patients and should be offered by trained practitioners. Many studies include the use of the home practice in the form of pre-recorded CDs or videos. Mind–body therapies are increasingly being successfully used in the pre-, intra-, and post-operative settings in both children and adults.

References

Ahmed, M., S. Modak, and S. Sequeira. 2014. Acute pain relief after Mantram meditation in children with neuroblastoma undergoing anti-GD2 monoclonal antibody therapy. *J Pediatr Hematol Oncol* 36 (2): 152–155. doi:10.1097/MPH.0000000000000024.

Birnie, K. A., M. Noel, J. A. Parker, C. T. Chambers, L. S. Uman, S. R. Kisely, and P. J. McGrath. 2014. Systematic review and meta-analysis of distraction and hypnosis for needle-related pain and distress in children and adolescents. *J Pediatr Psychol* 39 (8): 783–808. doi:10.1093/jpepsy/jsu029.

Black, D. S., C. Peng, A. G. Sleight, N. Nguyen, H. J. Lenz, and J. C. Figueiredo. 2017. Mindfulness practice reduces cortisol blunting during chemotherapy: A randomized controlled study of colorectal cancer patients. *Cancer* 123 (16): 3088–3096. doi:10.1002/cncr.30698.

Bluth, M. H., R. Thomas, C. Cohen, A. C. Bluth, and E. Goldberg. 2016. Martial arts intervention decreases pain scores in children with malignancy. *Pediatric Health Med Ther* 7: 79–87. doi:10.2147/PHMT.S104021.

Bower, J. E., G. Greendale, A. D. Crosswell, D. Garet, B. Sternlieb, P. A. Ganz, M. R. Irwin, R. Olmstead, J. Arevalo, and S. W. Cole. 2014. Yoga reduces inflammatory signaling in fatigued breast cancer survivors: A randomized controlled trial. *Psychoneuroendocrinology* 43: 20–29. doi:10.1016/j.psyneuen.2014.01.019.

Bragard, I., A. M. Etienne, M. E. Faymonville, P. Coucke, E. Lifrange, H. Schroeder, A. Wagener, G. Dupuis, and G. Jerusalem. 2017. A nonrandomized comparison study of self-hypnosis, yoga, and cognitive-behavioral therapy to reduce emotional distress in breast cancer patients. *Int J Clin Exp Hypn* 65 (2): 189–209. doi:10.1080/00207144.2017.1276363.

Campo, R. A., K. Bluth, S. J. Santacroce, S. Knapik, J. Tan, S. Gold, K. Philips, S. Gaylord, and G. N. Asher. 2017. A mindful self-compassion videoconference intervention for nationally recruited posttreatment young adult cancer survivors: Feasibility, acceptability, and psychosocial outcomes. *Support Care Cancer* 25 (6): 1759–1768. doi:10.1007/s00520-017-3586-y.

Carlson, L. E., E. Zelinski, K. Toivonen, M. Flynn, M. Qureshi, K. A. Piedalue, and R. Grant. 2017. Mind-body therapies in cancer: What is the latest evidence? *Curr Oncol Rep* 19 (10): 67. doi:10.1007/s11912-017-0626-1.

Charalambous, A., M. Giannakopoulou, E. Bozas, Y. Marcou, P. Kitsios, and L. Paikousis. 2016. Guided imagery and progressive muscle relaxation as a cluster of symptoms management intervention in patients receiving chemotherapy: A randomized control trial. *PLoS One* 11 (6): e0156911. doi:10.1371/journal.pone.0156911.

Chen, P. Y., Y. M. Liu, and M. L. Chen. 2017. The effect of hypnosis on anxiety in patients with cancer: A meta-analysis. *Worldviews Evid Based Nurs* 14 (3): 223–236. doi:10.1111/wvn.12215.

Danhauer, S. C., E. L. Addington, S. J. Sohl, A. Chaoul, and L. Cohen. 2017. Review of yoga therapy during cancer treatment. *Support Care Cancer* 25 (4): 1357–1372. doi:10.1007/s00520-016-3556-9.

Dionigi, A., and P. Gremigni. 2017. A combined intervention of art therapy and clown visits to reduce preoperative anxiety in children. *J Clin Nurs* 26 (5–6): 632–640. doi:10.1111/jocn.13578.

Doro, C. A., J. Z. Neto, R. Cunha, and M. P. Doro. 2017. Music therapy improves the mood of patients undergoing hematopoietic stem cells transplantation (controlled randomized study). *Support Care Cancer* 25 (3): 1013–1018. doi:10.1007/s00520-016-3529-z.

Greenlee, H., L. G. Balneaves, L. E. Carlson, M. Cohen, G. Deng, D. Hershman, M. Mumber et al. 2014. Clinical practice guidelines on the use of integrative therapies as supportive care in patients treated for breast cancer. *J Natl Cancer Inst Monogr* 2014 (50): 346–358. doi:10.1093/jncimonographs/lgu041.

Greenlee, H., M. J. DuPont-Reyes, L. G. Balneaves, L. E. Carlson, M. R. Cohen, G. Deng, J. A. Johnson et al. 2017. Clinical practice guidelines on the evidence-based use of integrative therapies during and after breast cancer treatment. *CA Cancer J Clin* 67 (3): 194–232. doi:10.3322/caac.21397.

Jacobs, S. S. 2014. Integrative therapy use for management of side effects and toxicities experienced by pediatric oncology patients. *Children (Basel)* 1 (3): 424–440. doi:10.3390/children1030424.

Jacobson, A. F., W. A. Umberger, P. A. Palmieri, T. S. Alexander, R. P. Myerscough, C. B. Draucker, S. Steudte-Schmiedgen, and C. Kirschbaum. 2016. Guided imagery for total knee replacement: A randomized, placebo-controlled pilot study. *J Altern Complement Med* 22 (7): 563–575. doi:10.1089/acm.2016.0038.

Kanitz, J. L., M. E. Camus, and G. Seifert. 2013. Keeping the balance—An overview of mind–body therapies in pediatric oncology. *Complement Ther Med* 21 (Suppl 1): S20–S25. doi:10.1016/j.ctim.2012.02.001.

Kazak, A. E., and C. Baxt. 2007. Families of infants and young children with cancer: A post-traumatic stress framework. *Pediatr Blood Cancer* 49 (Suppl 7): 1109–1113. doi:10.1002/pbc.21345.

King, N., L. G. Balneaves, G. T. Levin, T. Nguyen, J. G. Nation, C. Card, T. Truant, and L. E. Carlson. 2015. Surveys of cancer patients and cancer health care providers regarding complementary therapy use, communication, and information needs. *Integr Cancer Ther* 14 (6): 515–524. doi:10.1177/1534735415589984.

Klassen, A. F., R. Klaassen, D. Dix, S. Pritchard, R. Yanofsky, M. O'Donnell, A. Scott, and L. Sung. 2008. Impact of caring for a child with cancer on parents' health-related quality of life. *J Clin Oncol* 26 (36): 5884–5889. doi:10.1200/JCO.2007.15.2835.

Lee, C. E., S. Kim, S. Kim, H. M. Joo, and S. Lee. 2017. Effects of a mindfulness-based stress reduction program on the physical and psychological status and quality of life in patients with metastatic breast cancer. *Holist Nurs Pract* 31 (4): 260–269. doi:10.1097/HNP.0000000000000220.

Liossi, C., and P. Hatira. 1999. Clinical hypnosis versus cognitive behavioral training for pain management with pediatric cancer patients undergoing bone marrow aspirations. *Int J Clin Exp Hypn* 47 (2): 104–116. doi:10.1080/00207149908410025.

Liossi, C., and P. Hatira. 2003. Clinical hypnosis in the alleviation of procedure-related pain in pediatric oncology patients. *Int J Clin Exp Hypn* 51 (1): 4–28. doi:10.1076/iceh.51.1.4.14064.

Liossi, C., P. White, and P. Hatira. 2006. Randomized clinical trial of local anesthetic versus a combination of local anesthetic with self-hypnosis in the management of pediatric procedure-related pain. *Health Psychol* 25 (3): 307–315. doi:10.1037/0278-6133.25.3.307.

Liossi, C., P. White, and P. Hatira. 2009. A randomized clinical trial of a brief hypnosis intervention to control venepuncture-related pain of paediatric cancer patients. *Pain* 142 (3): 255–263. doi:10.1016/j.pain.2009.01.017.

Marusak, H. A., F. Elrahal, C. A. Peters, P. Kundu, M. V. Lombardo, V. D. Calhoun, E. K. Goldberg, C. Cohen, J. W. Taub, and C. A. Rabinak. 2018. Mindfulness and dynamic functional neural connectivity in children and adolescents. *Behav Brain Res* 336: 211–218. doi:10.1016/j.bbr.2017.09.010.

Mondanaro, J. F., P. Homel, B. Lonner, J. Shepp, M. Lichtensztein, and J. V. Loewy. 2017. Music therapy increases comfort and reduces pain in patients recovering from spine surgery. *Am J Orthop (Belle Mead NJ)* 46 (1): E13–E22.

Montgomery, G. H., D. H. Bovbjerg, J. B. Schnur, D. David, A. Goldfarb, C. R. Weltz, C. Schechter et al. 2007. A randomized clinical trial of a brief hypnosis intervention to control side effects in breast surgery patients. *J Natl Cancer Inst* 99 (17): 1304–1412. doi:10.1093/jnci/djm106.

Ndao, D. H., E. J. Ladas, Y. Bao, B. Cheng, S. N. Nees, J. M. Levine, and K. M. Kelly. 2013. Use of complementary and alternative medicine among children, adolescent, and young adult cancer survivors: A survey study. *J Pediatr Hematol Oncol* 35 (4): 281–288. doi:10.1097/MPH.0b013e318290c5d6.

Nelson, E. A., M. M. Dowsey, S. R. Knowles, D. J. Castle, M. R. Salzberg, K. Monshat, A. J. Dunin, and P. F. Choong. 2013. Systematic review of the efficacy of pre-surgical mind–body based therapies on post-operative outcome measures. *Complement Ther Med* 21 (6): 697–711. doi:10.1016/j.ctim.2013.08.020.

Nelson, K., M. Adamek, and C. Kleiber. 2017. Relaxation training and postoperative music therapy for adolescents undergoing spinal fusion surgery. *Pain Manag Nurs* 18 (1): 16–23. doi:10.1016/j.pmn.2016.10.005.

Oh, B., P. Butow, B. Mullan, S. Clarke, P. Beale, N. Pavlakis, E. Kothe, L. Lam, and D. Rosenthal. 2010. Impact of medical Qigong on quality of life, fatigue, mood and inflammation in cancer patients: A randomized controlled trial. *Ann Oncol* 21 (3): 608–614. doi:10.1093/annonc/mdp479.

Oh, B., P. N. Butow, B. A. Mullan, S. J. Clarke, P. J. Beale, N. Pavlakis, M. S. Lee, D. S. Rosenthal, L. Larkey, and J. Vardy. 2012. Effect of medical Qigong on cognitive function, quality of life, and a biomarker of inflammation in cancer patients: a randomized controlled trial. *Support Care Cancer* 20 (6): 1235–1242. doi:10.1007/s00520-011-1209-6.

Puetz, T. W., C. A. Morley, and M. P. Herring. 2013. Effects of creative arts therapies on psychological symptoms and quality of life in patients with cancer. *JAMA Intern Med* 173 (11): 960–969. doi:10.1001/jamainternmed.2013.836.

Robb, S. L., A. A. Clair, M. Watanabe, P. O. Monahan, F. Azzouz, J. W. Stouffer, A. Ebberts et al. 2008. A non-randomized [corrected] controlled trial of the active music engagement (AME) intervention on children with cancer. *Psychooncology* 17 (7): 699–708. doi:10.1002/pon.1301.

Shockey, D. P., V. Menzies, D. F. Glick, A. G. Taylor, A. Boitnott, and V. Rovnyak. 2013. Preprocedural distress in children with cancer: An intervention using biofeedback and relaxation. *J Pediatr Oncol Nurs* 30 (3): 129–138. doi:10.1177/1043454213479035.

Siegel, D. A., J. King, E. Tai, N. Buchanan, U. A. Ajani, and J. Li. 2014. Cancer incidence rates and trends among children and adolescents in the United States, 2001–2009. *Pediatrics* 134 (4): e945–e955. doi:10.1542/peds.2013-3926.

Thrane, S. 2013. Effectiveness of integrative modalities for pain and anxiety in children and adolescents with cancer: A systematic review. *J Pediatr Oncol Nurs* 30 (6): 320–332. doi:10.1177/1043454213511538.

Tsitsi, T., A. Charalambous, E. Papastavrou, and V. Raftopoulos. 2017. Effectiveness of a relaxation intervention (progressive muscle relaxation and guided imagery techniques) to reduce anxiety and improve mood of parents of hospitalized children with malignancies: A randomized controlled trial in Republic of Cyprus and Greece. *Eur J Oncol Nurs* 26: 9–18. doi:10.1016/j.ejon.2016.10.007.

Van der Gucht, K., K. Takano, V. Labarque, K. Vandenabeele, N. Nolf, S. Kuylen, V. Cosyns, N. Van Broeck, P. Kuppens, and F. Raes. 2017. A mindfulness-based intervention for adolescents and young adults after cancer treatment: Effects on quality of life, emotional distress, and cognitive vulnerability. *J Adolesc Young Adult Oncol* 6 (2): 307–317. doi:10.1089/jayao.2016.0070.

Wakefield, C. E., U. M. Sansom-Daly, B. C. McGill, M. McCarthy, A. Girgis, M. Grootenhuis, B. Barton et al. 2015. Online parent-targeted cognitive-behavioural therapy intervention to improve quality of life in families of young cancer survivors: Study protocol for a randomised controlled trial. *Trials* 16: 153. doi:10.1186/s13063-015-0681-6.

Wild, M. R., and C. A. Espie. 2004. The efficacy of hypnosis in the reduction of procedural pain and distress in pediatric oncology: A systematic review. *J Dev Behav Pediatr* 25 (3): 207–213.

Wurz, A., C. Chamorro-Vina, G. M. Guilcher, F. Schulte, and S. N. Culos-Reed. 2014. The feasibility and benefits of a 12-week yoga intervention for pediatric cancer out-patients. *Pediatr Blood Cancer* 61 (10): 1828–1834. doi:10.1002/pbc.25096.

Zeltzer, L., and S. LeBaron. 1982. Hypnosis and nonhypnotic techniques for reduction of pain and anxiety during painful procedures in children and adolescents with cancer. *J Pediatr* 101 (6): 1032–1035.

Zernicke, K. A., T. S. Campbell, M. Speca, K. McCabe-Ruff, S. Flowers, and L. E. Carlson. 2014. A randomized wait-list controlled trial of feasibility and efficacy of an online mindfulness-based cancer recovery program: The eTherapy for cancer applying mindfulness trial. *Psychosom Med* 76 (4): 257–267. doi:10.1097/PSY.0000000000000053.

13 Gastroenterology

INTRODUCTION

The use of complementary and integrative therapies is common in patients with gastrointestinal (GI) conditions (Korzenik et al. 2017). In part, this is due to gaps in conventional treatment options and to a growing recognition of the potential influence of mind–body therapies on the gut–brain connection (Edman et al. 2017). Desire to reduce medication use is another driver for the use of complementary and integrative therapies in GI conditions, particularly in the pediatric population (Yeh et al. 2017). Use of these approaches may be especially relevant in adults and children suffering from chronic GI conditions, in individuals whose symptoms are impacted by stress, and in those with functional gastrointestinal disorders (FGIDs) as classified by the Rome IV criteria, most recently revised in 2016. The current criteria classifications take into account the neurobiology of pain and age-developmental stage appropriate pain perception and recognize the importance of the brain–gut axis in pain perception (Koppen et al. 2017).

One example of stress-related GI pain is seen in adults with a history of adverse childhood experiences (ACE). In this population, studies have consistently shown a high correlation between increased ACE score, irritable bowel syndrome (IBS) diagnosis, and a range of other medical conditions (Park et al. 2016).

Other factors, such as personality traits similar to neuroticism, or introversion, and mental health diagnoses such as anxiety or depression can influence GI conditions and have been shown to be amenable to intervention with mind–body therapies in certain patients (Muscatello et al. 2016).

Similarly, mind–body therapies have shown efficacy in modulating the physiologic function of immune, inflammatory, autonomic, and endocrine systems which are intimately involved in gut health and functioning (Bonaz et al. 2017).

Disruption of lifestyle factors such as sleep, physical activity, and decreased quality of life can also impact those living with GI conditions, resulting in a negative feedback loop. The mind–body therapies can also be used to introduce and reinforce healthy lifestyle habits such as healthy diet and exercise which impact gut health (Patel et al. 2016).

The up-regulation of inflammation associated with GI conditions also makes them uniquely susceptible to the influence of mind–body therapies. The mechanisms involved in these interactions are the subject of active research. For example, in one uncontrolled pilot study in 19 patients with IBS and 29 with inflammatory bowel disease (IBD) enrolled in a 9-week relaxation-response-based mindfulness group intervention designed to teach participants how to elicit the relaxation response and build cognitive skills around stress management, specific alterations in gene expression in peripheral blood mononuclear cells that impacted inflammatory pathways related to IBD were induced by the use of a relaxation-response-directed mind—body interaction. This included a full set of genes linked to interferon regulation and signaling, genes associate with inflammation, endothelial barrier functions, vascular permeability, neutrophil recruitment, leukocyte adhesion and extravasation, innate immune response genes, and T-cell differentiation genes. These changes suggest that NF-kB activity led to the increase in expression of multiple cytokines directly linked to onset and expression of IBD. The intervention showed that most of the target genes for key molecules were down-regulated by the relaxation response intervention, likely triggering a corresponding decrease in inflammation (Kuo et al. 2017).

This chapter will review several of the most common GI conditions in adults, adolescents, and children and an update on the use of mind—body therapies in these patient populations. Conditions covered include gastrointestinal reflux disease (GERD), IBD, IBS, and pediatric functional abdominal pain disorders (FAPDs). The intent is not to present an exhaustive list of GI conditions but rather to offer an overview of those that currently have a body of supporting research for the use of mind—body therapies.

GASTROESOPHAGEAL REFLUX DISEASE

One classic working definition of gastroesophageal reflux disease (GERD) published by Moraes-Filho et al. (2002) describes GERD as a "chronic disorder related to the retrograde flow of gastroduodenal contents into the esophagus and other organs, resulting in a variable spectrum of symptoms, with or without tissue damage." It is seen in both adults and children and can manifest as heartburn, regurgitation of acidic stomach contents, chronic cough, asthma, or recurrent pneumonia in certain cases. It can be precipitated by a variety of factors, including obesity, stress, acidic foods, pregnancy, late-night meals, constipation, and reclining body position, especially during sleep. Stress has been shown to have multiple effects on the gut, including changes in motility, microbiome, permeability, lower esophageal sphincter pressure, delayed gastric emptying, and esophageal motility, among other things. Stress should be considered in cases of treatment failure in GERD treated with medication (Jones et al. 2005; Mujakovic et al. 2009; Usai Satta et al. 2017).

An estimated 7% of school-aged children and a slightly higher percentage of adolescents (up to 8%) report upper GI discomfort. Functional dyspepsia in children is defined as persistent upper abdominal pain or discomfort, not related to bowel movements, and without any organic cause—that persists for at least 2 months prior to diagnosis. This has been correlated with delayed gastric emptying in up to 70% of children studied (Yeh and Golianu 2014).

MIND—BODY THERAPIES IN GASTROESOPHAGEAL REFLUX DISEASE

To date, small studies indicate the benefit of mind—body interventions in GERD, including the use of clinical hypnosis and relaxation training (Maradey-Romero et al. 2014).

For example, in one randomized controlled trial of diaphragmatic breathing exercises in 19 patients with non-erosive GERD, 4 weeks of 30 minutes daily practice accompanied by recorded instructions and relaxing music in the treatment group ($n = 10$) correlated with significant improvement in the quality of life ($p < 0.05$) and decrease in esophageal acid exposure versus no change in the control group ($p < 0.05$). Of interest, patients who continued diaphragmatic breathing exercises showed a significant decrease in proton pump inhibitor use at 9-month follow-up (Eherer et al. 2012).

Another randomized controlled trial in 126 patients with functional dyspepsia used hypnotherapy ($n = 26$), placebo and supportive treatment ($n = 24$), or medical treatment ($n = 29$) for 56 weeks. Results at 16 weeks showed more symptom improvement in the hypnosis group (59% median) than in supportive (41%) or medical treatment (33%). The hypnosis group also showed significant improvement in overall quality of life at 16 weeks. At long-term follow-up, the hypnosis group showed even greater symptom improvement (73%) compared to supportive (34%) or medical treatment (43%). Quality of life improved significantly in the hypnosis group compared to medication group ($p < 0.001$), and none of the hypnosis group began medication during long-term follow-up versus 90% in the medical treatment group and 82% of the supportive care–placebo group. Overall visits to a general practitioner were also significantly reduced in the hypnosis group (Calvert et al. 2002).

INFLAMMATORY BOWEL DISEASE

IBD refers to a spectrum of illness that can range from ulcerative colitis which involves only the large intestine to Crohn's disease which can involve the entire GI tract from mouth to anus. There is also a range of indeterminate conditions along the spectrum that do not fit either diagnostic category and may require repeated diagnostic testing and therapeutic trials to establish the best-fit diagnosis and therapeutic approach. General pathophysiology is still a subject of active research and is thought to involve complex interactions between genetic, environmental, infectious, nutrition, stress, gut microbiome, and gut mucosal factors. There is a robust literature supporting the connection between the brain–gut axis in IBD disease course, particularly between ulcerative colitis and depression (Maunder and Levenstein 2008).

Multiple lines of physiologic communication, including the autonomic nervous system, central nervous system, hypothalamic–pituitary–adrenal axis, gastrointestinal corticotropin-releasing factor, and the inherent intestinal immune-microbiota-mucosal barrier response all play important roles in development and course of the disease. These connections highlight the potential influence of mood disorder, perceived stress, and inadequate or misdirected coping strategies and the potential for addressing psychological needs with mind–body therapies as appropriate (Bonaz and Bernstein 2013).

Also relevant is the overlap of IBS symptoms experienced by adults and children with IBD, even when in remission. These patients can experience a variety of physical symptoms such as bloating, pain, diarrhea, urgency, constipation, gas, and cramping that can be amplified by a variety of factors, including visceral hyperalgesia, strictures or adhesions, and dysmotility, among other things, and can be worsened by stress, sleep disruption, anxiety, depression, and other social stressors (Srinath et al. 2014).

One of the hallmarks of modern treatment of IBD is a *whole-person* approach to care that includes multidisciplinary expertise in gut inflammation, nutrition, and psychosocial and lifestyle factors to maximize health in every dimension (Day et al. 2012).

MIND–BODY THERAPIES IN INFLAMMATORY BOWEL DISEASE

It has been established that the use of integrative therapies, including mind–body therapies, is high in youth with IBD (Yeh et al. 2017) and is mirrored in the adult population (Gerbarg et al. 2015; Kuo et al. 2015). Mind–body therapies with solid supporting literature in IBD include cognitive behavioral therapy (CBT) (Levy et al. 2016), combined progressive muscle relaxation and guided imagery (Mizrahi et al. 2012).

In children, an approach combining CBT with PMR and imagery was found to show promise in a small study of 24 child–parent dyads. This intervention used a 1-day seminar on CBT that included education on disease-related elements such as pain management, stress, coping skills, limit setting, communication, and relaxation skills reinforced by a 6-week web-based skill review with homework and group chat portals for both children and parents (McCormick et al. 2010).

MINDFULNESS IN INFLAMMATORY BOWEL DISEASE

Mindfulness, especially in the form of mindfulness-based stress reduction has been shown to be effective and well accepted in adult patients with IBD (Ballou and Keefer 2017; Hood and Jedel 2017).

Mindfulness can be used to address stress, decrease anxiety and depression, adapt to unexpected setbacks, reduce pain, enhance coping skills, and improve overall quality of life. Mindfulness skills can help individuals with IBD modify pain perception and tolerance, help with adherence to healthy lifestyle habits, and modulate immune and inflammatory function. Most of the studies have used a classic 8-week MBSR program with the typical home practice component. One study in 60 adults with IBD which used a series of eight weekly 2.5-hour sessions and one 7-hour weekend retreat with weekly homework assignments, all tailored to patients with IBD, included discussions about the gut–brain connection and the impact of mindfulness meditation on bowel symptoms, life with IBD, and guided meditations that focused on physical symptoms, emotions, and thoughts associated with IBD symptoms. The treatment group showed a decrease in anxiety, depression ($p < 0.05$) and improvement in the quality of life ($P < 0.01$) and in mindfulness ($p < 0.001$) with sustained improvements in both depression and mindfulness at 6-month follow-up (Neilson et al. 2016).

In adults, mindfulness has also been combined with CBT in patients with IBD and was correlated with overall improvement in the quality of life ($p = 0.021$) in those participating in a 16-week program (Berrill et al. 2014).

To date, studies on the efficacy of mindfulness in children specifically targeting those living with IBD are lacking, although some pilot feasibility studies are in process in children living with chronic pain and functional somatic symptoms that show good acceptance of the intervention with the added benefit of peer group support (Ali et al. 2017).

CLINICAL HYPNOSIS IN INFLAMMATORY BOWEL DISEASE

To date, the bulk of studies on clinical hypnosis in GI conditions have been done in patients with IBS, although some supporting research is available in IBD. A review by Szigethy examining the use of hypnotherapy in IBD concludes the bulk of evidence relates to its utility in the reduction of inflammation and in improvement in health-related quality of life (Szigethy 2015).

Support exists for the role of hypnosis in modulating inflammation in patients with active IBD. For example, a controlled study by Mawdsley et al. in 17 adults with active ulcerative colitis, eight underwent a single 50-minute session of gut-focused hypnotherapy while a control group listened to music. The inflammatory response was measured before and after each session and was found to decrease serum IL-6 concentrations by 53% ($p = 0.001$) and rectal mucosal release of substance-P by 81% ($p = 0.001$), histamine by 35% ($p = 0.002$) and IL-13 by 53% ($p = 0.003$) in the hypnotherapy group (Mawdsley et al. 2008).

Another study in adults evaluated gut-directed hypnotherapy and time in clinical remission in a randomized controlled trial of 54 adults with ulcerative colitis. The treatment group ($n = 26$) received seven gut-directed hypnotherapy sessions versus controls ($n = 29$) who received training in attention control. The primary outcome measure was time in clinical remission over the course of 1 year. Time in remission in the treatment group was statistically significant ($p = 0.04$) compared to controls, marking the first prospective study to evaluate the use and benefit of gut-directed hypnosis in patients with ulcerative colitis in clinical remission. The exact mechanism of the effect of hypnotherapy on inflammation remains to be established (Keefer et al. 2013).

A relatively small literature exists supporting the use of hypnotherapy in pediatric IBD patients. One example is a case series involving six children who received between 4 and 12 sessions of hypnosis over 12 weeks who experienced a decrease in inflammatory markers and physical symptoms, although numbers were too small to be considered statistically significant (Shaoul et al. 2009).

Clinical hypnosis delivered by a trained practitioner shows promise as a safe and useful therapy for reduction of inflammation, improvement in symptoms and quality of life, and in supporting remission in some patients with IBD. Further studies are needed in both children and adults.

BIOFEEDBACK IN INFLAMMATORY BOWEL DISEASE

A small supporting literature exists on the use of biofeedback in adult IBD patients, primarily in the treatment of pelvic floor and anorectal disorders associated with defecation. This is an area of evolving research (Bondurri et al. 2015).

Biofeedback studies are lacking in pediatric IBD patients, although it has been shown to be helpful in children with IBS which is discussed in more detail below. Portability, non-invasiveness, and engaging child-friendly modern technology are features that make biofeedback attractive for future study in the pediatric IBD population.

YOGA IN INFLAMMATORY BOWEL DISEASE

The majority of current studies on yoga in GI disorders have been done in patients with IBS, where it has been shown to be of benefit and is discussed in more detail below. One randomized study in 100 IBD patients in remission ($n = 60$, ulcerative colitis and $n = 40$, Crohn's disease) used a yoga intervention for eight weekly 1-hour sessions that combined yoga postures, breathing exercises, and meditation combined with home practice using audio recordings. The treatment group ($n = 30$, ulcerative colitis and $n = 20$, Crohn's disease) reported a significant reduction in arthralgia and in abdominal pain after the 8-week intervention and decrease in state and trait anxiety levels were seen in the ulcerative colitis treatment group. No adverse events were reported (Sharma et al. 2015).

CLINICAL APPLICATION: PEDIATRIC GASTROENTEROLOGY

Nethia is a 9-year-old girl in second grade who immigrated to the United States with her mother to join extended family. Her father did not join the family, and they have faced serious economic challenges along the way. At her aunt's house, Nethia shares a room with her older female cousins and was enrolled in the local elementary school where she has struggled to make friends. In addition to the language barrier, she is small and very thin for her age and has become the target of repeated bullying. Her mother works two jobs and is constantly fatigued. Her aunt is an engaged caretaker but also works long hours, leaving the girls to prepare dinners as best they can. Nethia is unused to the processed foods she is now eating and has complained of a stomachache to her mother since they arrived. There has been no weight loss, no fevers, rashes, bloody stools, or other warning signs—but she has started to have intermittent diarrhea, especially on Sunday evenings and before school tests. Her mother and aunt took her to the local community health center where a basic exam and screening labs were found to be normal. The doctor there asked about stressors, but Nethia was unable to articulate all that was going on to the young male physician. After speaking with the mother and aunt, the physician felt that her symptoms were quite consistent with IBS and recommended a change of diet to reduce processed food, a food diary, and a pain diary to help better understand any connections between food and her symptoms. He also suggested a trial of progressive muscle relaxation coupled with imagery and music and gave them a recommendation for the free Kaiser guided imagery recordings (Permanente 2012).

He asked if the family practiced any sort of relaxation techniques at home such as yoga—but they did not. He also suggested Nethia take a look online with her cousins to see if there were any interesting yoga resources for children on YouTube, such as Cosmic Kids Yoga. The community center had limited classes for children, and the family was not able to attend any programs due to the mother's work schedule. The doctor also suggested speaking with Nethia's teacher and principal to address the bullying behaviors and stressed the importance of breaking this pattern, even if it meant changing schools.

CLINICAL APPLICATION: PATIENT FOLLOW-UP

The family did their best to upgrade the quality of Nethia's diet on a lean budget and ended up following a more traditional diet overall which did bring her some symptom relief. She found one recording online that she liked that used breath work and child-friendly graphics to teach belly breathing and overall relaxation. It helped her fall asleep, and she felt some increase in energy. Her mother and aunt talked to the teacher who was not overly invested in intervening in the bullying behavior because she had not seen it first-hand. She said she would follow the issue more closely and remain in touch with the mother. Over the next few weeks, there was slight improvement in Nethia's GI symptoms which she tracked on the simple diary, then just before the semester break, she began to wake in the night with urgency and diarrhea. The mother was able to take Nethia into the clinic a week later where she was found to have weight loss and anemia. Subsequently, she was referred to the pediatric GI clinic at the Children's Hospital downtown where she was admitted for further workup due to ongoing symptoms.

A full workup revealed a diagnosis of IBD with overlying symptoms of IBS. The family was told that Nethia would need long-term treatment, which initially completely overwhelmed the mother. The Social Work team stepped in to help with insurance and resources. As the mother's stress levels gradually decreased, Nethia began to calm down and began to process what was happening. A Child Life worker came to visit her, and Nethia shared some of the things she has learned about breathing and imagery and relaxation which the Child Life worker found very powerful. She and Nethia talked about how she could use these skills to help her get through the procedures and how she could use these to help her adjust to the new diagnosis.

One of the things Nethia found the most helpful was to make friends with another girl her age in the playroom. They were able to connect on many levels, as were the mothers of the girls. Both families enrolled in the support group and made plans to keep in touch after discharge which Nethia and her friend did online and by telephone. Over time, Nethia became a regular at the Children's Hospital clinics and made the adjustment to living with a chronic illness. She expanded her skill set in mind–body therapies, and although she continued to have an overlay of IBS symptoms when she was tired or stressed, she learned to cope with discomfort by using her mind–body therapies so that they did not become unmanageable. It took time, but she started to have normal linear growth which also increased her comfort at the school where she had changed to a new classroom which was a much better fit.

IRRITABLE BOWEL SYNDROME

The heterogeneous nature of IBS makes it important to take a *whole person* approach to the pain and functional disability that can be life limiting in some patients. The complex interactions of the gut–brain axis in IBS lend itself to a multidisciplinary approach to treatment. Diverse elements such as personality, emotional regulation skills, autonomic nervous system balance, endocrine system functioning, socioeconomic factors, quality of life, work stressors, diet, pain processing, inflammation, and microbiome are all areas associated with IBS and under active study (Muscatello et al. 2016).

Somatization is one example of behavioral influencers of IBS, characterized by a tendency to report multiple unexplained physical symptoms without evidence of medical condition to support or explain the feelings. Somatization is an independent risk factor for IBS and has been shown to influence how patients with IBS perceive their symptoms, their treatments, and their overall quality of life. Although challenging for both patient and practitioner, this state offers many avenues for the use of mind–body therapies to address a range of emotional and physical discomfort. Catastrophizing is another relevant behavior trait in IBS and is defined as "a negative cognitive process of exaggerated rumination and worry" (Muscatello et al. 2016).

Pain catastrophizing is a subset that describes the tendency to magnify seriousness of pain or the anticipation of painful stimuli. Individuals with depression and IBS have been shown to have a greater tendency to catastrophize through anticipation of pain and perception of greater limitations due to pain. Hypervigilance is another characteristic that can add complexity to IBS treatment (Muscatello et al. 2016; Surdea-Blaga et al. 2016; Ballou and Keefer 2017).

Suppressed emotions and a desire for social acceptance are the focus of other work, which has shown some correlation between the emotional state and severity of IBS symptoms.

Authors propose a pathway for patients become more adept and assertive in healthy self-expression as an approach to reduction of symptoms over time (Sibelli et al. 2017).

CLINICAL HYPNOSIS IN IRRITABLE BOWEL SYNDROME

Clinical hypnosis is one of the best studied mind–body therapies in IBS in both children and adults. A specific type of hypnotherapy called gut-directed hypnotherapy was developed in 1984 by Whorwell and colleagues, which has proven highly effective in a variety of patients (Whorwell et al. 1984).

It involves description of basic gut physiology, education about visualization and tactile techniques and therapeutic suggestions to normalize GI functioning and reduce unwanted GI symptoms. The original approach developed involved 10–12 weekly sessions of approximately 45 minutes each (Whorwell 2011).

A study by Vlieger et al. examined the efficacy of gut-directed hypnotherapy in 53 pediatric patients aged 8–18 years with functional abdominal pain ($n = 31$) or IBS ($n = 22$), randomized to receive either hypnosis or standard medical therapy. The hypnosis group received six sessions over a 3-month period. Results showed that the hypnosis group had a statistically significant decrease in pain scores than the control group ($P < 0.001$). At 1-year follow-up, 85% of patients in the hypnosis group had successful treatment versus 25% of the control group ($p < 0.001$) (Vlieger et al. 2007).

Follow-up of 52 of the patients in the initial study by Vlieger et al. showed that children in the original treatment group ($n = 27$) maintained efficacy with 68% of patients maintaining remission at 4.8 years as opposed to 20% receiving conventional therapy ($p = 0.005$). Somatization scores and pain intensity and frequency scores were all lower in the hypnosis group (Vlieger et al. 2012).

Over time, the technique has been adapted to various populations using fewer sessions with good success in both children and adults (Palsson and Whitehead 2013; Rutten et al. 2013).

The effectiveness of gut-directed home-based versus therapist-led hypnotherapy has been evaluated in 303 children 8–18 years with either IBS or functional abdominal pain. Immediately after treatment, 36.8% of children in the home hypnosis group ($n = 132$) had symptom resolution compared to 50% of those in the therapist-directed sessions. At 1-year follow-up, 62% in home-based therapy were in remission versus 71% in therapist-directed group ($p = 0.002$), suggesting that home-based therapy holds excellent potential for some children with IBS and functional abdominal pain (Rutten et al. 2017).

Extended positive results have also been seen in some adult studies. For example, a systematic review and meta-analysis on the use of clinical hypnosis in IBS involved seven randomized controlled trials and 374 adult patients. Results were evaluated at 3 and 12 months post-treatment. Change in abdominal pain score was found to be statistically significant at 3 months in the hypnotherapy group ($p = 0.05$). Improvements extended to 12 months follow-up in two of the studies, but study design variation was noted by authors as a compounding factor (Lee et al. 2014).

How does hypnosis work in irritable bowel syndrome?

Emerging research on the mechanism of action of hypnosis in IBS using fMRI suggests that hypnosis has a normalizing effect on the central processing abnormality (enhanced perception of visceral stimuli) seen in the areas of the brain associated with gut discomfort in a randomized controlled trial of 44 women with IBS.

The treatment group ($n = 25$) received seven 1-hour-long sessions of individual hypnotherapy using gut-directed hypnotherapy which included suggestions to reduce threat perception, lessen gut symptoms, and to deepen overall physical relaxation. The subjects received a pre-recorded CD for daily home practice. Those in the treatment group showed a clinically significant decrease in gut-related anxiety and improvement in symptoms and were able to modulate visceral stimuli centrally (Lowen et al. 2013).

Perhaps one of the most significant identified drawbacks in the use of clinical hypnosis in GI conditions is a lack of qualified providers. This, in part, has prompted development of other approaches, including the use of relaxation paired with guided imagery.

GUIDED IMAGERY AND IRRITABLE BOWEL SYNDROME

A randomized trial comparing home-based guided imagery using audio recordings versus standard medical care for functional abdominal pain in 34 children found that 64% of those in the guided imagery group were responders with significant improvement in symptoms versus 27% of control group. In this study, when control group participants received the guided imagery treatment, 61.5% became responders. Of those who were responders, 62.5% maintained improvement at 6-month follow-up (van Tilburg et al. 2009).

An important caveat in both children and adult patients is for clinicians to be aware of the high prevalence of IBS and functional abdominal pain in those with a history of early adverse life events. Use of the ACE questionnaire may be useful in this patient population, an area of active study (Park et al. 2016).

CLINICAL APPLICATION: ADULT IRRITABLE BOWEL SYNDROME

Colin is a 26-year-old man who is 3 months into his first job out of college. He is slightly overweight and experiencing an increase in abdominal pain, bloating, gas, and indigestion which has bothered him intermittently since high school. He is finding the job much more challenging than he anticipated. He is in a financial firm and unused to the level of competition he is experiencing from his new colleagues. He will be paid by productivity measures and by new accounts, so part of his work is to approach new clients. He is embarrassed by his GI symptoms and has been hanging back from social outings, which his boss has both noticed and commented on.

At his mother's urging, he comes into the clinic. His vital signs are normal, and other than a BMI consistent with *overweight*, his exam is normal. He repeatedly describes his extreme level of pain and discomfort and tells you his work stress is *through the roof*. On questioning about how he has met challenges in the past, he references his parents coming to his aid. He states he has always felt overweight and has struggled with self-esteem issues. His father used family connections to get him his job due to his below average college grades, and he is feeling substantial pressure to be successful.

Despite his level of anxiety, he prefers to avoid medication because of the random drug screen policy at work. He has heard of some of the mind–body therapies and is interested in exploring these. On reflection, it appears that he may be a good fit for gut-directed hypnotherapy given the overlay of symptoms, self-esteem issues, underlying anxiety, and desire to avoid any type of medication. In addition to counseling about diet and exercise, referral is given to a trained practitioner experienced in GI conditions. Colin attends weekly sessions after work for 6 weeks and learns to focus on creating a deeply relaxed physical and mental state where he can allow the therapeutic suggestions to decrease pain and reduce symptoms of bloating and gas. The therapist also gives suggestions to reinforce Colin's feeling of confidence and self-efficacy, which he finds very helpful. The therapist suggests daily home practice, but Colin's time is quite limited due to work demands. After discussion, the therapist proposes recording the weekly sessions onto Colin's smartphone so he can listen to them on the train commute. This turns out to be an excellent solution and allows Colin to arrive at work in a relaxed and comfortable state of mind.

In addition to lowering his baseline anxiety levels, Colin uses the suggestions to make healthier food choices and feels more confident in social settings. Over time, he found himself able to connect with new clients and gradually began to feel that he was indeed in the right job. He continued to see the therapist monthly and began to work on other issues in his life he felt needed work.

MINDFULNESS IN IRRITABLE BOWEL SYNDROME

Meditation and mindfulness-based stress reduction have both been shown to be of benefit, primarily in adults with IBS (Aucoin et al. 2014; Kuo et al. 2017), with MBSR and MBCT showing the highest benefit in subgroup analysis for pain, symptom severity, and quality of life ($p < 0.001$) in one meta-analysis that included 13 studies on the use of mindfulness in somatization disorders (Lakhan and Schofield 2013).

A lack of studies on the utility of mindfulness in pediatric IBS points to an area of rich research potential (Coakley and Wihak 2017).

PEDIATRIC FUNCTIONAL ABDOMINAL PAIN DISORDER

Pediatric functional abdominal pain disorder (FAPD) is defined as recurrent pain with no explanatory organic cause that persists 2 months prior to diagnosis as per Rome IV criteria. The pathogenesis of the pain remains under study. Some associated factors include altered gut motility, visceral hypersensitivity, psychosocial stressors, low socioeconomic status, parental GI complaints, and single parent and immigrant households (Korterink et al. 2015).

BIOFEEDBACK IN FUNCTIONAL ABDOMINAL PAIN DISORDER

Heart rate variability biofeedback has been studied for potential benefit in pediatric functional abdominal pain, a condition in which autonomic dysregulation has been documented. In one study evaluating the use of non-invasive heart rate variability monitors correlated to relaxation and video reward in the form of color and detail appearing on an engaging screen, children in the treatment group who undertook six sessions were able to significantly reduce symptoms and improve autonomic balance ($p = 0.019$) (Sowder et al. 2010).

A second study in 27 children with functional abdominal pain and IBD used a 30-minute heart rate variability biofeedback intervention for an average of eight sessions and found significant improvement in both groups. Full remission, defined as symptom free for 2 full weeks, was achieved by 63% of functional abdominal pain patients and 70% IBD patients in this study. The modality was well accepted overall (Stern et al. 2014).

YOGA IN ADULT AND PEDIATRIC IRRITABLE BOWEL SYNDROME

The use of yoga in children and adults with IBS has shown benefit, and its use has been found to be safe, well accepted, and associated with significant improvement in quality of life, although a systematic review (six studies and 273 patients) in adult IBS patients identified limitations in several studies such as small sample size and variable study design (Schumann et al. 2016).

The use of yoga in adolescents with IBS has been associated with improvement in gastrointestinal symptoms as well as with lower anxiety and avoidance behaviors, and lower levels of functional disability compared to controls in a study of 25 adolescents 11–18 years of age (Kuttner et al. 2006).

A meta-analysis of yoga in IBS that included six randomized controlled trials and 273 patients found evidence for benefit of yoga over conventional treatment in IBS patients in terms of quality of life, physical functioning, and global improvement—but was limited by small study size and methodologic concerns precluding the author's ability to make definitive recommendations (Schumann et al. 2016).

SUMMARY

Given the wealth of supporting literature for a range of mind–body therapies in patients with GI conditions, clinicians should be familiar with the options available. The complex interactions of the brain–gut axis make patients with GI disorders promising candidates for consideration of these therapies. Ideally, treatment of patients with GI conditions will receive a *whole person* approach to care involving counseling on nutrition, physical activity, sleep, and stress management along with discussion of the mind–body therapies. Resource limitations (time, personnel, funding) are common in GI clinics, and therefore consideration of group visits, home therapy, and self-directed therapies where appropriate should be considered. Educational online curriculum and home based interventions such as the gut-directed hypnotherapy CDs discussed earlier are other creative and practical options (Dossett et al. 2017).

References

Ali, A., T. R. Weiss, A. Dutton, D. McKee, K. D. Jones, S. Kashikar-Zuck, W. K. Silverman, and E. D. Shapiro. 2017. Mindfulness-based stress reduction for adolescents with functional somatic syndromes: A pilot cohort study. *J Pediatr* 183: 184–190. doi:10.1016/j.jpeds.2016.12.053.

Aucoin, M., M. J. Lalonde-Parsi, and K. Cooley. 2014. Mindfulness-based therapies in the treatment of functional gastrointestinal disorders: A meta-analysis. *Evid Based Complement Alternat Med* 2014: 140724. doi:10.1155/2014/140724.

Ballou, S., and L. Keefer. 2017. Psychological interventions for irritable bowel syndrome and inflammatory bowel diseases. *Clin Transl Gastroenterol* 8 (1): e214. doi:10.1038/ctg.2016.69.

Berrill, J. W., M. Sadlier, K. Hood, and J. T. Green. 2014. Mindfulness-based therapy for inflammatory bowel disease patients with functional abdominal symptoms or high perceived stress levels. *J Crohns Colitis* 8 (9): 945–955. doi:10.1016/j.crohns.2014.01.018.

Bonaz, B. L., and C. N. Bernstein. 2013. Brain–gut interactions in inflammatory bowel disease. *Gastroenterology* 144 (1): 36–49. doi:10.1053/j.gastro.2012.10.003.

Bonaz, B., V. Sinniger, and S. Pellissier. 2017. The vagus nerve in the neuro-immune axis: Implications in the pathology of the gastrointestinal tract. *Front Immunol* 8: 1452. doi:10.3389/fimmu.2017.01452.

Bondurri, A., A. Maffioli, and P. Danelli. 2015. Pelvic floor dysfunction in inflammatory bowel disease. *Minerva Gastroenterol Dietol* 61 (4): 249–259.

Calvert, E. L., L. A. Houghton, P. Cooper, J. Morris, and P. J. Whorwell. 2002. Long-term improvement in functional dyspepsia using hypnotherapy. *Gastroenterology* 123 (6): 1778–1785. doi:10.1053/gast.2002.37071.

Coakley, R., and T. Wihak. 2017. Evidence-based psychological interventions for the management of pediatric chronic pain: New directions in research and clinical practice. *Children (Basel)* 4 (2). doi:10.3390/children4020009.

Day, A. S., O. Ledder, S. T. Leach, and D. A. Lemberg. 2012. Crohn's and colitis in children and adolescents. *World J Gastroenterol* 18 (41): 5862–5869. doi:10.3748/wjg.v18.i41.5862.

Dossett, M. L., E. M. Cohen, and J. Cohen. 2017. Integrative medicine for gastrointestinal disease. *Prim Care* 44 (2): 265–280. doi:10.1016/j.pop.2017.02.002.

Edman, J. S., J. M. Greeson, R. S. Roberts, A. B. Kaufman, D. I. Abrams, R. J. Dolor, and R. Q. Wolever. 2017. Perceived stress in patients with common gastrointestinal disorders: Associations with quality of life, symptoms and disease management. *Explore (NY)* 13 (2): 124–128. doi:10.1016/j.explore.2016.12.005.

Eherer, A. J., F. Netolitzky, C. Hogenauer, G. Puschnig, T. A. Hinterleitner, S. Scheidl, W. Kraxner, G. J. Krejs, and K. M. Hoffmann. 2012. Positive effect of abdominal breathing exercise on gastroesophageal reflux disease: A randomized, controlled study. *Am J Gastroenterol* 107 (3): 372–378. doi:10.1038/ajg.2011.420.

Gerbarg, P. L., V. E. Jacob, L. Stevens, B. P. Bosworth, F. Chabouni, E. M. DeFilippis, R. Warren, M. Trivellas, P. V. Patel, C. D. Webb, M. D. Harbus, P. J. Christos, R. P. Brown, and E. J. Scherl. 2015. The effect of breathing, movement, and meditation on psychological and physical symptoms and inflammatory biomarkers in inflammatory bowel disease: A randomized controlled trial. *Inflamm Bowel Dis* 21 (12): 2886–2896. doi:10.1097/MIB.0000000000000568.

Hood, M. M., and S. Jedel. 2017. Mindfulness-based interventions in inflammatory bowel disease. *Gastroenterol Clin North Am* 46 (4): 859–874. doi:10.1016/j.gtc.2017.08.008.

Jones, M. P., L. K. Sharp, and M. D. Crowell. 2005. Psychosocial correlates of symptoms in functional dyspepsia. *Clin Gastroenterol Hepatol* 3 (6): 521–528.

Keefer, L., T. H. Taft, J. L. Kiebles, Z. Martinovich, T. A. Barrett, and O. S. Palsson. 2013. Gut-directed hypnotherapy significantly augments clinical remission in quiescent ulcerative colitis. *Aliment Pharmacol Ther* 38 (7): 761–771. doi:10.1111/apt.12449.

Koppen, I. J., S. Nurko, M. Saps, C. Di Lorenzo, and M. A. Benninga. 2017. The pediatric Rome IV criteria: What's new? *Expert Rev Gastroenterol Hepatol* 11 (3): 193–201. doi:10.1080/17474124.2017.1282820.

Korterink, J. J., K. Diederen, M. A. Benninga, and M. M. Tabbers. 2015. Epidemiology of pediatric functional abdominal pain disorders: A meta-analysis. *PLoS One* 10 (5): e0126982. doi:10.1371/journal.pone.0126982.

Korzenik, J., A. K. Koch, and J. Langhorst. 2017. Complementary and integrative gastroenterology. *Med Clin North Am* 101 (5): 943–954. doi:10.1016/j.mcna.2017.04.009.

Kuo, B., M. Bhasin, J. Jacquart, M. A. Scult, L. Slipp, E. I. Riklin, V. Lepoutre et al. 2015. Genomic and clinical effects associated with a relaxation response mind–body intervention in patients with irritable bowel syndrome and inflammatory bowel disease. *PLoS One* 10 (4): e0123861. doi:10.1371/journal.pone.0123861.

Kuo, B., M. Bhasin, J. Jacquart, M. A. Scult, L. Slipp, E. I. Riklin, V. Lepoutre et al. 2017. Correction: Genomic and clinical effects associated with a relaxation response mind–body intervention in patients with irritable bowel syndrome and inflammatory bowel disease. *PLoS One* 12 (2): e0172872. doi:10.1371/journal.pone.0172872.

Kuttner, L., C. T. Chambers, J. Hardial, D. M. Israel, K. Jacobson, and K. Evans. 2006. A randomized trial of yoga for adolescents with irritable bowel syndrome. *Pain Res Manag* 11 (4): 217–223.

Lakhan, S. E., and K. L. Schofield. 2013. Mindfulness-based therapies in the treatment of somatization disorders: A systematic review and meta-analysis. *PLoS One* 8 (8): e71834. doi:10.1371/journal.pone.0071834.

Lee, H. H., Y. Y. Choi, and M. G. Choi. 2014. The efficacy of hypnotherapy in the treatment of irritable bowel syndrome: A systematic review and meta-analysis. *J Neurogastroenterol Motil* 20 (2): 152–162. doi:10.5056/jnm.2014.20.2.152.

Levy, R. L., M. A. van Tilburg, S. L. Langer, J. M. Romano, L. S. Walker, L. A. Mancl, T. B. Murphy et al. 2016. Effects of a cognitive behavioral therapy intervention trial to improve disease outcomes in children with inflammatory bowel disease. *Inflamm Bowel Dis* 22 (9): 2134–2148. doi:10.1097/MIB.0000000000000881.

Lowen, M. B., E. A. Mayer, M. Sjoberg, K. Tillisch, B. Naliboff, J. Labus, P. Lundberg, M. Strom, M. Engstrom, and S. A. Walter. 2013. Effect of hypnotherapy and educational intervention on brain response to visceral stimulus in the irritable bowel syndrome. *Aliment Pharmacol Ther* 37 (12): 1184–1197. doi:10.1111/apt.12319.

Maradey-Romero, C., H. Kale, and R. Fass. 2014. Nonmedical therapeutic strategies for nonerosive reflux disease. *J Clin Gastroenterol* 48 (7): 584–589. doi:10.1097/MCG.0000000000000125.

Maunder, R. G., and S. Levenstein. 2008. The role of stress in the development and clinical course of inflammatory bowel disease: Epidemiological evidence. *Curr Mol Med* 8 (4): 247–252.

Mawdsley, J. E., D. G. Jenkins, M. G. Macey, L. Langmead, and D. S. Rampton. 2008. The effect of hypnosis on systemic and rectal mucosal measures of inflammation in ulcerative colitis. *Am J Gastroenterol* 103 (6): 1460–1469. doi:10.1111/j.1572-0241.2008.01845.x.

McCormick, M., B. Reed-Knight, J. D. Lewis, B. D. Gold, and R. L. Blount. 2010. Coping skills for reducing pain and somatic symptoms in adolescents with IBD. *Inflamm Bowel Dis* 16 (12): 2148–2157. doi:10.1002/ibd.21302.

Mizrahi, M. C., R. Reicher-Atir, S. Levy, S. Haramati, D. Wengrower, E. Israeli, and E. Goldin. 2012. Effects of guided imagery with relaxation training on anxiety and quality of life among patients with inflammatory bowel disease. *Psychol Health* 27 (12): 1463–1479. doi:10.1080/08870446.2012.691169.

Moraes-Filho, J., I. Cecconello, J. Gama-Rodrigues, L. Castro, M. A. Henry, U. G. Meneghelli, E. Quigley, and Group Brazilian Consensus. 2002. Brazilian consensus on gastroesophageal reflux disease: Proposals for assessment, classification, and management. *Am J Gastroenterol* 97 (2): 241–248. doi:10.1111/j.1572-0241.2002.05476.x.

Mujakovic, S., N. J. de Wit, C. J. van Marrewijk, G. A. Fransen, R. J. Laheij, J. W. Muris, M. Samsom et al. 2009. Psychopathology is associated with dyspeptic symptom severity in primary care patients with a new episode of dyspepsia. *Aliment Pharmacol Ther* 29 (5): 580–588. doi:10.1111/j.1365-2036.2008.03909.x.

Muscatello, M. R., A. Bruno, C. Mento, G. Pandolfo, and R. A. Zoccali. 2016. Personality traits and emotional patterns in irritable bowel syndrome. *World J Gastroenterol* 22 (28): 6402–6415. doi:10.3748/wjg.v22.i28.6402.

Neilson, K., M. Ftanou, K. Monshat, M. Salzberg, S. Bell, M. A. Kamm, W. Connell et al. 2016. A controlled study of a group mindfulness intervention for individuals living with inflammatory bowel disease. *Inflamm Bowel Dis* 22 (3): 694–701. doi:10.1097/MIB.0000000000000629.

Palsson, O. S., and W. E. Whitehead. 2013. Psychological treatments in functional gastrointestinal disorders: A primer for the gastroenterologist. *Clin Gastroenterol Hepatol* 11 (3): 208–216; quiz e22–e23. doi:10.1016/j.cgh.2012.10.031.

Park, S. H., E. J. Videlock, W. Shih, A. P. Presson, E. A. Mayer, and L. Chang. 2016. Adverse childhood experiences are associated with irritable bowel syndrome and gastrointestinal symptom severity. *Neurogastroenterol Motil* 28 (8): 1252–1260. doi:10.1111/nmo.12826.

Patel, A., S. Hasak, B. Cassell, M. A. Ciorba, E. E. Vivio, M. Kumar, C. P. Gyawali, and G. S. Sayuk. 2016. Effects of disturbed sleep on gastrointestinal and somatic pain symptoms in irritable bowel syndrome. *Aliment Pharmacol Ther* 44 (3): 246–258. doi:10.1111/apt.13677.

Permanente, K. 2012. Kaiser Guided Imagery Resources in cooperation with Health Journeys. Retrieved from https:// healthy.kaiserpermanente.org.

Rutten, J. M., J. B. Reitsma, A. M. Vlieger, and M. A. Benninga. 2013. Gut-directed hypnotherapy for functional abdominal pain or irritable bowel syndrome in children: A systematic review. *Arch Dis Child* 98 (4): 252–257. doi:10.1136/archdischild-2012-302906.

Rutten, J. M. T. M., A. M. Vlieger, C. Frankenhuis, E. K. George, M. Groeneweg, O. F. Norbruis, A. Ten et al. 2017. Home-based hypnotherapy self-exercises vs individual hypnotherapy with a therapist for treatment of pediatric irritable bowel syndrome, functional abdominal pain, or functional abdominal pain syndrome: A randomized clinical trial. *JAMA Pediatr* 171 (5): 470–477. doi:10.1001/jamapediatrics.2017.0091.

Schumann, D., D. Anheyer, R. Lauche, G. Dobos, J. Langhorst, and H. Cramer. 2016. Effect of yoga in the therapy of irritable bowel syndrome: A systematic review. *Clin Gastroenterol Hepatol* 14 (12): 1720–1731. doi:10.1016/j.cgh.2016.04.026.

Shaoul, R., I. Sukhotnik, and J. Mogilner. 2009. Hypnosis as an adjuvant treatment for children with inflammatory bowel disease. *J Dev Behav Pediatr* 30 (3): 268. doi:10.1097/DBP.0b013e3181a7eeb0.

Sharma, P., G. Poojary, S. N. Dwivedi, and K. K. Deepak. 2015. Effect of yoga-based intervention in patients with inflammatory bowel disease. *Int J Yoga Therap* 25 (1): 101–112. doi:10.17761/1531-2054-25.1.101.

Sibelli, A., T. Chalder, H. Everitt, P. Workman, F. L. Bishop, and R. Moss-Morris. 2017. The role of high expectations of self and social desirability in emotional processing in individuals with irritable bowel syndrome: A qualitative study. *Br J Health Psychol* 22 (4): 737–762. doi:10.1111/bjhp.12264.

Sowder, E., R. Gevirtz, W. Shapiro, and C. Ebert. 2010. Restoration of vagal tone: A possible mechanism for functional abdominal pain. *Appl Psychophysiol Biofeedback* 35 (3): 199–206. doi:10.1007/s10484-010-9128-8.

Srinath, A., E. Young, and E. Szigethy. 2014. Pain management in patients with inflammatory bowel disease: Translational approaches from bench to bedside. *Inflamm Bowel Dis* 20 (12): 2433–2449. doi:10.1097/MIB.0000000000000170.

Stern, M. J., R. A. Guiles, and R. Gevirtz. 2014. HRV biofeedback for pediatric irritable bowel syndrome and functional abdominal pain: A clinical replication series. *Appl Psychophysiol Biofeedback* 39 (3–4): 287–291. doi:10.1007/s10484-014-9261-x.

Surdea-Blaga, T., A. Baban, L. Nedelcu, and D. L. Dumitrascu. 2016. Psychological interventions for irritable bowel syndrome. *J Gastrointestin Liver Dis* 25 (3): 359–366. doi:10.15403/jgld.2014.1121.253.ibs.

Szigethy, E. 2015. Hypnotherapy for inflammatory bowel disease across the lifespan. *Am J Clin Hypn* 58 (1): 81–99. doi:10.1080/00029157.2015.1040112.

Usai Satta, P., F. Oppia, and F. Cabras. 2017. Overview of pathophysiological features of GERD. *Minerva Gastroenterol Dietol* 63 (3): 184–197. doi:10.23736/S1121-421X.17.02390-X.

van Tilburg, M. A., D. K. Chitkara, O. S. Palsson, M. Turner, N. Blois-Martin, M. Ulshen, and W. E. Whitehead. 2009. Audio-recorded guided imagery treatment reduces functional abdominal pain in children: A pilot study. *Pediatrics* 124 (5): e890–e897. doi:10.1542/peds.2009-0028.

Vlieger, A. M., C. Menko-Frankenhuis, S. C. Wolfkamp, E. Tromp, and M. A. Benninga. 2007. Hypnotherapy for children with functional abdominal pain or irritable bowel syndrome: A randomized controlled trial. *Gastroenterology* 133 (5): 1430–1436. doi:10.1053/j.gastro.2007.08.072.

Vlieger, A. M., J. M. Rutten, A. M. Govers, C. Frankenhuis, and M. A. Benninga. 2012. Long-term follow-up of gut-directed hypnotherapy vs. standard care in children with functional abdominal pain or irritable bowel syndrome. *Am J Gastroenterol* 107 (4): 627–631. doi:10.1038/ajg.2011.487.

Whorwell, P. J. 2011. IBS: Hypnotherapy—A wasted resource? *Nat Rev Gastroenterol Hepatol* 9 (1): 12–13. doi:10.1038/nrgastro.2011.235.

Whorwell, P. J., A. Prior, and E. B. Faragher. 1984. Controlled trial of hypnotherapy in the treatment of severe refractory irritable-bowel syndrome. *Lancet* 2 (8414): 1232–1234.

Yeh, A. M., and B. Golianu. 2014. Integrative treatment of reflux and functional dyspepsia in children. *Children (Basel)* 1 (2): 119–133. doi:10.3390/children1020119.

Yeh, A. M., A. Wren, and B. Golianu. 2017. Mind–body interventions for pediatric inflammatory bowel disease. *Children (Basel)* 4 (4). doi:10.3390/children4040022.

14 Pain

INTRODUCTION

Pain management has become a central issue in modern health care, with an estimated annual cost of $560–$635 billion in the United States alone, exceeding the combined costs of care for cardiovascular diseases, cancers, and diabetes (Institute of Medicine 2011).

Globally, chronic pain is estimated to impact 2 of every 10 people and is not limited to adults or seniors—although an aging population is a factor (Hoy et al. 2012). A review by King et al. (2011) estimates the range of global prevalence of chronic pain in children to range from 25% to 46%. Increasing pain prevalence correlates approximately with age progression to adolescence and is linked to lower socioeconomic status. Headache, abdominal, and musculoskeletal pain are the most frequently identified drivers in this population.

In the U.S. adults, low back pain, neck pain, joint pain, arthritis, gout, and fibromyalgia are the diagnoses most frequently associated with the use of integrative therapies, including the mind–body approaches (Clarke et al. 2016). Increasing prevalence of chronic pain parallels the rise of many lifestyle-driven disorders in adult and pediatric populations, including obesity and overweight, which now impact nearly one in three adults, adolescents, and children (Urquhart et al. 2011; Smith et al. 2014; Calenzani et al. 2017). Unhealthy lifestyle, socioeconomic stressors, and chronic pain often manifest in a punishing negative feedback loop where inflammation, functional limitation, and peripheral and central nervous system pathology combine, presenting complex treatment challenges (Huang et al. 2018).

The exploding opioid crisis is a testament to the complexity of chronic pain management and a reflection of the pressures faced by clinicians to provide patients quick relief, an approach whose cost has become self-evident. Although research in many approaches to pain, including psychological interventions, are still evolving (Markozannes et al. 2017), the multiple facets of chronic pain and its reach into an individual's personal, professional, social, and/or academic arenas provide unique levers for the use of mind–body therapies. The ability to address intangible factors such as pain perception, perceived stress, hope, resilience, coping and relaxation skills, motivation, and perseverance highlight the flexibility and power of the mind–body therapies and provide clinician's important new tools (Hsu et al. 2010).

Even the vocabulary of pain lends itself to use of the mind–body therapies. For example, a skilled clinician can teach patients ways to blunt the *sting*, cool the *burning*, soften the *pressure*, and calm the *throbbing* sensations. Unlike reliance on a prescription medication, mind–body skills can also be cultivated to help patients harness inner resources needed to initiative lifestyle change, for example: increased physical activity, upgrade nutrition, or weight loss—all of which have potential to enhance self-efficacy, sense of agency, and self-confidence while potentially reducing perceived pain.

Flexibility of offerings is another important component of the use of mind–body therapies in pain. Interventions such as mindfulness have shown benefit in a variety of pain patients (discussed later in the chapter) and allow for tailoring to specific conditions for optimal result. For example, a systematic review by Reiner et al. (2013) included 16 papers, 10 of which involved controlled trials and six uncontrolled. A significant reduction in perception of pain intensity was seen in the mindfulness-based intervention groups across studies with sustained improvements in many of the groups. Creative use of online education, for example, in mindfulness-based stress reduction (MBSR), has allowed patients wider access to self-directed training (Gardner-Nix et al. 2008).

The ability to expand therapeutic options and partner with the patient also has the potential to reduce clinician stress and burnout. As seen in evolving practice models, an integrative team approach in chronic pain patients may help clinicians distribute responsibility for patient care and expand treatment options. The 2012 National Health Interview Survey indicated that more than 50% of adults using integrative approaches for low back pain reported significant benefit from integrative therapy use, which includes a range of practitioners (Ghildayal et al. 2016).

New guidelines on the non-pharmacologic management of low back pain by the American College of Physicians reinforce the growing awareness of the usefulness of integrative therapies in chronic pain and recommend consideration of a range of approaches, including multidisciplinary rehabilitation, acupuncture, MBSR, tai chi, yoga, progressive muscle relaxation (PMR), EMG biofeedback, and cognitive behavioral therapy (CBT) for chronic pain with grade *strong recommendation* (Qaseem et al. 2017).

Although theoretically mind–body approaches could be applied in nearly any pain condition, research support is currently strongest in a handful of conditions, among them: low back pain, musculoskeletal pain, headache, functional abdominal pain, end of life pain, and arthritis and central sensitization patterns seen in fibromyalgia and related illnesses. The following material will review literature on the use of mind–body therapies in selected conditions. The intent is not to give an exhaustive overview of research in mind–body therapies in pain, or to imply that the mind–body therapies are recommended in all chronic pain patients, but rather to raise awareness of work going in this area and provide an underpinning of data that will hopefully motivate clinicians to consider the use of mind–body therapies in pain patients if they have not already done so. As in any medical condition, organic causes should be ruled out in any patient with pain, and any progression of symptoms should be promptly addressed.

ADVANCES IN UNDERSTANDING PAIN PHYSIOLOGY

One of the newest theories in our understanding of chronic pain has been termed central sensitization, which describes generalized hypersensitivity of the somatosensory system.

Characteristics include disproportionate pain, the presence of diffuse pain distribution, allodynia, and hyperalgesia, and hypersensitivity of senses unrelated to the musculoskeletal system (Nijs et al. 2014).

This classification covers a broad array of conditions not previously linked, such as fibromyalgia, chronic low back pain, migraine headache, functional abdominal pain, and others. Neuroplastic changes in both central and peripheral nervous systems are a hallmark of central sensitization and are an area of intense study which lies beyond the scope of the chapter. One of the key elements of the condition is a malfunction of the endogenous descending nociceptive modulatory systems (Malfliet et al. 2017).

This descending system interacts with and influences pain perception through intricate connections with areas of the brain, including the periaqueductal gray matter, prefrontal cortex, limbic system, and others, that have been linked with abnormal pain processing in various patient chronic pain populations. This can be influenced by certain personality traits and cognitive patterns which may in turn influence treatment outcomes (Vadivelu et al. 2017).

Of special note is the research showing the reversible nature of these changes and the inherent plasticity of both central and peripheral nervous systems (Tajerian and Clark 2017). Emerging research efforts to identify effective treatments are focusing on the pathophysiology of central sensitization and how best to modify abnormal pain processing pathways. The utility of the mind–body therapies in this condition is highlighted by research showing the connection between the stress response and pain processing (Martenson et al. 2009) and how dysregulation of the stress response can play a role in the progression from acute to chronic pain (Li and Hu 2016).

LOW BACK PAIN

Estimated to impact 8 of 10 adults at some point, low back pain may be one of the most researched pain subtypes (Hoy et al. 2012), with the majority of cases occurring without identified specific underlying cause (Chou et al. 2007).

The complexity occurs when acute back pain becomes chronic, which can lead to loss of function and high levels of psychological distress. Central nervous system changes have also been documented; for example, imaging studies in 111 patients with chronic back pain and 432 controls without pain show striking changes in brain architecture in areas associated with pain processing and emotional demands. Atrophy of gray matter in associated brain areas is another consistent finding (Fritz et al. 2016).

Predictors of the development of persistent disabling back pain have been examined by Chou et al. (2007) and include several factors that may be amenable to mind–body therapies. Examples include maladaptive coping behaviors such as excessive fear and catastrophizing, depression and anxiety, and overreaction to external stimuli (Chou and Shekelle 2010).

Supervised physical activity to build strength, increase function, maintain or build flexibility, reduce inflammation, and decrease the risk of deconditioning associated with comorbidities such as overweight, obesity, and cardiovascular disease are important as first-line approaches in low back pain in addition to the use of mind–body therapies.

MIND–BODY THERAPIES IN CHRONIC LOW BACK PAIN

Some of the best studied mind–body approaches to chronic low back pain include CBT and MBSR. For example, a 2017 systematic review and analysis evaluated seven randomized controlled trials involving 864 patients with low back pain who underwent MBSR training. Compared to studies using usual care as control (4RCTs) MBSR was associated with a statistically significant improvement in pain intensity at short-term follow-up. Compared to an active comparator (CBT), MBSR interventions did not show statistically significant improvements in short- or long-term follow-up. Authors conclude that larger rigorous randomized controlled trials are needed to further clarify effectiveness and safety of MBSR in low back pain patients (Anheyer et al. 2017).

In a randomized controlled trial evaluating the effectiveness of MBSR in adults age 20–70 years living with chronic back pain, participants were assigned to MBSR ($n = 116$) or CBT ($n = 113$) or usual care ($n = 113$). The MBSR and CBT training was given in group settings in eight 2-hour sessions. Clinically meaningful improvements were seen in 43.6% of the MBSR group and in 44.9% of CBT group at 26 weeks versus 26.6% in those getting usual care. The improvements in the MBSR group continued to 52-week follow-up (Cherkin et al. 2016).

And a study by Tan et al. (2015) evaluated 100 male veterans with long-standing severe low back pain in a randomized four-group study. Groups received either eight-session hypnosis training without home audio resources; eight-session self-hypnosis training with audio resources for home use; two-session self-hypnosis training with audio recordings and weekly telephone check-in; or eight-session active biofeedback control intervention. Results showed that all groups experienced improvement in pain intensity, interference with activity, and sleep quality. Hypnotic suggestions focused on deep relaxation, sensory substitution, reduction of pain intensity, imagined anesthesia, decreased pain unpleasantness, managing breakthrough pain, and post-hypnotic suggestions for effective self-hypnosis. Groups who received hypnosis training had significantly more reduction in pain intensity than the control biofeedback group, and more than 50% of hypnosis participants maintained reductions in pain intensity for at least 6 months. In this study, two sessions of self-hypnosis training with home access to audio recordings was as effective as eight sessions of hypnosis treatment.

MINDFUL MOVEMENT IN LOW BACK PAIN

Mindful movement in the form of yoga and tai chi also show promise in the treatment of chronic low back pain. Yoga and tai chi are discussed below.

Yoga

A 2017 Cochrane Database Review evaluating 12 trials and 1,080 participants concluded that low-to-moderate evidence supports the efficacy of yoga compared to usual treatment and non-exercise controls in improving back-related function at 3- and 6-month follow-up. No serious adverse events were reported in participants (Wieland et al. 2017).

And an overview of yoga research in a range of psychiatric and other medical conditions, including pain perception, depression, and anxiety also touches on its potential usefulness in addressing the full spectrum of factors that can influence duration and intensity of experiencing chronic low back pain (Field 2016).

Tai chi

One randomized controlled trial in adults with low back pain ($n = 160$) used a 10-week intervention of tai chi ($n = 80$ treatment group) that consisted of eighteen 40-minute sessions delivered in a group format by an experienced instructor. Results showed that tai chi was superior to usual care in the reduction of pain intensity and improvement in self-report disability (Hall et al. 2011).

A 2017 systematic review and meta-analysis of the effect of tai chi and fatigue included 10 trials and ($n = 689$) participants and, although not specific to back pain, found significant improvements in a range of patient groups (cancer, fibromyalgia, multiple sclerosis, and others) experiencing fatigue with no adverse events reported (Xiang et al. 2017).

Web-based app for low back pain

Web-based technology has also been developed and tested for use in adults with non-specific low back pain. A mobile web app called FitBack was tested in 597 adults randomized into three groups: a treatment group with email prompts, an alternative care group who received email prompts to Internet resources on back pain, and a control group. Results showed that the treatment group using the FitBack app had significant improvement over the other groups in physical, behavioral, and work-site outcome at 4-month follow-up, including decreased recurrence of pain and improvement in overall quality of life (Irvine et al. 2015).

CLINICAL APPLICATION: CHRONIC LOW BACK PAIN

Walter is a 65-year-old retired railroad worker who has suffered low back pain since an on-the-job injury 15 years ago. He was in and out of occupational health services while he was still working and was told that he would probably always have pain, although no specific abnormality was ever found. Walter lost his wife of 50 years to cancer not long after he retired and has one son who lives across the country. He has a very limited social life and watches TV most evenings. He used to keep up with his friends from work but finds it too much trouble to get out of the house now. When his wife was alive, they attended church regularly and he enjoyed the men's group there. He has not been to church in 2 years and feels it has now been too long to go back. He has gained weight and has noticed some stiffness in his hips and knees. He has had worsening back pain over the last 3 months and comes to the clinic at the urging of his neighbor who had to help him into the house after a back spasm when he was bringing in groceries.

On questioning, Walter states that he is as out of shape as he ever has ever been in his life and getting back into shape feels like an overwhelming proposition. Workup in the clinic ruled out underlying pathology, and the discussion moved to rehabilitative and preventive measures. Tai chi and yoga were discussed, and a brief overview of the promising research was given, but Walter fully rejected the idea of yoga class, even chair yoga. He was referred to physical therapy to begin an organized strength and flexibility rehabilitation program.

He needed help with transportation initially, and this was arranged through a community service. In the first several sessions Walter was shocked to see how much function and strength he had lost—and decided that he wanted to regain his mobility and avoid use of prescription pain medications (which he had been repeatedly offered).

In the physical therapy waiting room, Walter saw a flyer for tai chi and made a wisecrack about the unfamiliar therapy to another man waiting to be seen. It turned out that the man had been enrolled in a tai chi class by his physician after a fall and enjoyed the slow balancing movements. He and Walter started talking, and it turned out they had been in the military around the same time. The man said to Walter, "My philosophy about the class was, you don't have to like it, you just have to do it." Then, he said, "It gets easier and the teacher is great—he is 80 years old but you would never know it." Walter's curiosity was piqued, and he decided he had little to lose by trying it.

Walter continued to go to physical therapy and initially he did not mention to his therapist that he was trying tai chi. Over time, he began to enjoy the tai chi class, as much for the social aspect as for the exercise. He gradually began to notice some flexibility and some core strength returning. His physical therapist was pleased with his progress, and once his course of therapy was completed, Walter continued in the tai chi class and went on to make steady progress over the rest of the year.

HEADACHE

The 2015 Global Burden of Disease Study lists migraine headache as the third cause of disability in those under 50 years of age, and collectively migraine, tension-type, and medication overuse headache were ranked sixth in 2015. In the younger age group (15–49 years) collectively, the headache categories rank in third place (Steiner et al. 2016). The societal cost of all types of headaches is substantial in terms of overall reduced quality of life, impact on family, and lost productivity.

The multifactorial nature of headaches and their significant comorbidities present a powerful argument for the use of an integrative approaches, especially with regards to migraine prophylaxis. Preventive measures such as healthy nutrition, effective stress management, regular enjoyable physical activity, and restorative sleep have all been shown to reduce migraine headache frequency and severity.

There is also a strong potential role for mind–body therapies, especially in the treatment of migraine, in part due to the interplay between emotional distress and migraine symptoms. Behavioral treatments (e.g., relaxation, biofeedback, hypnosis, and CBT) currently have the best supporting evidence for successful headache management. They are considered first-line preventive options, especially in those who have a significant headache-related disability, comorbid mood or anxiety disorder, difficulty managing stress or other triggers, and medication overuse (Nicholson et al. 2011). Although survey studies have shown that many clinicians are unaware of the range of non-pharmacologic approaches to headache (Minen et al. 2016), partnering with patients can assist them in identifying personal triggers and help to identify the best treatment options.

Various mind–body therapies can be combined, for example, biofeedback with relaxation training, and have been shown to be more effective than solo therapy in reducing headache frequency, muscle tension, anxiety, depression, and medication usage in migraine patients in some studies (Nestoriuc and Martin 2007).

PROGRESSIVE MUSCLE RELAXATION (PMR) IN HEADACHE

PMR has been shown to be highly efficacious in migraine prevention and has been shown to be as effective as a pharmacological migraine prophylaxis (Nestoriuc and Martin 2007). In a study on the effectiveness of PMR as a preventive treatment, 35 migraine patients and 46 healthy controls were selected and 16 migraineurs and 21 healthy participants underwent the study with the remaining serving as controls. Those in the study received 6-week training in PMR with pre- and post-measures of evoked potentials, contingent negative variation (CNV), which reflects central information processing. CNV has been shown to be altered in migraine patients who show higher amplitudes and reduced habituation—findings that have been shown to be modifiable with some prophylactic migraine treatments such as beta-blockers and behavioral therapy. In this study, the effects of PMR were measured.

Post-PMR training, the migraine patients had a statistically significant reduction in migraine frequency and normalization of the early component CNV amplitude as opposed to controls. No changes in habituation were seen. The authors suggest further studies and were confident confirming the clinical efficacy of PMR in migraine prophylaxis (Meyer et al. 2016).

HYPNOSIS IN HEADACHE

Multiple studies support the efficacy of clinical hypnosis in migraine treatment, including the use of self-hypnosis in producing significant reductions in frequency, duration, and intensity of headaches in both pediatric and adult populations. For example, in one study of 144 pediatric patients, headache frequency was reduced from an average of 4.5 per week to 1.4 per week ($p < 0.01$) with a significant reduction in intensity and duration. No adverse effects were noted (Kohen and Zajac 2007).

Hypnosis also has a long history of use in tension-type headache and has been found to have efficacy similar to that in migraine treatment (Hammond 2007).

MINDFULNESS IN HEADACHE

MBSR has been found to be effective in multiple studies of patients experiencing various types of chronic pain, including headache (Rosenzweig et al. 2010), and an MBSR course was found to be safe and feasible in a small randomized controlled trial of 19 migraineurs. The small study size limited conclusive findings, although an overall reduction in migraine frequency and severity was seen. Further study is warranted in this emerging area (Wells et al. 2014).

Mindfulness was shown to be equally as effective as medical prophylaxis after supervised medication withdrawal in a small study of 44 patients suffering from chronic migraine associated with medication overuse. Patients in the mindfulness group ($n = 22$) received MBSR training in weekly sessions and did not receive any medical prophylaxis. Results were comparable, and the authors suggest larger randomized studies to further non-pharmaceutical options (Grazzi et al. 2017).

MBSR has also shown promise in a pilot study of a 6-week MBSR course in tension-type headache patients who showed a significant decrease in headache frequency (Day et al. 2014).

YOGA IN HEADACHE

Yoga has been shown to be helpful for headache relief in several studies. In one study, yoga therapy was contrasted with self-care for 72 randomized migraineurs over 3 months. Headache intensity, frequency, pain, medication use, and anxiety and depression scores were statistically lower in the yoga group ($p < 0.001$ all categories) (John et al. 2007).

BIOFEEDBACK IN HEADACHE

Electromyographic biofeedback has shown efficacy in tension-type headache, as have CBT and relaxation training (autogenics, PMR) (Nestoriuc et al. 2008; Bendtsen and Jensen 2011; Sun-Edelstein and Mauskop 2012).

CLINICAL APPLICATION: MIGRAINE HEADACHE

Pooja is a 30-year-old woman who is a survivor of childhood sexual abuse. She is in ongoing therapy and does not manifest PTSD symptoms. She has struggled to complete her college degree due to a variety of disruptive factors, including chronic migraine headache. She has tried a variety of preventive and abortive medications without consistent benefit and is interested in exploring her treatment options. A friend in her support group had success with the use of clinical hypnosis for smoking cessation, and she is interested in learning more about it.

Prior to introducing hypnosis to Pooja, it will be important to communicate with and obtain clearance from her therapist to avoid inadvertently provoking symptoms related to past traumas.

Once this step was cleared, Pooja was introduced to clinical hypnosis with a focus on the multisensory aspect of her migraine symptoms. The session started with a brief relaxation exercise using breath work and PMR, then she was asked to describe the migraine in detail, from its earliest symptoms to resolution. She described the headache as a red circle that began as a small dot behind her right eye and gradually expanded in size to encompass the right side of her head. She described the color as increasing in intensity, with wave-like pulsations. She also described the intermittent appearance of zigzag patterns along her peripheral vision that were black and yellow in color. Her description of the pain relayed a vivid sense of pressure and constriction and a very heightened sensitivity to noise, light, and smell. She also relayed an overwhelming sense of fatigue that usually accompanied the migraines and a desire to recline in a dark, quiet room.

Pooja's vivid description provided a rich vocabulary that could be used to modify the symptoms with therapeutic suggestions while in hypnotic trance. For example, she was invited to visualize the headache in its earliest stages, and while in a deeply relaxed and focused state (trance) use her imagination to shrink the size of the red circle behind her eye, and to gradually lessen the intensity of the color from red to a light pink, and perhaps to see if the light pink dot resembled something she might find pleasant or comforting, such as a wildflower or a small token of support from a loved one. She was invited to imagine this as a gentle reminder from her body that she was experiencing stress and to take this as a signal to implement relaxation strategies to redirect the potential headache. She was then invited to use a combination of breath work and PMR involving her shoulders, neck, jaw muscles, and face and scalp muscles to soften and interrupt any developing muscle tension and to reground herself in the moment. If in the future she were to experience any sensation of pressure or constriction related to the headache, she was reminded that she could work with the sensations to lighten pressure, open constricted areas, and allow a feeling of cool gentle comfort to replace the uncomfortable sensations as they faded away.

Pooja undertook weekly sessions with a practitioner certified in clinical hypnosis and learned self-hypnosis which she practiced daily. Based on her description of the headache symptoms, the practitioner recorded a 10-minute session onto Pooja's smartphone to facilitate practice of her new skills. Over time, the frequency and intensity of the migraine headaches decreased significantly, and Pooja benefited from a growing sense of confidence in her ability to problem solve. She went on to complete her college degree over the next few years and maintained steady momentum toward her career goals.

FIBROMYALGIA

Fibromyalgia has been classified under the *central pain disorder* category that includes diagnoses such as irritable bowel syndrome, reflex neurovascular dystrophy, chronic daily headache, and others, correlating with persistent central nervous system sensitization. Modern imaging has facilitated understanding of the brain and nervous system involvement in these conditions and demonstrated atrophy of gray matter and changes in functional brain connectivity of specific networks in patients with fibromyalgia (Lin et al. 2016; Hsiao et al. 2017).

The pain has been described as *central sensitization* resulting in "amplification of neural signaling within the central nervous system eliciting pain hypersensitivity." It has been shown that a variety of types of stimuli can trigger central sensitization pain (pressure, light, cold, sound, heat, stress, etc.). The effect of brain derived neurotrophic factor, a key driver of synaptic plasticity, is an area of active study in pain (Nijs et al. 2015).

Imaging studies in patients with fibromyalgia have shown increased functional connectivity in brain areas associated with sensory discrimination of pain and the anterior insula associated with the evaluation of nociceptive processing that has been associated with high rates of pain catastrophizing. Some studies have correlated participation in CBT training with reduction of connectivity in this area (Lazaridou et al. 2017).

Conditions in these categories often require a multipronged approach to address elevated pain levels, hypersensitivity to stimuli, and associated comorbidities such as depression, anxiety, sleep disorders, and fatigue. Upregulation of proinflammatory cytokines has also been reported in numerous studies (Adler-Neal and Zeidan 2017).

One of the most important approaches on the part of the clinician may be to acknowledge the patient's pain, recognize and inquire about the presence of common comorbidities, and partner with the patient to craft an effective multidisciplinary approach to symptom management (Harris 2011). Introduction of the mind–body therapies can prove valuable for some patients. For example, a group of 177 female adult fibromyalgia patients was randomized to one of three study arms: classic MBSR; active control group used PMR and stretching, weekly support and education but no mindfulness component; wait-list control. Of the interventions, only MBSR in post-hoc analysis resulted in a statistically significant improvement in the main outcome measure, health-related quality of life ($p = 0.02$). The effect sizes in the study were too small to make generalized recommendations. No adverse events were reported.

A 2017 review of fibromyalgia treatment highlights CBT and exercise as approaches with the strongest evidence supporting short-term improvement to date and explores approaches to the use of mindfulness in fibromyalgia (Adler-Neal and Zeidan 2017). For example, a study comparing CBT in a group setting ($n = 74$) with MBSR adapted to what was called mindfulness awareness training. Meditation awareness training (MAT) group ($n = 74$) used eight-weekly 2-hour sessions, guided meditation homework, facilitated group discussions, and two one-on-one sessions with an instructor. This study arm focused on non-attachment and was modified to address fibromyalgia-specific symptoms, incorporating objectifying somatic pain, compassion-empathy training, and altruism promoting techniques. The MAT group showed statistically significant and sustained improvement over controls in pain perception, sleep quality, non-attachment, stress perception, and civic engagement. The authors concluded that an approach to mindfulness that developed concepts of pain acceptance non-judgmental awareness, and non-attachment to concepts related to self, symptoms, or environment may be effective in fibromyalgia treatment (Van Gordon et al. 2017).

HYPNOSIS AND GUIDED IMAGERY IN FIBROMYALGIA

Relatively few studies in the use of imagery or hypnosis currently exist in fibromyalgia treatment. One review by Zech et al. (2017) included seven randomized trials with a total of 387 participants. Studies compared hypnosis versus CBT and hypnosis with CBT versus control and the use of guided imagery and hypnosis versus controls in the home or group settings. Results showed that hypnosis combined with CBT was superior to CBT alone, and a clinically relevant benefit of guided imagery and hypnosis over controls was seen, with over 50% improvement in pain relief and psychological distress. No adverse events were reported.

YOGA IN FIBROMYALGIA

Small studies on the use of mindful movement therapies in fibromyalgia have not shown substantive benefits. One review that included seven papers and 362 subjects involved qi gong, tai chi, and yoga. Only the yoga interventions showed benefit in this review with improvements in pain, fatigue, depression, and health-related quality of life seen in short-term follow-up, median range 4.5 months. No adverse events were seen and a need for larger randomized trials is noted (Langhorst et al. 2013).

ARTHRITIS AND OTHER RHEUMATIC DISEASES

Relatively few studies on mind–body interventions in arthritis and other rheumatic diseases are currently available. One systematic review of randomized controlled trials included seven studies and 287 participants who used guided imagery as either sole or partial intervention. All of the interventions used recorded guided imagery scripts and ranged from a one-time session to a 16-week program. Statistically significant results supporting the use of imagery were observed in all studies although study design and size were variable (Giacobbi et al. 2015).

YOGA IN ARTHRITIS

An emerging literature on the benefits of yoga in arthritis finds that gentle-relaxation-based yoga has been found to be feasible in small studies (Ward et al. 2017). Yoga has also been shown to be well accepted in group classes in a community-based setting in a small study in adults with rheumatoid arthritis (Greysen et al. 2017) and when delivered in a chair yoga class in twice-weekly 45-minute sessions to seniors in community settings ($n = 131$) where it was associated with reduction in pain, fatigue, and improvement in gait speed (Park et al. 2017).

CLINICAL APPLICATION: FIBROMYALGIA

Junelle is a 40-year-old woman with a 10-year history of diffuse pain and accompanying fatigue. She has had multiple extensive workups that have all been considered *negative* for pathology. She is viewed as a hypochondriac and drug seeker in her current health care system, a stigma that has caused her significant distress. She has become progressively more depressed, is sleeping poorly, and lives with the fear that a serious medical issue such as cancer is going undiagnosed. Few of her friends remain in contact, and she has recently applied for disability benefits.

The multifactorial components of Junelle's case mirror that seen in many chronic pain patients in that nearly every aspect of their lives is impacted by pain symptoms. In an initial evaluation, it is important to acknowledge the scope of the problem, recognize that the person is feeling real pain despite lack of abnormal test results, provide reassurance that their concerns are taken seriously, and provide hope that they have the potential to improve.

In addition to a whole person approach to her health, mind–body therapies can provide ways for Junelle to address a range of symptom, including the nature and intensity of pain, fatigue, and catastrophizing, and may be helpful in increasing motivation to address healthy lifestyle habits.

Due to her extreme discomfort and fatigue, the initial approach in Junelle included introduction to MBSR, distributed through an online course and home-based CDs and workbook that allowed her to establish a sense of connection with others living with chronic health issues (Toivonen et al. 2017).

Over time, she was able to achieve an objective relationship with the pain and tentatively expanded her physical activity to include gentle chair yoga as part of her home-based activities. She repeated the MBSR course twice and gradually expanded her daily meditation time to 30 minutes.

At the recommendation of her clinician, she restarted therapy and received information on new research in fibromyalgia that gave her an understanding of its pathophysiology. She felt validated by the research advancements and realized that the clinicians she had seen in the past were treating her as best they could, guided by research available at the time. She began CBT with an experienced practitioner who wove a variety of mind–body skills into the treatment, including relaxation, ongoing mindfulness practice, and dampening of hypersensitivity to external stimuli.

Over the course of a year, Junelle gradually reduced her days with pain, expanded her yoga practice to include standing yoga, and deepened her meditation practice. This helped her to gain insights and perspective into her experiences and helped her to begin to identify life events that may have been involved in triggering her condition. She was able to avoid prescription medication, which was important to her, and she was eventually able to restart her job in a company with a much more supportive culture.

PEDIATRIC PAIN

Introduction

Pain in children has multiple facets, including the pain's primary source, pain memory, fear and anticipation of pain, disability, coexisting conditions such as anxiety or depression, and familial influence. In the chronic form, pediatric pain touches every area of a child's life, including social and emotional well-being, school attendance and performance, long-term academic achievement, sleep, family dynamics, and family finances, making finding an individualized treatment approach very important (Brown et al. 2017).

The use of complementary therapies in children with chronic pain was studied in an academic pain center in 1,175 children from 7 to 18 years of age. Predictors of complementary medicine use included female gender, a higher level of parental education, higher pain intensity, and more functional disability. In the sample, 42% of patients had used a complementary therapy to address their pain (acupuncture 22%, massage 22%, biobehavioral 15%) (Vinson et al. 2014).

An earlier survey study by Lin et al. (2005) of pediatric anesthesia training programs in the United States found that 38 of 43 national programs (86%) offered one or more complementary therapy. These included: biofeedback 65%, guided imagery 49%, relaxation therapy 33%, massage 35%, hypnosis 44%, acupuncture 33%, art therapy 21%, and meditation 21%.

A 2011 systematic review on the epidemiology of chronic pain in children included 41 papers and found a high range of prevalence estimates for various conditions seen in children and adolescents with wide variability in study quality and size.

Headache was one of the most common studies complaints, mentioned in nine papers ($n = 24{,}230$) with prevalence rates estimated at between 26% and 69% in children 7 and 16 years of age. Weekly headaches in this study group had a prevalence rate ranging from 6% to 31% with daily headache ranging from 1% to 9% in ages 10–18. Estimated mean prevalence was 23%. Headache prevalence increased with age and was more prevalent in girls. Lower socioeconomic status and positive family history of a headache were also predictive factors, as were depression, anxiety, and low self-esteem.

Abdominal pain was reviewed in five studies ($n = 27{,}526$) and recurrent abdominal pain (now functional abdominal pain) showed a range of prevalence rates with a mean of 12%. Four studies looked at the prevalence of weekly abdominal pain which had rates ranging from 8% to 22%. Girls showed a higher prevalence than males in most studies, and lower socioeconomic status was also predictive.

Back pain was evaluated in two studies ($n = 7{,}262$) and was found to have a median prevalence of 21%. Gender differences were not found to be as significant in this category.

Musculoskeletal pain was evaluated in four studies ($n = 3{,}842$) and was found to have prevalence rates of 9%–39%, higher in those participating in sports. In general, musculoskeletal pain increased with age and was more prevalent in girls.

Overall conclusions emphasize the high prevalence of persistent and recurrent pain in children and adolescents and the need to explore etiologies and design effective interventions, especially in high-risk groups that include those living in low socioeconomic conditions (King et al. 2011).

CHRONIC PAIN IN PEDIATRICS

Chronic pain in children living with chronic diseases can be persistent or recurrent and is often seen in children with inflammatory bowel disease, sickle cell disease, and inflammatory conditions such as juvenile arthritis, migraine headache, and in oncology patients among other groups (Friedrichsdorf et al. 2016).

A 5-year retrospective study of 2,249 children with chronic pain by Zernikow et al. (2012) showed distribution of pain as follows: tension headache (48%), migraine (43%), functional abdominal pain (11%), and these had a high rate of overlap; 55% of children had more than one pain diagnosis. Somatic and psychiatric findings were common. Clinically significant depression was seen in 24% and generalized anxiety in 19%, with girls over age 13 years most likely to seek higher levels of care. Almost one in two children had significant daily pain, and 43% were taking analgesics with no specific indication for treatment.

Untreated pain in childhood can persist into adult life. A study by Hassett et al. (2013) in 1,045 adults seen in an academic tertiary pain clinic showed that approximately 17% had a history of chronic pain in childhood or adolescence, and nearly 80% of those reported continuing pain. Chronic pain in children and adolescents is also associated with higher rates of mental health disorders in adulthood, including increased risk for suicidal ideation and suicide attempt.

Given the prevalence of chronic pain in the pediatric population and its significant toll on children's development and quality of life, new approaches are needed. One tool is a rapid (1–2 minute) Pediatric Pain Screening Tool under development that may be very useful in identifying at-risk youth. Screening questions address the areas: comorbid pain, ambulating, attending school, sleep, pain catastrophizing, pain-related fear, general anxiety, depression, and pain *bothersomeness*. Development and validation of the tool is discussed in this review by Simons et al. (2015).

Other advances are seen in an innovative program described by Friedrichsdorf et al. (2016) at Children's Hospitals and Clinics of Minnesota that emphasizes early return to normal function and implementation of a multipronged approach that includes: physical therapy, integrative medicine emphasizing active mind–body techniques, including guided imagery, hypnosis, biofeedback, yoga, and distraction. These have been shown to modulate the release of endogenous opioids and suppress pain transmission in the dorsal horn of the spinal cord, as well as increasing activity of areas in the brain involved in pain modulation. In the Minnesota program, self-directed techniques are taught to both children and parents for home use. Psychological consult to address anxiety, depression, and behavioral disorders is also addressed to restore baseline function. Normalizing life through reengagement with *sports, school, socializing and sleep* is prioritized, and parent coaching around pain response is an integral part of the program to assist the child in succeeding.

MIND–BODY THERAPIES IN PEDIATRIC HEADACHE

In addition to finding effective, age, and developmental ways to explain to and educate children and families about pain, training in self-regulation skills have been used to address a variety of pain symptoms in children and adolescents. Catastrophizing behavior, seen in both children and their parents, can complicate treatment, making the reduction of fear and anticipation of pain particularly important targets for mind–body therapies in pediatric pain patients and their families (Simons et al. 2016). CBT is one approach that has been used extensively in pediatric pain and studies have been widely published elsewhere on the topic.

Breath work

Breath work and PMR are commonly used in children, as discussed earlier in Chapters 5 and 7, and do not require special training on the part of the clinician to introduce to children.

Progressive muscle relaxation

PMR has been used successfully for both tension-type and migraine headache in adolescents. In one review of seven randomized controlled trials in 288 adolescents from age 10 to 18 years, children with tension-type headaches responded well overall to school nurse-administered relaxation training, but those with migraine headache had better response with therapist-directed training with reduced pain intensity and fewer number of days with headache (Larsson et al. 2005).

Biofeedback

Biofeedback has been reported to be helpful in children to tune into their body's headache signals since the early 1980s (Hermann and Blanchard 2002). A retrospective study involving 132 children was shown to reduce headache frequency from an average of 3.5 to 2 headaches per week. In this review, treatment response was correlated with the child's success at raising hand temperature, correlating with vasodilation (Blume et al. 2012).

Psychological therapies, including CBT, biofeedback, and relaxation therapy, have been shown to be effective in a pediatric headache with clinically relevant improvement seen in approximately 70% of the treated children at follow-up examination (Kroner-Herwig 2011).

Combining biofeedback with virtual reality has also been shown to be successful and well accepted in small studies. In a study by Shiri et al., 10 patients with chronic headache (nine completers) showed improvement in pain, daily functioning, and overall quality of life at both 1- and 3-month follow-up in a pilot study that involved 10 outpatient sessions (Shiri et al. 2013). An excellent overview of virtual reality in pediatrics can be found in a review by Won et al. (2017).

Hypnosis

In one study of 144 pediatric patients, headache frequency was reduced from an average of 4.5 per week to 1.4 per week ($p < 0.01$) with a significant reduction in intensity and duration. No adverse effects were noted (Kohen and Zajac 2007).

Self-hypnosis is a skill readily learned by children and adolescents that has proven effective in the treatment of chronic daily headache (Kohen 2011).

PEDIATRIC ABDOMINAL PAIN

Functional gastrointestinal disorders (FGIDs), including irritable bowel syndrome, are common in children of all ages. An estimated 6%–14% of children have IBS symptoms, with higher prevalence estimates in adolescents of 22%–35.5%. Centrally mediated abdominal pain (CAPS) is a revised term for functional abdominal pain based on the 2016 revision of the Rome Criteria, 4th Revision (Koppen et al. 2017).

This terminology is based on the mechanism of central sensitization with disinhibition of pain signals as described earlier in the chapter and furthers our understanding of why the mind–body therapies show such promise in previously unexplained abdominal pain and in irritable bowel syndrome in children (Keefer et al. 2016).

Gut health in children rests on many factors, just as in adults. Factors such as stress and its impact on the HPA axis, gut microbiome, diet, genetics and epigenetics, and environmental factors all play roles and are areas of intense study (Caes et al. 2017).

HYPNOSIS IN PEDIATRIC FGIDs

Gut-directed hypnosis has been used successfully and is discussed in more detail in Chapter 13—"Gastroenterology." Several randomized controlled trials in children with either functional abdominal pain or irritable bowel syndrome have shown its benefit in both therapist-directed and home-based approaches (Rutten et al. 2013; Rutten et al. 2014).

MEDITATION AND MINDFULNESS IN PEDIATRIC FGIDs

Specific studies are lacking on the use of mindfulness for pain in children and adolescents, although an accruing literature supports its use in the school setting and in urban youth to reduce psychological distress (Sibinga et al. 2016).

YOGA IN PEDIATRIC FGIDs

Yoga has been studied in pediatric pain with data in small studies showing encouraging effects. A pilot study in pediatric patients ($n = 20$) with irritable bowel syndrome and functional abdominal pain who received 10 yoga lessons resulted in statistically significant reduction in pain frequency ($p = 0.031$ and $p = 0.004$) in 8–11 year olds and 11–18 year olds, respectively, and intensity ($p = 0.015$) and in parent-reported improvement in quality of life (Brands et al. 2011).

Another small study of yoga in eight pediatric patients with rheumatic arthritis investigated the feasibility of a 6-week, biweekly Iyengar yoga program, with five patients completing the study. Improvements in pain, depression, pain-related disability, and self-efficacy were reported. Overall, the course was found to be well accepted, and larger studies were recommended (Evans et al. 2010).

Emerging areas of pediatric pain treatment research include (Simons and Basch 2016; Coakley and Wihak 2017):

* Group-based CBT for patient and family
* Internet-based CBT for patient and family
* Motivational interviewing for patient and family
* Treatment of pain and comorbid obesity
* Intensive interdisciplinary treatment programs
* Matching disease to psychological treatment
* Use of pediatric pain screening tool
* Addressing pain-related fear
* Addressing lifestyle comorbidities

CLINICAL APPLICATION: PEDIATRIC PAIN

Soon-Li is a 10-year-old boy with a history of chronic pain related to a serious burn injury involving both legs. He spent several months at a regional trauma center where he received regular medication for pain control. He has recently been transferred to a rehabilitation center closer to home where he is gradually being weaned off his high-dose pain medication. Despite a comprehensive approach to his medication management and satisfactory external wound healing, he has developed severe anticipatory anxiety surrounding wound care and dressing changes related to prior painful experiences. His family is very concerned about his distress yet also realizes the importance of gradual weaning of the narcotics.

At a team meeting, a variety of approaches are discussed, including acupuncture and mind–body therapies to address both pain and anxiety. The family is very receptive to both suggestions, and the initial acupuncture session is scheduled for that week. Soon-Li has seen his grandparents receive acupuncture treatment but has never experienced it himself.

The first session is designed as an introduction using a mix of acupressure and small fine gauge needles. Soon-Li was given the chance to place a needle in his father, which reassured him before experiencing a short treatment himself. In addition to the acupuncture, Soon-Li was introduced to a *buffet* of mind—body therapies to see which might interest him. He expressed interest in the game-based biofeedback program and quickly mastered the technology. Over the next week, he was able to play the biofeedback game in the early afternoon in the hour prior to his dressing change. This allowed him to build his relaxation skills while almost fully distracted from pain and significantly reduced his anticipatory anxiety. He was able to try a virtual reality program during one dressing change but disliked the feeling of not being able to see what was happening, which increased his anxiety.

With ongoing support of his family and the Child Life team and continued use of the biofeedback game, Soon-Li was able to master his fear and found that when he was calm the dressing changes were actually not that painful anymore. He continued to heal well and was successfully weaned off the majority of his medications while regaining his strength, flexibility, and conditioning. Importantly, he was able to continue school in the rehabilitation center and connected with other children his age who were experiencing a wide variety of challenges. He was eventually discharged home with good function and range of motion in both legs and no longer needed the biofeedback program.

SUMMARY

Chronic pain presents a complex challenge in modern medicine. Clinicians of all specialties require expanded treatment options to address its multifactorial components, including the underlying elements of emotional and spiritual pain that may contribute to physical symptoms. Pain cuts across age group, gender, socioeconomic level, and profession and therefore requires the clinician to be aware, flexible, and creative in therapeutic approaches. Mind—body therapies in chronic pain patients offer powerful non-pharmacologic options with potential to engage the inner resources of patients, enhancing sense of self-efficacy, confidence, and hope in what are often very challenging situations.

References

Adler-Neal, A. L., and F. Zeidan. 2017. Mindfulness meditation for fibromyalgia: Mechanistic and clinical considerations. *Curr Rheumatol Rep* 19 (9): 59. doi:10.1007/s11926-017-0686-0.

Anheyer, D., H. Haller, J. Barth, R. Lauche, G. Dobos, and H. Cramer. 2017. Mindfulness-based stress reduction for treating low back pain: A systematic review and meta-analysis. *Ann Intern Med* 166 (11): 799–807. doi:10.7326/M16-1997.

Bendtsen, L., and R. Jensen. 2011. Treating tension-type headache—An expert opinion. *Expert Opin Pharmacother* 12 (7): 1099–1109. doi:10.1517/14656566.2011.548806.

Blume, H. K., L. N. Brockman, and C. C. Breuner. 2012. Biofeedback therapy for pediatric headache: Factors associated with response. *Headache* 52 (9): 1377–1386. doi:10.1111/j.1526-4610.2012.02215.x.

Brands, M. M., H. Purperhart, and J. M. Deckers-Kocken. 2011. A pilot study of yoga treatment in children with functional abdominal pain and irritable bowel syndrome. *Complement Ther Med* 19 (3): 109–114. doi:10.1016/j.ctim.2011.05.004.

Brown, M. L., E. Rojas, and S. Gouda. 2017. A mind-body approach to pediatric pain management. *Children (Basel)* 4 (6). doi:10.3390/children4060050.

Caes, L., A. Orchard, and D. Christie. 2017. Connecting the mind-body split: Understanding the relationship between symptoms and emotional well-being in chronic pain and functional gastro-intestinal disorders. *Healthcare (Basel)* 5 (4). doi:10.3390/healthcare5040093.

Calenzani, G., F. F. D. Santos, V. L. Wittmer, G. K. F. Freitas, and F. M. Paro. 2017. Prevalence of musculoskeletal symptoms in obese patients candidates for bariatric surgery and its impact on health related quality of life. *Arch Endocrinol Metab* 61 (4): 319–325. doi:10.1590/2359-3997000000237.

Cherkin, D. C., K. J. Sherman, B. H. Balderson, A. J. Cook, M. L. Anderson, R. J. Hawkes, K. E. Hansen, and J. A. Turner. 2016. Effect of mindfulness-based stress reduction vs cognitive behavioral therapy or usual care on back pain and functional limitations in adults with chronic low back pain: A randomized clinical trial. *JAMA* 315 (12): 1240–1249. doi:10.1001/jama.2016.2323.

Chou, R., A. Qaseem, V. Snow, D. Casey, J. T. Cross, Jr., P. Shekelle, D. K. Owens, Physicians Clinical Efficacy Assessment Subcommittee of the American College of, Physicians American College of, and Panel American Pain Society Low Back Pain Guidelines. 2007. Diagnosis and treatment of low back pain: A joint clinical practice guideline from the American College of Physicians and the American Pain Society. *Ann Intern Med* 147 (7): 478–491.

Chou, R., and P. Shekelle. 2010. Will this patient develop persistent disabling low back pain? *JAMA* 303 (13): 1295–1302. doi:10.1001/jama.2010.344.

Clarke, T. C., R. L. Nahin, P. M. Barnes, and B. J. Stussman. 2016. Use of complementary health approaches for musculoskeletal pain disorders among adults: United States, 2012. *Natl Health Stat Report* (98): 1–12.

Coakley, R., and T. Wihak. 2017. Evidence-based psychological interventions for the management of pediatric chronic pain: New directions in research and clinical practice. *Children (Basel)* 4 (2). doi:10.3390/children4020009.

Day, M. A., B. E. Thorn, L. C. Ward, N. Rubin, S. D. Hickman, F. Scogin, and G. R. Kilgo. 2014. Mindfulness-based cognitive therapy for the treatment of headache pain: A pilot study. *Clin J Pain* 30 (2): 152–161. doi:10.1097/AJP.0b013e318287a1dc.

Evans, S., M. Moieni, R. Taub, S. K. Subramanian, J. C. Tsao, B. Sternlieb, and L. K. Zeltzer. 2010. Iyengar yoga for young adults with rheumatoid arthritis: Results from a mixed-methods pilot study. *J Pain Symptom Manage* 39 (5): 904–913. doi:10.1016/j.jpainsymman.2009.09.018.

Field, T. 2016. Yoga research review. *Complement Ther Clin Pract* 24: 145–161. doi:10.1016/j.ctcp.2016.06.005.

Friedrichsdorf, S. J., J. Giordano, K. Desai Dakoji, A. Warmuth, C. Daughtry, and C. A. Schulz. 2016. Chronic pain in children and adolescents: Diagnosis and treatment of primary pain disorders in head, abdomen, muscles and joints. *Children (Basel)* 3 (4). doi:10.3390/children3040042.

Fritz, H. C., J. H. McAuley, K. Wittfeld, K. Hegenscheid, C. O. Schmidt, S. Langner, and M. Lotze. 2016. Chronic back pain is associated with decreased prefrontal and anterior insular gray matter: Results from a population-based cohort study. *J Pain* 17 (1): 111–118. doi:10.1016/j.jpain.2015.10.003.

Gardner-Nix, J., S. Backman, J. Barbati, and J. Grummitt. 2008. Evaluating distance education of a mindfulness-based meditation programme for chronic pain management. *J Telemed Telecare* 14 (2): 88–92. doi:10.1258/jtt.2007.070811.

Ghildayal, N., P. J. Johnson, R. L. Evans, and M. J. Kreitzer. 2016. Complementary and alternative medicine use in the US adult low back pain population. *Glob Adv Health Med* 5 (1): 69–78. doi:10.7453/gahmj.2015.104.

Giacobbi, P. R., Jr., M. E. Stabler, J. Stewart, A. M. Jaeschke, J. L. Siebert, and G. A. Kelley. 2015. Guided imagery for arthritis and other rheumatic diseases: A systematic review of randomized controlled trials. *Pain Manag Nurs* 16 (5): 792–803. doi:10.1016/j.pmn.2015.01.003.

Grazzi, L., E. Sansone, A. Raggi, D. D'Amico, A. De Giorgio, M. Leonardi, L. De Torres, F. Salgado-Garcia, and F. Andrasik. 2017. Mindfulness and pharmacological prophylaxis after withdrawal from medication overuse in patients with chronic migraine: An effectiveness trial with a one-year follow-up. *J Headache Pain* 18 (1): 15. doi:10.1186/s10194-017-0728-z.

Greysen, H. M., S. R. Greysen, K. A. Lee, O. S. Hong, P. Katz, and H. Leutwyler. 2017. A qualitative study exploring community yoga practice in adults with rheumatoid arthritis. *J Altern Complement Med* 23 (6): 487–493. doi:10.1089/acm.2016.0156.

Hall, A. M., C. G. Maher, P. Lam, M. Ferreira, and J. Latimer. 2011. Tai chi exercise for treatment of pain and disability in people with persistent low back pain: A randomized controlled trial. *Arthritis Care Res (Hoboken)* 63 (11): 1576–1583. doi:10.1002/acr.20594.

Hammond, D. C. 2007. Review of the efficacy of clinical hypnosis with headaches and migraines. *Int J Clin Exp Hypn* 55 (2): 207–219. doi:10.1080/00207140601177921.

Harris, R. E. 2011. Central pain states: A shift in thinking about chronic pain. *J Fam Pract* 60 (9 Suppl): S37–S42.

Hassett, A. L., P. E. Hilliard, J. Goesling, D. J. Clauw, S. E. Harte, and C. M. Brummett. 2013. Reports of chronic pain in childhood and adolescence among patients at a tertiary care pain clinic. *J Pain* 14 (11): 1390–1397. doi:10.1016/j.jpain.2013.06.010.

Hermann, C., and E. B. Blanchard. 2002. Biofeedback in the treatment of headache and other childhood pain. *Appl Psychophysiol Biofeedback* 27 (2): 143–162.

Hoy, D., C. Bain, G. Williams, L. March, P. Brooks, F. Blyth, A. Woolf, T. Vos, and R. Buchbinder. 2012. A systematic review of the global prevalence of low back pain. *Arthritis Rheum* 64 (6): 2028–2037. doi:10.1002/art.34347.

Hsiao, F. J., S. J. Wang, Y. Y. Lin, J. L. Fuh, Y. C. Ko, P. N. Wang, and W. T. Chen. 2017. Altered insula-default mode network connectivity in fibromyalgia: A resting-state magnetoencephalographic study. *J Headache Pain* 18 (1): 89. doi:10.1186/s10194-017-0799-x.

Hsu, C., J. Bluespruce, K. Sherman, and D. Cherkin. 2010. Unanticipated benefits of CAM therapies for back pain: An exploration of patient experiences. *J Altern Complement Med* 16 (2): 157–163. doi:10.1089/acm.2009.0188.

Huang, X., K. M. Keyes, and G. Li. 2018. Increasing prescription opioid and heroin overdose mortality in the United States, 1999–2014: An age-period-cohort analysis. *Am J Public Health* 108 (1): 131–136. doi:10.2105/AJPH.2017.304142.

Institute of Medicine. 2011. *Relieving Pain in America: A Blueprint for Transforming Prevention, Care, Education, and Research*. Washington, DC: The National Academies Press.

Irvine, A. B., H. Russell, M. Manocchia, D. E. Mino, T. Cox Glassen, R. Morgan, J. M. Gau, A. J. Birney, and D. V. Ary. 2015. Mobile-Web app to self-manage low back pain: Randomized controlled trial. *J Med Internet Res* 17 (1): e1. doi:10.2196/jmir.3130.

John, P. J., N. Sharma, C. M. Sharma, and A. Kankane. 2007. Effectiveness of yoga therapy in the treatment of migraine without aura: A randomized controlled trial. *Headache* 47 (5): 654–661. doi:10.1111/j.1526-4610.2007.00789.x.

Keefer, L., D. A. Drossman, E. Guthrie, M. Simren, K. Tillisch, K. Olden, and P. J. Whorwell. 2016. Centrally mediated disorders of gastrointestinal pain. *Gastroenterology*. doi:10.1053/j.gastro.2016.02.034.

King, S., C. T. Chambers, A. Huguet, R. C. MacNevin, P. J. McGrath, L. Parker, and A. J. MacDonald. 2011. The epidemiology of chronic pain in children and adolescents revisited: A systematic review. *Pain* 152 (12): 2729–2738. doi:10.1016/j.pain.2011.07.016.

Kohen, D. P. 2011. Chronic daily headache: Helping adolescents help themselves with self-hypnosis. *Am J Clin Hypn* 54 (1): 32–46. doi:10.1080/00029157.2011.566767.

Kohen, D. P., and R. Zajac. 2007. Self-hypnosis training for headaches in children and adolescents. *J Pediatr* 150 (6): 635–639. doi:10.1016/j.jpeds.2007.02.014.

Koppen, I. J., S. Nurko, M. Saps, C. Di Lorenzo, and M. A. Benninga. 2017. The pediatric Rome IV criteria: What's new? *Expert Rev Gastroenterol Hepatol* 11 (3): 193–201. doi:10.1080/17474124.2017.1282820.

Kroner-Herwig, B. 2011. Psychological treatments for pediatric headache. *Expert Rev Neurother* 11 (3): 403–410. doi:10.1586/ern.11.10.

Langhorst, J., P. Klose, G. J. Dobos, K. Bernardy, and W. Hauser. 2013. Efficacy and safety of meditative movement therapies in fibromyalgia syndrome: A systematic review and meta-analysis of randomized controlled trials. *Rheumatol Int* 33 (1): 193–207. doi:10.1007/s00296-012-2360-1.

Larsson, B., J. Carlsson, A. Fichtel, and L. Melin. 2005. Relaxation treatment of adolescent headache sufferers: Results from a school-based replication series. *Headache* 45 (6): 692–704. doi:10.1111/j.1526-4610.2005.05138.x.

Lazaridou, A., J. Kim, C. M. Cahalan, M. L. Loggia, O. Franceschelli, C. Berna, P. Schur, V. Napadow, and R. R. Edwards. 2017. Effects of cognitive-behavioral therapy (CBT) on brain connectivity supporting catastrophizing in fibromyalgia. *Clin J Pain* 33 (3): 215–221. doi:10.1097/AJP.0000000000000422.

Li, X., and L. Hu. 2016. The role of stress regulation on neural plasticity in pain chronification. *Neural Plast* 2016: 6402942. doi:10.1155/2016/6402942.

Lin, C., S. H. Lee, and H. H. Weng. 2016. Gray matter atrophy within the default mode network of fibromyalgia: A meta-analysis of voxel-based morphometry studies. *Biomed Res Int* 2016: 7296125. doi:10.1155/2016/7296125.

Lin, Y. C., A. C. Lee, K. J. Kemper, and C. B. Berde. 2005. Use of complementary and alternative medicine in pediatric pain management service: A survey. *Pain Med* 6 (6): 452–458. doi:10.1111/j.1526-4637.2005.00071.x.

Malfliet, A., L. Leysen, R. Pas, K. Kuppens, J. Nijs, P. Van Wilgen, E. Huysmans, L. Goudman, and K. Ickmans. 2017. Modern pain neuroscience in clinical practice: Applied to post-cancer, paediatric and sports-related pain. *Braz J Phys Ther* 21 (4): 225–232. doi:10.1016/j.bjpt.2017.05.009.

Markozannes, G., E. Aretouli, E. Rintou, E. Dragioti, D. Damigos, E. Ntzani, E. Evangelou, and K. K. Tsilidis. 2017. An umbrella review of the literature on the effectiveness of psychological interventions for pain reduction. *BMC Psychol* 5 (1): 31. doi:10.1186/s40359-017-0200-5.

Martenson, M. E., J. S. Cetas, and M. M. Heinricher. 2009. A possible neural basis for stress-induced hyperalgesia. *Pain* 142 (3): 236–244. doi:10.1016/j.pain.2009.01.011.

Meyer, B., A. Keller, H. G. Wohlbier, C. H. Overath, B. Muller, and P. Kropp. 2016. Progressive muscle relaxation reduces migraine frequency and normalizes amplitudes of contingent negative variation (CNV). *J Headache Pain* 17: 37. doi:10.1186/s10194-016-0630-0.

Minen, M., A. Shome, A. Halpern, L. Tishler, K. C. Brennan, E. Loder, R. Lipton, and D. Silbersweig. 2016. A migraine management training program for primary care providers: An overview of a survey and pilot study findings, lessons learned, and considerations for further research. *Headache* 56 (4): 725–740. doi:10.1111/head.12803.

Nestoriuc, Y., and A. Martin. 2007. Efficacy of biofeedback for migraine: A meta-analysis. *Pain* 128 (1–2): 111–127. doi:10.1016/j.pain.2006.09.007.

Nestoriuc, Y., A. Martin, W. Rief, and F. Andrasik. 2008. Biofeedback treatment for headache disorders: A comprehensive efficacy review. *Appl Psychophysiol Biofeedback* 33 (3): 125–140. doi:10.1007/s10484-008-9060-3.

Nicholson, R. A., D. C. Buse, F. Andrasik, and R. B. Lipton. 2011. Nonpharmacologic treatments for migraine and tension-type headache: How to choose and when to use. *Curr Treat Options Neurol* 13 (1): 28–40. doi:10.1007/s11940-010-0102-9.

Nijs, J., M. Meeus, J. Versijpt, M. Moens, I. Bos, K. Knaepen, and R. Meeusen. 2015. Brain-derived neurotrophic factor as a driving force behind neuroplasticity in neuropathic and central sensitization pain: A new therapeutic target? *Expert Opin Ther Targets* 19 (4): 565–576. doi:10.1517/14728222.2014.994506.

Nijs, J., R. Torres-Cueco, C. P. van Wilgen, E. L. Girbes, F. Struyf, N. Roussel, J. van Oosterwijck et al. 2014. Applying modern pain neuroscience in clinical practice: Criteria for the classification of central sensitization pain. *Pain Physician* 17 (5): 447–457.

Park, J., R. McCaffrey, D. Newman, P. Liehr, and J. G. Ouslander. 2017. A pilot randomized controlled trial of the effects of chair yoga on pain and physical function among community-dwelling older adults with lower extremity osteoarthritis. *J Am Geriatr Soc* 65 (3): 592–597. doi:10.1111/jgs.14717.

Qaseem, A., T. J. Wilt, R. M. McLean, M. A. Forciea, and Physicians Clinical Guidelines Committee of the American College of. 2017. Noninvasive treatments for acute, subacute, and chronic low back pain: A clinical practice guideline from the American College of Physicians. *Ann Intern Med* 166 (7): 514–530. doi:10.7326/M16-2367.

Reiner, K., L. Tibi, and J. D. Lipsitz. 2013. Do mindfulness-based interventions reduce pain intensity? A critical review of the literature. *Pain Med* 14 (2): 230–242. doi:10.1111/pme.12006.

Rosenzweig, S., J. M. Greeson, D. K. Reibel, J. S. Green, S. A. Jasser, and D. Beasley. 2010. Mindfulness-based stress reduction for chronic pain conditions: Variation in treatment outcomes and role of home meditation practice. *J Psychosom Res* 68 (1): 29–36. doi:10.1016/j.jpsychores.2009.03.010.

Rutten, J. M., J. B. Reitsma, A. M. Vlieger, and M. A. Benninga. 2013. Gut-directed hypnotherapy for functional abdominal pain or irritable bowel syndrome in children: A systematic review. *Arch Dis Child* 98 (4): 252–257. doi:10.1136/archdischild-2012-302906.

Rutten, J. M., A. M. Vlieger, C. Frankenhuis, E. K. George, M. Groeneweg, O. F. Norbruis, W. Tjon a Ten et al. 2014. Gut-directed hypnotherapy in children with irritable bowel syndrome or functional abdominal pain (syndrome): A randomized controlled trial on self exercises at home using CD versus individual therapy by qualified therapists. *BMC Pediatr* 14: 140. doi:10.1186/1471-2431-14-140.

Shiri, S., U. Feintuch, N. Weiss, A. Pustilnik, T. Geffen, B. Kay, Z. Meiner, and I. Berger. 2013. A virtual reality system combined with biofeedback for treating pediatric chronic headache—A pilot study. *Pain Med* 14 (5): 621–627. doi:10.1111/pme.12083.

Sibinga, E. M., L. Webb, S. R. Ghazarian, and J. M. Ellen. 2016. School-based mindfulness instruction: An RCT. *Pediatrics* 137 (1). doi:10.1542/peds.2015-2532.

Simons, L. E., and M. C. Basch. 2016. State of the art in biobehavioral approaches to the management of chronic pain in childhood. *Pain Manag* 6 (1): 49–61. doi:10.2217/pmt.15.59.

Simons, L. E., L. Goubert, T. Vervoort, and D. Borsook. 2016. Circles of engagement: Childhood pain and parent brain. *Neurosci Biobehav Rev* 68: 537–546. doi:10.1016/j.neubiorev.2016.06.020.

Simons, L. E., A. Smith, C. Ibagon, R. Coakley, D. E. Logan, N. Schechter, D. Borsook, and J. C. Hill. 2015. Pediatric pain screening tool: Rapid identification of risk in youth with pain complaints. *Pain* 156 (8): 1511–1518. doi:10.1097/j.pain.0000000000000199.

Smith, S. M., B. Sumar, and K. A. Dixon. 2014. Musculoskeletal pain in overweight and obese children. *Int J Obes (London)* 38 (1): 11–15. doi:10.1038/ijo.2013.187.

Steiner, T. J., L. J. Stovner, and T. Vos. 2016. GBD 2015: Migraine is the third cause of disability in under 50s. *J Headache Pain* 17 (1): 104. doi:10.1186/s10194-016-0699-5.

Sun-Edelstein, C., and A. Mauskop. 2012. Complementary and alternative approaches to the treatment of tension-type headache. *Curr Pain Headache Rep* 16 (6): 539–544. doi:10.1007/s11916-012-0295-6.

Tajerian, M., and J. D. Clark. 2017. Nonpharmacological interventions in targeting pain-related brain plasticity. *Neural Plast* 2017: 2038573. doi:10.1155/2017/2038573.

Tan, G., D. H. Rintala, M. P. Jensen, T. Fukui, D. Smith, and W. Williams. 2015. A randomized controlled trial of hypnosis compared with biofeedback for adults with chronic low back pain. *Eur J Pain* 19 (2): 271–280. doi:10.1002/ejp.545.

Toivonen, K. I., K. Zernicke, and L. E. Carlson. 2017. Web-based mindfulness interventions for people with physical health conditions: Systematic review. *J Med Internet Res* 19 (8): e303. doi:10.2196/jmir.7487.

Urquhart, D. M., P. Berry, A. E. Wluka, B. J. Strauss, Y. Wang, J. Proietto, G. Jones, J. B. Dixon, and F. M. Cicuttini. 2011. 2011 young investigator award winner: Increased fat mass is associated with high levels of low back pain intensity and disability. *Spine (Phila Pa 1976)* 36 (16): 1320–1325. doi:10.1097/BRS.0b013e3181f9fb66.

Vadivelu, N., A. M. Kai, G. Kodumudi, K. Babayan, M. Fontes, and M. M. Burg. 2017. Pain and psychology-A reciprocal relationship. *Ochsner J* 17 (2): 173–180.

Van Gordon, W., E. Shonin, T. J. Dunn, J. Garcia-Campayo, and M. D. Griffiths. 2017. Meditation awareness training for the treatment of fibromyalgia syndrome: A randomized controlled trial. *Br J Health Psychol* 22 (1): 186–206. doi:10.1111/bjhp.12224.

Vinson, R., G. Yeh, R. B. Davis, and D. Logan. 2014. Correlates of complementary and alternative medicine use in a pediatric tertiary pain center. *Acad Pediatr* 14 (5): 491–496. doi:10.1016/j.acap.2014.04.003.

Ward, L., S. Stebbings, J. Athens, D. Cherkin, and G. David Baxter. 2017. Yoga for the management of pain and sleep in rheumatoid arthritis: A pilot randomized controlled trial. *Musculoskeletal Care.* doi:10.1002/msc.1201.

Wells, R. E., R. Burch, R. H. Paulsen, P. M. Wayne, T. T. Houle, and E. Loder. 2014. Meditation for migraines: A pilot randomized controlled trial. *Headache* 54 (9): 1484–1495. doi:10.1111/head.12420.

Wieland, L. S., N. Skoetz, K. Pilkington, R. Vempati, C. R. D'Adamo, and B. M. Berman. 2017. Yoga treatment for chronic non-specific low back pain. *Cochrane Database Syst Rev* 1: CD010671. doi:10.1002/14651858.CD010671.pub2.

Won, A. S., J. Bailey, J. Bailenson, C. Tataru, I. A. Yoon, and B. Golianu. 2017. Immersive virtual reality for pediatric pain. *Children (Basel)* 4 (7). doi:10.3390/children4070052.

Xiang, Y., L. Lu, X. Chen, and Z. Wen. 2017. Does Tai Chi relieve fatigue? A systematic review and meta-analysis of randomized controlled trials. *PLoS One* 12 (4): e0174872. doi:10.1371/journal.pone.0174872.

Zech, N., E. Hansen, K. Bernardy, and W. Hauser. 2017. Efficacy, acceptability and safety of guided imagery/hypnosis in fibromyalgia–A systematic review and meta-analysis of randomized controlled trials. *Eur J Pain* 21 (2): 217–227. doi:10.1002/ejp.933.

Zernikow, B., J. Wager, T. Hechler, C. Hasan, U. Rohr, M. Dobe, A. Meyer, B. Hubner-Mohler, C. Wamsler, and M. Blankenburg. 2012. Characteristics of highly impaired children with severe chronic pain: A 5-year retrospective study on 2249 pediatric pain patients. *BMC Pediatr* 12: 54. doi:10.1186/1471-2431-12-54.

Conclusion

The primary goals of this book are to explore the use of mind–body therapies in the clinical setting and to raise awareness of the rapidly accruing research in the field. Although many of the therapies have their roots in ancient practices such as meditation and yoga, the mind–body therapies are still viewed with some trepidation by conventionally trained practitioners who have not had a chance to familiarize themselves with the rich body of evidence that exists to support their safe use in a range of clinical conditions. Modern imaging techniques such as fMRI have allowed reassuring new insights into physiologic mechanisms, for example, how clinical hypnosis positively impacts neural connectivity or which areas of the brain benefit both structurally and functionally from mindfulness meditation—breakthroughs that both pique scientific curiosity and offer tremendous hope for those suffering with chronic conditions.

Adult and pediatric research updates and clinical applications are covered throughout the work, and emphasis is placed on the benefit of early acquisition of mind–body skills, not only early in the lifecycle but early in the course of a patient's diagnosis and treatment course so that they are equipped with expanded treatment options if unexpected challenges arise and needs exceed the scope of conventional care. The power of the mind–body therapies in children and adolescents should not be underestimated. Proactively equipping young patients with non-pharmacologic tools that build self-efficacy and self-confidence and help reduce pain perception, fear, and stress is technically easy, cost-effective, compassionate, and wise to help minimize long-term sequelae associated with living with a chronic medical condition, especially pain.

One outstanding benefit of the mind–body therapies is their flexibility to act as either complementary or sole therapies. For example, consider their use in a patient undergoing chemotherapy where guided imagery during infusions may be of great benefit in reducing anxiety—similarly guided imagery may be of use in reinforcing healthy lifestyle behaviors throughout the same patient's survivorship.

Potential use of the mind–body therapies requires a shift in perspective on the part of the clinician (and perhaps the patient) and may require an initial step out of one's comfort zone. Some may be skeptical, worried about other's perceptions, or simply afraid of ridicule. Hopefully, many more will be open to learning about new techniques and curious about the incredible body of supporting research in the field.

Part I reviews an introduction to mind–body medicine and explores a brief history of the field's development, including research breakthroughs such as the relaxation response that underpinned its gradual acceptance into conventional medical practice. An overview of emerging research in stress physiology is covered to emphasize the physiologic cost of unmitigated stress, and an update on the complex research in the field of placebo–nocebo response is reviewed to raise awareness of potential opportunities to engage the patient's healing response. Clinician self-care is introduced early to update the reader on emerging research about the potential benefit of the mind–body therapies to buffer burnout and cultivate healthy resilience. Immediately applicable resources and recommendations to help protect one's health and well-being are included. Part I also introduces the critical topic of language use in medicine, and its ability to inadvertently harm as well as to encourage, an area rarely covered in traditional medical training. Clinical examples in Part I include Dr. Johnson, a colleague struggling with burnout, and a young patient and his family who experience an unexpected conversation in a clinic visit. The overarching goal of Part I is to increase awareness of the strong research base that underpins the field of mind–body medicine, to demonstrate its immediate relevance to the clinician, and to raise awareness of how the clinician's attitude, behavior, and language can convey long-lasting benefits, or harm, to their patients.

Part II reviews selected mind–body therapies, providing background on their development and physiologic mechanisms, and provides an update on adult and pediatric research for each. The mind–body therapies covered include: breath work, autogenics, progressive muscle relaxation, biofeedback, clinical hypnosis, guided imagery, mindfulness and compassion-based therapy, creative arts therapies, and movement therapies such as yoga and tai chi. The intent was not to provide an exhaustive review of therapies but to focus on those with sufficient supporting research in the clinical setting. Some therapies were not covered as they have been extensively reviewed elsewhere. An example is massage, which has substantial supporting data and is more typically considered a manual medicine therapy. Others were not covered due to a current lack of robust supporting research. Clinical application examples in Part II are given in every modality in a range of patients to demonstrate the flexibility of the therapies and to hopefully stimulate the reader's curiosity about how they might be used in their particular practice setting or in their own lives.

Part III builds on the material presented in Parts I and II and explores the use of mind–body therapies in a group of common conditions where research on their use in the clinical setting shows promise. These conditions include adult and pediatric anxiety and depression; various oncologic and surgical diagnoses; gastroenterologic conditions, including GERD, IBD, IBS, and pediatric functional abdominal pain disorders; and pain—including low back pain, headache, fibromyalgia, arthritis, and pediatric chronic pain. Emphasis is placed on the fact that, although accruing research can be used to guide clinical choices, there are no hard and fast rules for the application of mind–body therapies. And these are certainly not the only conditions where mind–body therapies may be useful. Curiosity and creativity in partnership with the patient are required to find the best therapeutic fit within the scope of available resources. The wide margin of safety of the mind–body therapies in most patients generally allows room for trial with minimal downside.

The adult, adolescent, and pediatric cases woven throughout Part III are real stories of patients who in many cases overcame daunting odds to heal. They are introduced to put human faces on the application of the mind–body therapies and to remind us all of the complexity of challenges faced by our patients every day—that too often remain unspoken. The final chapter in Part III covers pain and is designed to demonstrate the sobering reach of chronic pain and its impact on nearly every element of a patient's life. Remaining open to the introduction of mind–body therapies in these challenging, suffering patients has potential to benefit patients and providers in a myriad of ways.

Despite their many benefits, it is undeniable that cost and lack of insurance reimbursement can be prohibitive factors in the use of mind–body therapies for many patients. Hopefully, as their value is recognized, especially in reducing use of pain medication, buffering the physiologic toll of stress, and shortening length of hospital stay, forward-looking health care executives will acquaint themselves with the accruing research in the field and partner with clinicians to accelerate the introduction of the mind–body therapies into the mainstream of health care.

Resources

PART II

Chapter 5 Breath work, autogenics, progressive muscle relaxation

Simple breath work exercises

- 10 to 1 (slowly count breaths down from 10 to 1).
- Breath count 4 up, 4 down (slowly count breaths 1,2,3,4—4,3,2,1).
- Count in the gap (slow inhale, slow exhale, hold and count 1,2,3 after each out breath before next inhalation).
- Square breath (inhale for count of 4, hold for 4, exhale for 4, pause for count of 4).

- 4-7-8 breath (in for a count of 4, hold for 7, exhale for 8) up to four repetitions.
- Belly breath or diaphragmatic breath (inhale while relaxing belly, allowing the abdomen to protrude while lungs fully inflate, exhale, and relax abdomen) repeat for 1–2 minutes.

Mantras or word prompts can be added to individualize the following exercises

- Breathe in "I am," breathe out "at peace."
- Breathe in "calm," breath out "worry" or "tension."
- A, B, C Breath: Bringing yourself to the moment, think "awareness," take a "breath," repeat "center" or "calm" with the exhale.

Apps of potential interest

- Breathe2Relax
- Breathe Deep—Personal Assistant for Breathing Meditation
- Relax & Rest Guided Meditations

Autogenics: Six classic phrases

1 My arms are heavy (heaviness, muscular relaxation).
2 My arms are warm (warmth, vascular dilation).
3 My heartbeat is calm and strong (heart function regulation).
4 My breathing is calm and relaxed (regulation of breathing).
5 My abdomen radiates warmth (regulation of the visceral organs).
6 My forehead is pleasantly cool (regulation of brain activity).

Finish by repeating a preferred mantra such as "I am at peace," or "I am calm."

Progressive muscle relaxation resources

- Apps: Autogenic Training and Progressive Muscle Relaxation—Guided Rest and Meditation Techniques
- Relaxation App—Guided Relaxation
- Free downloads—Student Wellness Center Dartmouth: http://www.dartmouth.edu/~healthed/relax/downloads.html
- Other resources: Audio CD Progressive Muscle Relaxation: 20 Minutes to Total Relaxation, B. Salcedo, MD

Chapter 6 Biofeedback

- Biofeedback Certification International Alliance: http://www.bcia.org/i4a/pages/index.cfm?pageid=1
- HeartMath LLC: https://www.heartmath.com
- Association for Applied Psychophysiology and Biofeedback (AAPB): https://www.aapb.org/i4a/pages/index.cfm?pageid=1
- International Society for Neurofeedback and Research (ISNR): https://www.isnr.org
- Muse portable personal neurofeedback device: http://www.choosemuse.com

Chapter 7 Hypnosis and guided imagery

Hypnosis

- American Society of Clinical Hypnosis: http://www.asch.net/
- The National Pediatric Hypnosis Training Institute offers ASCH certified pediatric specialization: http://www.nphti.org/
- Society for Clinical and Experimental Hypnosis: http://www.sceh.us/
- *American Journal of Clinical Hypnosis*: http://www.asch.net/Public/American JournalofClinicalHypnosis.aspx
- *International Journal of Clinical and Experimental Hypnosis*: http://www.ijceh.com/
- *Hypnosis and Hypnotherapy with Children* by Karen Olness and Daniel Kohen, 1996, Guilford Press, NY
- *Harry the Hypnopotomous: Metaphorical Tales for the Treatment of Children* by Linda Thompson, 2005, Crown House Publishing, Wales, UK

Guided imagery

- Academy for Guided Imagery—150-hour, mentored, long distance learning, certificate program for health professionals: http://www.academyforguidedimagery.com
- Health Journeys: http://www.healthjourneys.com
- Kaiser Guided Imagery Resources (free to all) in cooperation with Health Journeys Podcasts: https://healthy.kaiserpermanente.org

Chapter 8 Mindfulness

- Center for Mindfulness, University of Massachusetts Medical School, Jon Kabat-Zinn: http://www.umassmed.edu
- Center for Healthy Minds at the University of Wisconsin-Madison: https://centerhealthy-minds.org/join-the-movement/well-being-tips-for-children-and-their-families
- Child Mind Institute: https://childmind.org/article/the-power-of-mindfulness/
- The Chopra Center: http://www.chopra.com/articles/4-exercises-to-teach-your-kids-about-mindfulness-and-compassion
- Emory University, Emory-Tibet Partnership, Emory Tibet Science Initiative: https://tibet.emory.edu/emory-tibet-science-initiative/
- Stanford University's Center for Compassion and Altruism Research and Education, Stanford CCare: http://ccare.stanford.edu

Apps

- Stop, Breathe, Think
- Take a Chill
- Sleep Meditations for Kids
- Mindfulness for Children

Publications

- *Planting Seeds: Practicing Mindfulness with Children* by Thich Nhat Hanh.
- *A Still Quiet Place: A Mindfulness Program for Teaching Children and Adolescents to Ease Stress and Difficult Emotions* by Amy Saltzman and Saki Santorelli.

- *The Mindful Child* by Susan Kaiser Greenland
- *The Mindfulness Revolution* edited by Barry Boyce
- *Train Your Mind, Change Your Brain* by Sharon Begley
- *Stressed Teens*: http://stressedteens.com
- *Investigating Healthy Minds*: http://investigating healthyminds.org
- *Mindful Schools*: http://mindfulschools.org

Chapter 9 Creative arts therapies

- American Music Therapy Association
  8455 Colesville Road, Suite 1000
  Silver Spring, MD 20910
  Phone (301) 589-3300
  Fax (301) 589-5175
  Web: www.musictherapy.org/Email: info@musictherapy.org
- *Journal of Music Therapy*
- *Music Therapy Perspectives*
- *International Journal of Community Music*
- *International Society for Music Education*

National Coalition of Creative Arts Therapies Associations: http://www.nccata.org
    Founded in 1979, represents 15,000 individual members of seven creative arts therapies associations in the United States:

- American Music Therapy Association: https://www.musictherapy.org/
- American Dance Therapy Association: https://adta.org/
- American Art Therapy Association: https://arttherapy.org/
- North American Drama Therapy Association: http://www.nadta.org/
- National Association of Poetry Therapy: http://poetrytherapy.org/
- American Society for Group Psychotherapy and Psychodrama: http://www.asgpp.org/
- University of Florida General Arts in Medicine Program: http://arts.ufl.edu/academics/center-for-arts-in-medicine/

Chapter 10 Movement therapies

In the United States, the Yoga Alliance is a nonprofit 501(c)(6) membership professional and trade association: www.yogaalliance.org

Pediatric yoga

- International Association of Yoga Therapists: http://iayt.org/
- Kripalu Yoga in the Schools: http://kripalu.org/be_a_part_of_kripalu/812
- NCCAM Yoga for Health: http://nccam.nih.gov/health/yoga
- Yoga Alliance: http://www.yogaalliance.org/
- Yoga in Schools: http://yogainschools.org
- YogaKids: http://yogakids.com/
- Yoga for the Special Child: http://www.specialyoga.com/

PART III

Chapter 13 Gastroenterology

- IBSHypnosis.com A Public Information Website by Olafur S. Palsson, PhD, Professor of Medicine, University of North Carolina at Chapel Hill: http://www. ibshypnosis.com
- IBS Audio Program 100 for Irritable Bowel Syndrome Self-Hypnosis—Audio CD available commercially. By Michael Mahoney, Psychotherapist, Hypnotherapist, Cheshire, England

Index

Printed in the United States
by Baker & Taylor Publisher Services